AMA Education Consortium

HEALTH SYSTEMS SCIENCE

AMA Education Consortium

HEALTH SYSTEMS SCIENCE

Editors-in-Chief:

Susan E. Skochelak, MD, MPH

Richard E. Hawkins, MD

Editors:

Luan E. Lawson, MD, MAEd

Stephanie R. Starr, MD

Jeffrey M. Borkan, MD, PhD

Jed D. Gonzalo, MD, MSc

ELSEVIER

ELSEVIER

1600 John F. Kennedy Blvd.
St 1800
Philadelphia, PA 19103-2899

HEALTH SYSTEMS SCIENCE, FIRST EDITION   ISBN: 978-0-323-46116-0

Notices

Knowledge and best practice in this field are constantly changing. As new research and experience broaden our understanding, changes in research methods, professional practices, or medical treatment may become necessary.

Practitioners and researchers must always rely on their own experience and knowledge in evaluating and using any information, methods, compounds, or experiments described herein. In using such information or methods they should be mindful of their own safety and the safety of others, including parties for whom they have a professional responsibility.

With respect to any drug or pharmaceutical products identified, readers are advised to check the most current information provided (i) on procedures featured or (ii) by the manufacturer of each product to be administered, to verify the recommended dose or formula, the method and duration of administration, and contraindications. It is the responsibility of practitioners, relying on their own experience and knowledge of their patients, to make diagnoses, to determine dosages and the best treatment for each individual patient, and to take all appropriate safety precautions.

To the fullest extent of the law, neither the Publisher nor the authors, contributors, or editors assume any liability for any injury and/or damage to persons or property as a matter of products liability, negligence or otherwise, or from any use or operation of any methods, products, instructions, or ideas contained in the material herein.

Library of Congress Cataloging-in-Publication Data

Names: Skochelak, Susan E., editor. | Hawkins, Richard E., editor. | AMA Education Consortium, sponsoring body.
Title: Health systems science / AMA Education Consortium; editors-in-chief, Susan E. Skochelak, Richard E. Hawkins; editors, Luan E. Lawson, Stephanie R. Starr, Jeffrey M. Borkan, Jed D. Gonzalo.
Description: St. Louis, Missouri: Elsevier, [2016] | Includes bibliographical references and index.
Identifiers: LCCN 2016040074 | ISBN 9780323461160 (pbk.)
Subjects: | MESH: Delivery of Health Care | Health Services Administration| United States
Classification: LCC RA410.53 | NLM W 84 AA1 | DDC 362.110973--dc23
LC record available at https://lccn.loc.gov/2016040074

Executive Content Strategist: James Merritt
Director, Content Development: Rebecca Gruliow
Publishing Services Manager: Julie Eddy
Book Production Specialist: Clay S. Broeker
Design Direction: Ashley Miner

Printed in Canada

Last digit is the print number: 9   8   7   6   5   4   3   2

Contributors

Neera Agrwal, MD
Mayo Clinic
Chapter 4: Value in Health Care

Niti S. Armistead, MD
East Carolina University
Chapter 6: Quality Improvement

Jose Azar, MD
Indiana University
Chapter 13: Application of Foundational Skills to Health Systems Science

Elizabeth G. Baxley, MD
East Carolina University
Chapter 11: Socio-Ecologic Determinants of Health

Jeffrey M. Borkan, MD, PhD
Brown University
Chapter 2: What Is Health Systems Science? Building an Integrated Vision
Chapter 15: The Future of Health Systems Science

Brian Clyne, MD
Brown University
Chapter 8: Leadership in Health Care

Matthew M. Davis, MD, MAPP
Northwestern University
Chapter 12: Health Care Policy and Economics

Timothy Dempsey, MD, MPH
University of California, Davis
Chapter 4: Value in Health Care

Jesse M. Ehrenfeld, MD, MPH
Vanderbilt University
Chapter 5: Patient Safety
Chapter 9: Clinical Informatics

Victoria Stagg Elliott, MA
American Medical Association
Chapter 15: The Future of Health Systems Science

Tonya L. Fancher, MD, MPH
University of California, Davis
Chapter 11: Socio-Ecologic Determinants of Health

Paul George, MD, MHPE
Brown University
Chapter 10: Population Health

Daniel Goldberg, JD, PhD
University of Colorado
Chapter 11: Socio-Ecologic Determinants of Health

Jed D. Gonzalo, MD, MSc
Penn State College of Medicine
Chapter 1: Health Systems Science in Medical Education
Chapter 2: What Is Health Systems Science? Building an Integrated Vision

Sara Jo Grethlein, MD
Indiana University
Chapter 8: Leadership in Health Care
Chapter 13: Application of Foundational Skills to Health Systems Science

Karen E. Hauer, MD, PhD
University of California, San Francisco
Chapter 14: The Use of Assessment to Support Learning and Improvement in Health Systems Science

Richard E. Hawkins, MD
American Medical Association
Chapter 14: The Use of Assessment to Support Learning and Improvement in Health Systems Science

William Hersh, MD
Oregon Health & Science University
Chapter 9: Clinical Informatics

Jason Higginson, MD, MA
East Carolina University
Chapter 7: Principles of Teamwork and Team Science

Jill M. Huber, MD
Mayo Clinic
Chapter 10: Population Health

Jordan M. Kautz, MD
Mayo Clinic
Chapter 6: Quality Improvement

Donna M. Lake, PhD, RN, MEd
East Carolina University
Chapter 7: Principles of Teamwork and Team Science

Natalie Landman, PhD
Arizona State University
Chapter 4: Value in Health Care

Luan E. Lawson, MD, MAEd
East Carolina University
Chapter 5: Patient Safety

Kimberly D. Lomis, MD
Vanderbilt University
Chapter 14: The Use of Assessment to Support Learning and
Improvement in Health Systems Science

Erin McKean, MD, MBA
University of Michigan
Chapter 8: Leadership in Health Care

Robert E. Nesse, MD
Mayo Clinic
Chapter 3: The Health Care Delivery System

Mark D. Schwartz, MD
New York University School of Medicine
Chapter 12: Health Care Policy and Economics

Susan E. Skochelak, MD, MPH
American Medical Association
Chapter 1: Health Systems Science in Medical Education

Stephanie R. Starr, MD
Mayo Clinic
Chapter 2: What Is Health Systems Science? Building an
Integrated Vision
Chapter 3: The Health Care Delivery System
Chapter 6: Quality Improvement

Elizabeth Tobin-Tyler, JD, MA
Brown University
Chapter 12: Health Care Policy and Economics

Danielle Walsh, MD
East Carolina University
Chapter 5: Patient Safety

Donna Williams, MD
University of California, Davis
Chapter 4: Value in Health Care

Natalia Wilson, MD, MPH
Arizona State University
Chapter 10: Population Health

Daniel R. Wolpaw, MD
Penn State College of Medicine
Chapter 1: Health Systems Science in Medical Education

Therese M. Wolpaw, MD, MHPE
Penn State College of Medicine
Chapter 15: The Future of Health Systems Science

Foreword

Technology is changing our world and the practice of medicine at a pace unmatched in human history. Yet, for all the societal advancements and technological marvels over the last century, the way we train and educate new doctors is little changed.

Medical school curricula have, of course, expanded over the years to include important new medical breakthroughs and discoveries, but their focus and overall structure remain stubbornly captives of early twentieth-century thinking. The result is an ever-widening gap between how physicians in the United States are trained and educated and the realities of the modern health care environment.

Recognizing this gap, the American Medical Association (AMA) in 2013 set out to transform and modernize medical education in this country by creating and providing funding for a diverse network of medical schools to innovate, share practices, and push the boundaries of traditional medical education. In short, we inspired them to think big.

This reinvention of the medical school of the future was part of a strategic realignment at the AMA to further our mission to promote the art and science of medicine and the betterment of public health. The other pillars in our renewed strategic focus include creating the tools and resources to help physicians thrive in modern health care and developing new and better approaches to combat America's growing epidemic of chronic disease. Many opportunities for innovation were identified in these efforts; to address these, an AMA innovation ecosystem was created, with nodes including a Chicago-based health care start-up incubator (Matter) and a Silicon Valley–based prototyping and design studio (Health 2047). Together, these initiatives are foundational to the AMA's work to lead meaningful innovation and enable a better health care system for patients, physicians, and the nation.

Each of these three core focus areas is shaping health care today and long into the future. However, it is our efforts around medical education, our exciting Accelerating Change in Medical Education initiative, that may ultimately be the most far-reaching and impactful.

Two years into this program, the schools in our Accelerating Change in Medical Education Consortium regularly meet to share their different ideas on curricular innovation, which, when aggregated, form a vision of the medical school of the future: one that measures competency; one that responds to the needs of chronic disease through a team-based care approach, greater continuity, and more outpatient exposure; and one that adopts new technologies for education and creates new fields of medical science.

These are schools that will do more than simply prepare young doctors to care for patients. They will prepare physicians for a lifetime of training and learning. They will prepare them to take leadership roles in their practices while also exploring the most innovative ways to care for patients, populations, and communities.

The emergence of health systems science will be a key component of the medical school of the future, bridging the study of basic and clinical sciences and giving new physicians a broad view of the societal influences and administrative challenges that sometimes complicate patient care. Health systems science is that window into the lives of our patients and our communities that makes us more effective, compassionate, and knowledgeable doctors.

It's important to remember that the history of medicine is the history of innovation and change. For nearly 170 years, physicians have relied on the AMA to keep them informed, engaged, and at the forefront of technological advancements so that they can better meet the ever-changing needs of their patients.

By reinventing medical education and encouraging our doctors of tomorrow to rethink how we deliver care in this new digital age of medicine, the AMA is bringing the future of our profession into sharper focus and improving health care for generations to come.

James L. Madara, MD
Executive Vice President and CEO
American Medical Association

Preface

Over the last decade it has become clearer that trainees require knowledge, attitudes, and skills beyond the scope of and in addition to the basic and clinical sciences if they are to be prepared for practice in our current and future health care system. To meet this need, in 2013 the American Medical Association (AMA) asked medical schools across the United States to apply to become part of the Accelerating Change in Medical Education initiative. The 11 schools with the most innovative projects were chosen from 119 applications to become part of the initiative and form a consortium. After long debate, the concept of *health systems science* emerged from this collaboration as a required third pillar of medical education. Competency in this realm ensures medical school graduates can effectively translate and apply the basic and clinical sciences to become physicians who meaningfully improve patients' health at the individual, community, and population level.

More than a century ago, the Flexner report recommended significant changes to increase the scientific rigor and standardization of medical school curricula. The consortium is recommending health systems science as the third critical science required of physicians and other health professionals in order to prepare them for their future roles and for them to have the greatest impact on the health of patients and society. Basic science is about understanding the mechanisms and functions of the human body. Clinical science is focused on diagnosis, treatment, and prevention—obtaining histories, examining patients, and choosing interventions that maintain health, ameliorate decline, and maximize the function of the human body. Even if basic and clinical sciences are expertly learned and executed, without health systems science, physicians cannot realize their full potential on patients' health or on the population. Health systems science includes all of the factors in the lives of patients that influence their well-being (e.g., social determinants of health and health disparities); the structures and processes of the health system itself (e.g., patient access, financing, quality improvement); societal factors (e.g., health policy and advocacy); communication (e.g., verbal, written, team), and information technology (e.g., electronic health records, search engines). Incorporating an understanding of health systems science in medical education will improve the quality and value of care that physicians and other health professionals deliver and that patients and communities experience.

There are other textbooks that explore health systems science from the perspective of managers, administrators, or policymakers, and there are other textbooks that delve more fully into the subjects of each individual chapter of this book. This textbook is the first that aims to define the cannon of health systems science and elucidate the health systems science framework for educating health care professionals. We hope it will serve as the base for ever-expanding advancements in the teaching of health systems science and the incorporation of health systems science into practice.

While this textbook seeks to define health systems science, it is important to note that health systems science is an emerging discipline. We know health systems science is a dynamic, rapidly changing field. Our intention is that this textbook will serve as a platform on which changes can be made over time. We are just at the beginning of our health systems science journey.

The editors and authors would like to thank the members of the AMA Accelerating Change in Medical Education Consortium for their tireless work to transform medical education by implementing health systems science as well as other significant innovations. This textbook is dedicated to the patients, communities, and populations we serve.

Susan E. Skochelak, MD, MPH
Richard E. Hawkins, MD
Jeffrey M. Borkan, MD, PhD
Jed D. Gonzalo, MD, MSc
Luan E. Lawson, MD, MAEd
Stephanie R. Starr, MD

Contents

1

Health Systems Science in Medical Education

Jed D. Gonzalo, MD, MSc, Susan E. Skochelak, MD, MPH, and
Daniel R. Wolpaw, MD

LEARNING OBJECTIVES

1. Distinguish between several evolving concepts in health systems science.
2. Identify the need to align medical education with ongoing changes in health care delivery.
3. Review the traditional "two-pillar" model of medical education.
4. Examine the relationship between the two pillars and health systems science (the "third pillar") in medical education.

For over 100 years, medical education has relied upon two pillars for training physicians who are ready to practice medicine: basic science and clinical science. Health systems science—the understanding of how physicians deliver care to patients, how patients receive care, and how health systems function—has been part of the hidden curriculum or taught as part of elective courses. There have been many attempts to formalize the role of health systems science in medical school curriculum and make it the third pillar; to date these have had limited success.

Health systems science is intimately intertwined with the two pillars of medical education but also a subject in its own right requiring study by medical students. Additionally, physicians' roles in the health care system are changing significantly, and physicians need to understand health systems science in order to fulfill their changing roles. Health systems science training extends beyond the historically segregated boundaries of physician training and is applicable to all health professions students.

CHAPTER OUTLINE

"We will never transform the prevailing system of management without transforming our prevailing system of education. They are the same system."

Edwards Deming, an American engineer and quality improvement expert, believed that if people fail in their roles within their jobs it is because they are socialized in ways of thinking and acting that are embedded in their formative institutional experiences.[1,2] Although this philosophy was proposed for management in business and organizations outside of health care, this philosophy directly applies to both the urgent need for health care transformation as well as medical education reform. Rapidly evolving challenges in health care mandate changes in the way health care professionals are educated, and these educational systems will in turn directly impact the health of patients. This textbook is devoted to Health Systems Science (HSS), which is the fundamental understanding of how health care is delivered, how health care professionals work together to deliver that care, and how the health system can improve health. An understanding of HSS provides the building blocks for physicians and other health care professionals to improve all aspects of patient care and health care delivery. Additionally, awareness of HSS and mindfulness of its role in understanding health care delivery helps to ensure that significant advancements in basic and clinical science ultimately translate to improved patient outcomes and improved satisfaction for medical professionals.

I. THE NEED FOR A TEXTBOOK IN HEALTH SYSTEMS SCIENCE

Health systems are rapidly evolving in the face of substantial challenges. Health systems need to provide care to expanding and diverse patient populations, including the underserved, patients at the extremes of age, and those with chronic, often environmentally enabled, comorbid conditions. The exploding growth of health care–related knowledge and technology promises remarkable benefits, but also has the potential for compromising value and even doing harm. At the same time, social, economic, and political forces have become an integral part of the health care transformation. The successful alignment of all of these factors with our goals for the optimal health of people and populations will require that health professions students and medical education programs step up to the plate and engage in an entirely new game, one that requires increased focus on health care delivery and patient-centered care rather than just providers' skills in diagnosis and treatment. It is not just that the players, rules, and equipment in the health care game are new; more importantly, they are constantly changing and evolving. Old or static models of education and health care delivery simply will not work. In order to meet Deming's challenge to change the system through educational transformation, health professions students and medical educators must critically prioritize content to ensure adaptive thinking skills and the associated professional identity formation.

II. THE RAPIDLY CHANGING HEALTH CARE ENVIRONMENT

Health care is currently and will continue to undergo significant redesign and changes that will impact the ways in which patients receive care and how physicians and health care professionals "deliver" care. Although several paradigms have been proposed that reflect that ultimate goal of the ideal health care system, the Institute for Healthcare Improvement's Triple Aim goal of improved patient experience, improved care for patient populations, and decreased cost embodies the key points in all of these models, and reflects the overall goals of the evolving health care system in the United States (Fig. 1.1).[3] Additionally, Porter further defined value as the quality of care relative to the cost required for the care (value = quality/cost). Combined, these two principles form a unifying thread throughout the subsequent chapters in this textbook.[4]

There are four ongoing developments in US health care that highlight this rapidly changing health care environment: 1) health care policy initiatives, 2) payment reform and value, 3) health care delivery system innovation and transformation, and 4) transformative health information technology, data, and informatics. Identifying these four shifts allows for the elucidation of key implications for physicians and other health care professionals practicing in and leading change within these health systems.

A. Health Care Policy Initiatives

The recognition of the high cost and comparatively moderate quality of US health care has led to years of ongoing debate and policy initiatives to stimulate change and transformation. Signed into law in 2010, the Patient Protection and Affordable Care Act (PPACA) seeks to improve the quality and affordability of health insurance, lower the number of uninsured patients by increasing insurance coverage, and reduce health care costs. The Affordable Care Act (often referred to as "Obamacare" or the ACA), along with other policy initiatives, provides critical drivers for change in US health care at

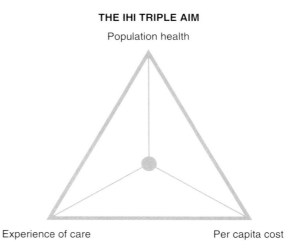

THE IHI TRIPLE AIM

Population health

Experience of care   Per capita cost

Fig. 1.1 The Triple Aim framework. The framework was developed by the Institute for Healthcare Improvement in Cambridge, Massachusetts *(ihi.org)*.

all levels. It seeks to transform health care by improving its value and efficiency, implementing preventive strategies, and refocusing on population health. However, these initiatives are insufficient by themselves to impact the health of patients and populations. The way forward will require professionals who are fluent in a new language and perspective of health care goals and systems.

B. Payment Reform and Value

For decades, the fee-for-service model of health care has been the predominant method of reimbursement. In this model, health systems and providers are provided reimbursement for health care delivery and services independent of the quality of the care delivered or the outcomes obtained. With the recognition of the need for change, there is an evolving push toward reimbursing high-value care rather than quantity of service provided.[5] Several strategies are being used to achieve this transformation. **Pay for Performance** (P4P) and Value-Based Purchasing seek to reimburse based on a reward model for meeting quality measures in care delivery. These strategies depend on utilization of electronic health records and patient registries, while shifting accountability to providers and systems to design and implement the best strategies to obtain quality outcomes. In this process, providers and systems must reduce inappropriate use of health care resources (e.g., laboratory tests, radiographic testing), understand and employ evidence-based strategies for best outcomes, and initiate health systems change to reach these goals. **Bundled payments** incorporate expected costs for a typical encounter or episode of care into a single payment. The team of physicians and other health care professionals is held accountable for the communication and coordination along the continuum of care to improve the outcomes of care interventions. For example, a knee replacement surgery for a patient involves numerous physicians and other health care professionals, including the orthopedic surgeon, anesthesiologists, physical therapists, nursing staff, and care coordinators, who collectively seek to provide safe and effective care from the hospital to home or rehabilitation facility, improving function and quality of life, and supporting seamless transitions of care within a collaborating team of physicians and other health care professionals. This "bundled" approach to organizing and reimbursing care requires an entirely new approach to the process of health care delivery. Lastly, **shared savings** plans seek to provide financial incentives to health plans and providers to improve quality while reducing cost. All of these payment reform initiatives and the predominant shift toward value require physicians and other health care professionals to understand and engage in the individual and team skills necessary to achieve best outcomes.

C. Health Care Delivery System Innovation and Transformation

With the need to implement new health care policies and value, US health systems must redesign and transform the structures and processes of health care to achieve the Triple Aim.[3] The current system is often fragmented, with inadequate processes for communication and collaboration. The result is one of high cost and inefficiency, unacceptable levels of patient safety events and medical errors, and a compromise in the kinds of authentic patient-provider partnerships required for shared-decision making and patient-centered care. Additionally, current health system design and delivery processes are not well aligned with the needs of the most vulnerable patient populations, specifically those with behavioral and mental health challenges, those from racial or ethnic minority groups, and those from rural and socioeconomically disadvantaged backgrounds.[6,7] The current shift in health care transformation seeks to drive the health system to operate more like an ideal system—one that aligns with person- and population-centered care goals, allowing for appropriate distribution of resources where they are most needed.

To this end, health systems will increasingly seek to develop team-based models of care that optimize interprofessional collaboration and communities of care. This will not only require a frameshift in how physicians and other health care professionals view all members of the health care team, but also in how teams coordinate care in the larger context of the health system, and how patients, families, and social networks are engaged as well. There is growing appreciation for the multiple social and ecological determinants of health that require health systems and provider teams to factor homes, neighborhoods, and communities into plans for health promotion and disease prevention. Health systems are transforming to add a focus on populations or groups of patients, expanding the traditional lens of one patient at any given time. This transition to population-based care requires a skill set not previously addressed in the education of most physicians and other health care professionals.

D. Transformative Health Information Technology and Data

The success of health care delivery innovation and transformation relies upon working expertise in health information technology and "big data." There has been an explosion of readily available clinical data and discovery, all of which require critical appraisal and thoughtful application in health systems and at the point of care. Electronic health records are currently a mixed blessing, offering up equal measures of timely information exchange and frustrating barriers.[8] Large databases are offering previously unavailable windows into health care at the practice level as well as the larger health system levels, but also carry their own set of pitfalls. These unprecedented opportunities and challenges require providers and health systems to understand, engage, and redesign system and point of care IT resources to improve health for patients and populations.

The "Iceberg" of health care transformation (Fig. 1.2) highlights the numerous concepts and factors that are intricately connected and interrelated to care provided to any one patient in any one episode of care. Traditionally, the focus of health care delivery has remained "above the water," on the provider-patient encounter within a clinic, hospital, or other health care setting. Patient care must continue to be a necessary focus of health care as well as medical education. Providers must be able to communicate with patients, pursue and make accurate diagnoses about medical issues, and determine best treatment modalities, all while using shared-decision–making processes. They must utilize the continuously updated knowledge cloud and contribute where appropriate to discovery. These are evolving perspectives on traditional physician-centric roles—almost all above the water. Medical education leaders, medical students, and those studying other health care professions can no longer ignore the complex network of processes, systems, and insights that lie beneath the surface of the individual patient encounter in order to be prepared to address the challenges and practice in the evolving health care environment of the 21st century. This is, in a nutshell, the focus of this textbook.

III. PROVIDER READINESS TO PRACTICE IN THE EVOLVING HEALTH CARE SYSTEM

This expanded view of this mandate for the medical education system translates directly into role expectations for providers in evolving health systems, and, in turn, highlights unmet needs in our current approach to training. Physicians and other health care providers will be expected to move beyond traditional narrowly-defined roles to participate in collaborative teams as both leaders and supporting players, and perhaps most importantly, to contribute to a systems view of meaningful patient outcomes beyond disease-specific diagnosis and treatment. The following reports highlight the "new" and emerging needs for learners who will soon be entering the health care workforce and need to learn HSS[9]:

- Chang and colleagues identified the essential skills needed for medical student graduates to better ably practice in 21st century health care, including leadership skills, understanding of organization norms and values, navigating of health care finances, quality improvement skills, information technology, and patient engagement.[10,11]
- Crosson and associates identified health systems leaders' perceptions regarding the unmet needs for graduates to practice in health systems, including office-based practice competencies, care coordination, continuity of care, familiarity with clinical information technology, leadership and management skills, systems thinking perspectives, and procedural skills.[12]
- Thibault highlighted the need for interprofessional collaboration skills to improve the undergraduate medical education to graduate medical education transition.[13]

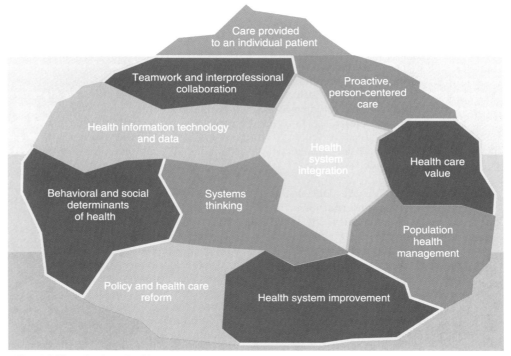

Fig. 1.2 **The "Iceberg" of health care concepts impacting health.** Numerous factors and concepts are often underappreciated in the provider-patient interaction within a clinic room. Traditionally, these concepts have not been included in the scope of medical education.

- Skochelak reviewed the recommendations for change in medical education and identified the common themes of better aligning providers' skills with the changes in the health care delivery system, emphasis on social accountability, and importance of leadership.[14]
- Lucey identified the need for future providers to embrace the knowledge and skills of clinical quality, patient safety, data-driven improvement, and innovation, all to improve the health system of today.[15]
- Combes and Arespacochaga, in a report from leaders in the American Hospital Association, identified a range of "deficits" encountered in graduates from US training programs, including cost-conscious care, care coordination, and interprofessional communication.[16]

IV. PROVIDERS AS HEALTH CARE "CHANGE AGENTS"

Physicians have traditionally been trained to care for one patient at a time in the office or hospital, making autonomous decisions and utilizing supporting personnel. Additionally, other health care providers have been trained to focus on their area of expertise, and contribute to a physician's ultimate decision in the hope of improving patient care. Political and business perspectives have increasingly affected how medicine is delivered and altered expectations of the providers within the system, resulting in many providers who are ill-equipped to venture outside of this model, migrating more and more to an "employee" approach to medical practice. The lack of training in systems and the complex determinants of care has become a self-fulfilling prophecy. As a result, change in health care

is often led by managers, accountants, and policymakers who are skilled in understanding the financial implications of potential change, but may not be well versed in understanding the needs of patient-centered care.[11] It is clearly the time for physicians to engage in this process. One of the key foundational principles of this textbook is that the goals of education in the health professions need to be broadened and rebalanced. Knowledge acquisition in basic and clinical science is not enough. Practicing in an increasingly limited box of diagnosis and treatment is not enough. Health care providers and physicians need to be collaborators and leaders in a system transformation that is already well on its way, and medical education must do its part to develop and support students for these new professional roles.

An interesting way to conceptualize this need for a different "type" of provider is through the constructive-developmental theory as set forth by Kegan.[17,18] In studying adult learning, Kegan describes "orders of mind," each with a qualitative shift in complexity. Most adults and health care providers live in a "socialized" or a self-authoring mindset. In the socialized mindset, providers have the ability to subordinate their desires to the desires of others (this very nicely describes the "employee" mentality alluded to earlier in the chapter). They are guided by others or institutions, and are focused on "getting along" rather than changing or confronting a problematic situation. Individuals exhibiting a "self-authoring" mind are inclined to "own" their work, exhibiting agency, self-motivation, and vision (though this may be fairly rigid and uncompromising). Though these qualities are often viewed as essential characteristics of leadership, they are also characteristics of the old model of the physician as an independent agent or "cowboy," acting alone in calling the shots and pointing the way. At the same time, the self-authoring mind often lacks the capacity for meaningful teamwork and collaboration, and falls short of the complexity of a "self-transforming" mind. A self-transforming mind is characterized by the ability to mediate conflicts, thoughtfully review and appropriately integrate input from multiple sources and perspectives, see the larger context and back stories, and flexibly lead in an environment of uncertainty and change. This aptly describes the environment in health care today, and the goal of our educational systems should be to support the development of self-transforming minds in our learners. Health professions students must begin to view this as a process and outcome of their own personal growth in medicine.

However, for health care professionals to be self-transforming leaders, they require the prerequisite knowledge and skills of HSS as elucidated in this textbook along with deliberate expertise in systems thinking.[1] This is an absolute requirement for change agents and leaders in the evolving world of health care, and represents a critical content and process challenge for medical education. In addition, the professional identity of future physicians will require a "native" fluency in collaborative care, a self-transforming mind that is fluent in the language of teams, collaboration, and value-based care.

V. THE CURRENT TWO-PILLAR MODEL OF MEDICAL EDUCATION

In 1910, Abraham Flexner published the first comprehensive review of American and Canadian medical education, effectively revolutionizing medical education in the US and Canada. The report established that medical education for physicians should include a rigorous grounding in biological sciences and scientific theory as the underpinning of medical practice.[19] The report called for training physicians to practice in a scientific manner and to engage in research. These recommendations have had a profound impact on medical education, with many core tenets of the report still in place over 100 years later, including a requirement for a certain number of years dedicated to medical education and a firm grounding in scientific theory. Specifically, the resulting 2 + 2 model of education, which includes 2 years of preclinical learning in the basic and clinical sciences, followed by 2 years of clinical education and apprenticeships, is still the norm in most US medical schools.[19] Until 2016, the primary framework for undergraduate medical education in the United States was based upon the two-pillar model (Fig. 1.3).

VI. CONCEPTUALIZING HEALTH SYSTEMS SCIENCE—THE "THIRD PILLAR" OF MEDICAL EDUCATION

Abraham Flexner recognized that basic and clinical sciences did not provide the complete picture of medicine and health care. His report fulfilled a critical need at that time, namely standardizing and elevating the rigor of science in medical training.[13] Additionally, the next century of medical educators in US medical schools understood that the basic and clinical sciences were not the entirety of medicine, although the underlying 2 + 2 structure remained the predominant structure for undergraduate

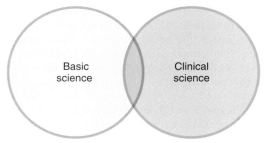

Fig. 1.3 The traditional two-pillar model of medical education. Basic science topic areas have included subjects such as biochemistry, anatomy, physiology, and/or pathology. Clinical science topic areas have included subjects such as physician examination skills, communication, and clinical diagnosis.

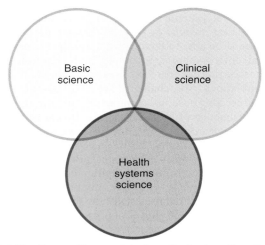

Fig. 1.4 The three-pillar model of medical education. Health Systems Science—the "third science"—complements and synergizes with basic and clinical science, and addresses subject areas including value-based care, teamwork, and health system improvement.

medical education. In the meantime, the landscape of health care has changed dramatically—foundational science along with diagnostic and therapeutic options have exploded in range and complexity, the understanding of the bio-psycho-social-environmental model of health and disease has progressed dramatically, and societal-economic-political pressures have emerged as major influencers, all supported by unprecedented data and information systems.

Knowledge and skills limited to the scientific basis of diseases, diagnoses, and treatments are necessary but not sufficient. Aligned with the evolving landscape of health care delivery (see Fig. 1.2), educators have proposed a "third pillar" of medical education, termed *Health Systems Science* (Fig. 1.4).[9,20] In this third science, physicians in training and health professions students must understand the broader system of health care, principles of policy and economics, population health management, interprofessional collaboration, behavioral and social determinants of health, and health system improvement (see Fig. 1.2). Currently, most medical education programs are not providing sufficient education of HSS content and concepts.[12,14,16,21,22] Chapter 2 outlines a comprehensive and synthetic framework of the knowledge and skill concept areas related to HSS.

The shifts in health care have a direct impact on the profession of medicine and are changing how doctors work and contribute to the health of society. The contemporary practice of medicine requires a fundamental adjustment for doctors trained in the Flexnerian model of rigorous education in the basic sciences followed by clinical application and research under the supervision of experienced professors.[13,23] Flexner's worldview revolved around the idea of sovereign physicians utilizing enlightened biomedical science to lead the way in curing disease. Although scientific discovery continues to enhance health care capabilities and opportunities, the world of medical practice and physician roles have changed and continue to evolve, and it is clear that basic and clinical science alone are insufficient to reach our goals in health care. Optimal health care in the 21st century requires the expertise and integration of multiple domains of HSS. It is no longer enough to know why and how biological systems work, or to prescribe and implement the latest medical or surgical therapy; health professionals must be able to factor in the multiple complexities of social, environmental, economic, and technical systems and translate this expertise to the care of individual patients and populations. The challenge for medical education is to introduce this system's complexity into the traditional bimodal sequence of biomedical and clinical science in a substantive, meaningful fashion. In order to achieve this goal, a range of attitudes, skills, and knowledge domains that had been previously marginalized or assumed, such as learning to function in interprofessional teams, communicating effectively across multiple mediums from cultural divides to electronic databases, linking the ability to make a difference in a situation with action and advocacy with professionalism, improving patient and population experience while reducing costs, and navigating fragmented social, economic, and policy gaps, will need to be incorporated into the foundations of educational curriculum. Whether pursuing the Triple Aim or preparing students to succeed in the 21st century, medical educators need to completely rethink how classroom and experiential learning is structured, while students must consider the prioritization of these topics in their learning. This will require not only significant re-engineering of classrooms and practice experiences, but also attention to how our learners view themselves as the professionals who will assume the reigns of this change, embrace it, and be the change agents required for the next wave of care.

VII. PROFESSIONAL IDENTITY FORMATION

As discussed earlier, the rapidly evolving health care landscape creates an immediate need to re-evaluate medical education curriculum and meaningfully incorporate HSS. The key here is "meaningful"; the two-pillar model is deeply embedded in our educational DNA and career pathways, and this will require no less than a transformative rebalancing of priorities and incentives. At the core of this transformation is a vital need to develop and educate a new generation of providers who view their role inherently differently than groups that have come earlier, who view themselves as part of an interprofessional care team, rather than an independent autonomous provider. They need to be fluent in the

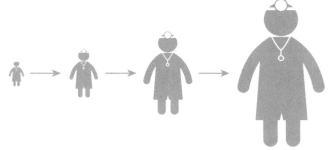

Fig. 1.5 Traditional view of medical student education and professional role identity formation. Student growth during medical school has traditionally focused on "physician-centric" education, which is, by and large, separated and divorced from authentic perspectives into health care processes and interprofessional collaboration.

"language" of collaboration and systems thinking, rather than hesitant "systems immigrants" who prefer an autonomous role.

The HSS consist of knowledge and concepts that are not "physician-centric" but rather are "patient-centered." The goal is not limited to the treatment of disease; it is guided by the health and outcomes of patients and populations, taking into account multiple complex factors. HSS fluency requires the provider to understand the challenges and successes encountered by patients as they traverse the health "system" to obtain care and achieve or sustain health. This understanding is independent of any one profession or health care role. This new professional identity is required by all health professionals to not only provide patient-centered care, but also to appropriately function in the rapidly evolving and increasingly collaborative care models needed to achieve the Triple Aim.

A. Physician-Centric Role Identity

In traditional models of medical education, students entered medical school and assumed the role of the "apprentice." A method adopted and advanced by Flexner in the early 1900s, students' learning occurred primarily from working with and observing more senior physicians. Physicians were viewed as an actively-practicing repository of knowledge, information, and decision-making prowess for nearly all aspects of a patient's care. In this model, students observed, or "shadowed" in the clinical environment, before developing more autonomy over time toward a path of independent practitioner. Fig. 1.5 depicts this traditional view of medical student education and professional role identity formation.

In this model, students are separated from the "wheel" of health care delivery and authentic participation in team-based care. As a result, students are often viewed as extraneous to the functions and process of patient care, making them feel devalued (Fig. 1.6). There are times, although infrequent, when students are active contributors to teams. But increasing regulatory and supervision requirements, including students' inability to contribute to meaningful documentation in the electronic health record, have effectively limited their ability to authentically contribute to patient care.

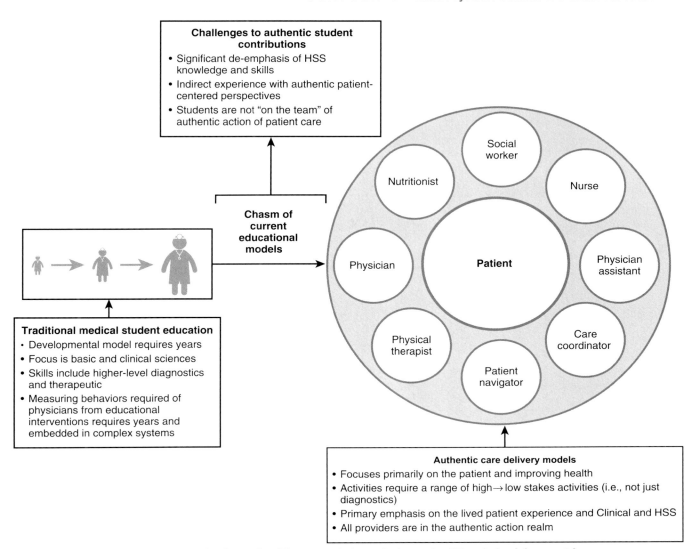

Fig. 1.6 Conceptual schematic of the current chasm between traditional physician-centric medical education and authentic patient-centered contributions impacting professional role identity.

A key analogy that captures the essence of the new professional role identity needed in evolving health care systems is one of the digital native versus the digital immigrant. A digital immigrant is an individual who was born into a culture of a system without all of the technological advances of current day. These individuals likely have acquired some of the customs and adopted some of the technology that is available, however they have not fully integrated technology into their rubric of everyday living; they are "immigrants" to this way. On the contrary, digital natives are those who are born into the technology environment, and therefore it becomes part of their "DNA" of living. For health care, medical education seeks to educate "HSS natives," those future providers who are aware of the key ideas of the HSS and see these areas as critical for their maturation, as well as the growth of our health care system into a more optimal and safe enterprise.

B. Patient-Centered, Systems Role Identity

For physicians in training to develop an early professional role identity that aligns with the needs of the 21st century health care system, students must be provided with early immersive experiences to learn about and engage in HSS. Akin to the need to perform clinical preceptorships to learn clinical skills such as cardiac and lung auscultation, communication, and history taking, students must authentically engage with HSS through clinical work. This involves students being embedded into interprofessional care teams and becoming a true "ball bearing" contributor to the health care teams (Fig. 1.7). In this model, students engage in HSS by participating in roles that are not traditionally physician-centric roles. When students serve in these collaborative team environments and provide value through engagement in concepts outside of the physician-patient interface (the tip of the iceberg in Fig. 1.2), students can

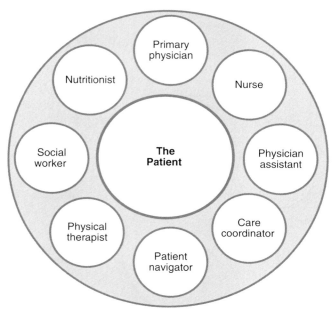

Fig. 1.7 Proposed "ball bearing" model for medical student education and professional role identity formation in the context of Health Systems Science. With Health Systems Science, medical students begin to view health care systems in new ways, and potentially undertake authentic systems roles (e.g., patient navigator). Through these roles, students fully engage with the health system and see first-hand the roles of other team members and health care processes. This proposed model provides students with opportunities to see their professional role as one within the health system and among other team members.

begin to understand the roles of other health professionals and have the opportunity to develop a new patient-centered systems role identity.

VIII. OVERVIEW OF BOOK CHAPTERS

In this textbook, the subsequent 14 chapters will address the key components of HSS. This textbook has been specifically designed for all health professions students, including students in medicine, physician assistant, nursing, and public health schools. However, these core concepts are applicable to all other health care providers with an interest in these areas and medical education faculty responsible for educating the next generation of health providers about HSS and the evolving frontier of health care education.

In Chapter 2, an explicit definition of HSS and the relationship between all the various aspects of HSS will be explored. In Chapters 3 to 13, each chapter will "take on" a critical component of HSS, with a discussion of the current key concepts that are applicable to current-day, and also factor in the evolving landscape of health care delivery. Chapter 14 will provide students with insights into assessment strategies and how they might utilize feedback from a variety of sources to help them understand how they are performing within health care systems in which they are learning and assisting in the provision of patient-centered care. Finally, Chapter 15 will address the next steps in delineating HSS concepts in medical education and raise provocative questions about the future of HSS.

Table 1.1 Chapter Template

Learning objectives

Chapter outline

Core chapter content

Summary

Questions for reflection

Annotated bibliography and references

IX. CHAPTER TEMPLATE

The goal of this textbook is to enhance the education of health professions students, faculty, and other individuals interested in advancing their knowledge and skills in HSS, with the aim of ultimately improving the health of patients. To this end, each chapter is intended to provide useful information and stimulating concepts for the reader to consider on a broad scale. Each chapter will highlight salient aspects of medicine that are deemed appropriate for the soon-to-be or currently practicing provider within the health care system. Each chapter will additionally seek to incorporate tables and case studies to stimulate further engagement with each of the concepts (Table 1.1). The authors fully anticipate, given the rapid transformation of health care redesign, specific content that could be included in such a textbook could quickly become "out of date." Each chapter has been purposefully designed to build a framework for subsequent knowledge and conceptual learning, so the anticipated changes could still be directly applied to this structure and therefore applicable across time. Readers are encouraged to supplement this reading and content with other resources that have the potential to build upon these concepts in a synergistic manner.

X. QUESTIONS

1. What is health systems science, and why is it important to 21st century health care delivery?
2. How will success in achieving the elements of the Triple Aim address some of the most serious problems confronting health care in the United States?
3. Describe three payment (reform) strategies that are designed to replace the current fee-for-service model and enhance the value of health care delivery?
4. How can development of the knowledge and skills necessary to function and lead change in our health care systems actually lead to enhanced patient-centered care?
5. What meaningful roles can students assume during immersive experiences in our health care systems that allow them to participate authentically as members of a health care team? How are these roles different than those previously available through an "apprenticeship model" of medical education?

Annotated Bibliography

Berwick DM, Nolan TW, Whittington J. The triple aim: care, health, and cost. *Health Aff (Millwood)*. 2008;27(3):759–769.
    Set the stage for the current quality movement.

Gonzalo JD, Haidet P, Papp KK, et al. Educating for the 21st-century healthcare system: an interdependent framework of basic, clinical, and systems sciences. *Acad Med.* 2015. [Epub ahead of print].
Outlines the framework for health systems science and forms the basis for this textbook.

Institute of Medicine (US) Committee on Quality of Health Care in America. *Crossing the quality chasm: a new health system for the 21st century.* Washington, D.C.: National Academy Press; 2001.
Landmark report that identified significant problems with the quality of health care provided in the United States.

Skochelak SE. A decade of reports calling for change in medical education: What do they say? *Acad Med.* 2010;85(suppl 9):S26–S33.
Important paper that summarizes the modern medical education reform movement.

References

1. Senge PM. *The Fifth Discipline: The Art and Practice of the Learning Organization.* Revised and updated edition. New York: Doubleday/ Currency; 2006.
2. Deming WE. *Out of the Crisis.* Cambridge: Massachusetts Institute of Technology, Center for Advanced Engineering Study; 1986.
3. Berwick DM, Nolan TW, Whittington J. The triple aim: care, health, and cost. *Health Aff (Millwood).* 2008;27(3):759–769.
4. Porter ME. What is value in health care? *New Engl J Med.* 2010;363(26):2477–2481.
5. Porter ME, Pabo EA, Lee TH. Redesigning primary care: a strategic vision to improve value by organizing around patients' needs. *Health Aff (Millwood).* 2013;32(3):516–525.
6. Hirmas Adauy M, Poffald Angulo L, Jasmen Sepúlveda AM, Aguilera Sanhueza X, Delgado Becerra I, Vega Morales J. [Health care access barriers and facilitators: a qualitative systematic review]. *Rev Panam Salud Publica.* 2013;33(3):223–229.
7. Institute of Medicine (US) Committee on Quality of Health Care in America. *Crossing the quality chasm: a new health system for the 21st century.* Washington, D.C.: National Academy Press; 2001.
8. Friedberg MW, RAND Health, American Medical Association. *Factors affecting physician professional satisfaction and their implications for patient care, health systems, and health policy.* Santa Monica, CA: Rand Corporation; 2013.
9. Gonzalo J, Dekhtyar M, Starr SR, et al. Healthcare delivery science curricula in undergraduate medical education: identifying and defining a potential curricular framework. *Acad Med.* 2016 Apr 5. [Epub ahead of print].
10. Chang A, Bowen JL, Buranosky RA, et al. Transforming primary care training—patient-centered medical home entrustable professional activities for internal medicine residents. *J Gen Intern Med.* 2013;28(6):801–809.
11. Chang A, Ritchie C. Patient-centered models of care: closing the gaps in physician readiness. *J Gen Intern Med.* 2015;30(7):870–872.
12. Crosson FJ, Leu J, Roemer BM, Ross MN. Gaps in residency training should be addressed to better prepare doctors for a twenty-first-century delivery system. *Health Aff (Millwood).* 2011;30(11):2142–2148.
13. Thibault GE. Reforming health professions education will require culture change and closer ties between classroom and practice. *Health Aff (Millwood).* 2013;32(11):1928–1932.
14. Skochelak SE. A decade of reports calling for change in medical education: what do they say? *Acad Med.* 2010;85(Suppl 9):S26–S33.
15. Lucey CR. Medical education: part of the problem and part of the solution. *JAMA Intern Med.* 2013;173(17):1639–1643.
16. Combes JR, Arespacochaga E. *Lifelong Learning: Physician Competency Development.* Chicago, IL: American Hospital Association's Physician Leadership Forum; June 2012.
17. Kegan R. *The Evolving Self: Problem and Process in Human Development.* Cambridge: Harvard University Press; 1982.
18. Kegan R, Lahey LL. *Immunity to Change: How to Overcome It and Unlock Potential in Yourself and Your Organization.* Boston: Harvard Business Press; 2009.
19. Flexner A. Medical education in the United States and Canada. From the Carnegie Foundation for the Advancement of Teaching, Bulletin Number Four, 1910. *B World Health Organ.* 2002;80(7):594–602.
20. Gonzalo JD, Haidet P, Papp KK, et al. Educating for the 21st-century healthcare system: an interdependent framework of basic, clinical, and systems sciences. *Acad Med.* 2015 Oct 16. [Epub ahead of print].
21. Patel MS, Lypson ML, Davis MM. Medical student perceptions of education in health care systems. *Acad Med.* 2009;84(9):1301–1306.
22. Greysen SR, Schiliro D, Curry L, Bradley EH, Horwitz LI. "Learning by doing"—resident perspectives on developing competency in high-quality discharge care. *J Gen Intern Med.* 2012;27(9):1188–1194.
23. Ludmerer KM. *Time to Heal: American Medical Education from the Turn of the Century to the Era of Managed Care.* New York: Oxford University Press; 1999.

2

What Is Health Systems Science? Building an Integrated Vision

Jed D. Gonzalo, MD, MSc, Stephanie R. Starr, MD, and
Jeffrey M. Borkan, MD, PhD

LEARNING OBJECTIVES

1. Describe the importance of Health Systems Science (HSS) and its integration with basic and clinical sciences to maximize health for patients and society.
2. Define HSS in medical education.
3. Describe an HSS curricular framework for medical education.
4. List the steps in moving from the HSS definition to an integrated HSS curriculum.
5. Identify and discuss barriers to HSS in undergraduate medical education, including challenges for the "third science" of medical education from the student perspective.

Chapter 2 builds on the definition of Health Systems Science (HSS) and provides a conceptual framework for understanding the history and importance of HSS in medical education and a roadmap for building HSS curricula. The framework recognizes HSS as a *third medical science* that must be integrated with the basic and clinical sciences if graduates of our health professional schools are to succeed in contributing to the achievement of the Triple Aim. The HSS curricular framework is rooted in the bio-psycho-social model proposed by Engel, with underpinnings in system theory. The chapter describes the HSS framework and content (the "what") and provides a glimpse into the subjects that will be covered in detail in subsequent chapters. Finally, this chapter examines barriers to HSS education in undergraduate medical education, and raises questions and potential solutions regarding the work that remains in HSS education.

CHAPTER OUTLINE

I. THE THIRD MEDICAL SCIENCE: HEALTH SYSTEMS SCIENCE

Chapter 1 describes gaps in clinical care, the focused areas for change in care delivery, and the need for medical education to align with these gaps. Filling in these gaps requires a new knowledge base and skillset for future physicians to both participate in and contribute to the transformation of the health care delivery system in order to achieve the Triple Aim. The third medical science in medical education, Health Systems Science (HSS), described in this chapter provides much of what is needed, particularly when it is seamlessly integrated with the basic and clinical sciences. The development of a new type of physician who is competent in all three medical sciences is critically required for both the patients for whom they will care and the health of society as a whole. To successfully prepare for and engage in HSS activities, such as interprofessional team-based care, health care quality improvement, or population health management, new curricula are needed at our nation's medical schools and training programs that will help future practitioners achieve these ends. Students must also be aware of the importance of this science in their own professional development.

A. Why Is a Conceptual Framework Needed?

There are several critical reasons for elucidating an HSS curriculum and conceptual framework. Medical and health professions students need a conceptual framework to understand the scope and overlap of HSS knowledge, attitudes, and skills. In addition, understanding how the basic sciences (e.g., physiology, anatomy), clinical sciences (e.g., history-taking, communication), and Health Systems Sciences (e.g., teamwork, quality improvement) interrelate is critical to achieve the Triple Aim of improved patient experience, population health, and decreased cost.[1]

Medical educators and clinical faculty need a conceptual framework for HSS to build educational experiences for students and assess student progress in mastering HSS competencies across their professional careers; for the medical profession, this includes pre-medical education, undergraduate medical education (UME), graduate medical education (GME), and continuous professional development/continuing medical education (CME). Education leaders in medical schools require an HSS curricular roadmap to design curricula that diminish confusion and ambiguity about content/objectives that are to be included in a curriculum, and better align curricula with key HSS objectives and outcomes, such as the **Core Entrustable Professional Activities for Entering Residency (CEPAER)** and competencies, and the relevant **Accreditation Council for Graduate Medical Education (ACGME) competency domains** (practice-based learning improvement and systems-based practice).[2-5] Last, a clear framework will allow for the identification of educational opportunities that allow for collaboration across health care professions at all points within the educational continuum at the interface of clinical practice and education.

B. What Is Health Systems Science?

Health Systems Science is defined as the principles, methods, and practice of improving quality, outcomes, and costs of health care delivery for patients and populations within systems of medical care. As identified in Chapter 1, HSS provides a comprehensive and holistic vision of topics, subjects, and competencies for individuals who are training and providing care within health care systems.[6-9] This third medical science should ideally synergize, complement, and be integrated with the core content and concepts of the traditional basic and clinical sciences. Using a patient-centered perspective that also reflects the Triple Aim, HSS can also be conceptualized as consisting of the factors that impact the health outcomes for individual patients and populations of patients beyond the basic and clinical sciences.

II. HSS IN MEDICAL EDUCATION: PAST TO PRESENT

The awareness and inclusion of HSS topics in medical education programs at the UME, GME, and practice level has been patchy at best, though the field has been rapidly evolving and advancing in recent years. There have been numerous publications and presentations addressing selected content areas within HSS domains, including novel curricular innovations and assessments of such curricula.[10-13] Multiple works have described ideal physician outcomes and/or curricula addressing content beyond the traditional basic and clinical sciences such as quality improvement, interprofessional teamwork, health care policy, transitions of care, and related areas of physician development.[14-16] Since 2000, several textbooks have been published that explore areas of education and care delivery that are related to specific HSS domains. For example, *Understanding Patient Safety, Understanding Value-Based Healthcare,* and *The Health Care Handbook* are three books that eloquently describe some of the core concepts in HSS.[17-19]

Collectively, these contributions are critical for advancing learners' knowledge, attitudes, behaviors, and skills in these areas. However, despite casting spotlights on previously underrepresented topics in medical education and providing some resources for curricular innovation, there is still a critical need to fully define the scope of the principles and application of HSS, identify a full range of critical HSS topics, make explicit the relationships across and between topics that could be included in HSS domains, and provide an integrated comprehensive model of HSS. Despite extra elements being added to local curricula—or perhaps because of them—there is no unified approach to building and exposing learners to a systematically designed HSS curriculum.

Two earlier initiatives are notable in their attempts to build a framework of topics that could be included in an HSS curriculum. The Undergraduate Medical Education (UME-21) collaborative was a consortium of US medical schools in the late 1990s sponsored by the Health Resources and Services Administration (HRSA).[20] The collaborative sought to advance medical education topics such as health care policy, financing, and teamwork. In the late 2000s, the R25 collaborative to "strengthen behavioral and social science in medical education" and an Association of American Medical Colleges (AAMC) collaborative panel of experts advanced the field of HSS curriculum by synthesizing several content domains of public health and the determinants of health.[21,22] Despite these initiatives, a synthesized and unified whole of all potential content and concepts that could be included in HSS has not been developed prior to this effort.

As noted in Chapter 1, HSS learning among health professions students, and specifically medical students, has ranged from "lacking" to "insufficient." Upon graduation from medical school, the AAMC asks medical student graduates to report their degree of learning in numerous content areas, some of which relate to HSS. In 2012, when HSS-related concepts began appearing on the questionnaire, students reported a paucity of exposure to HSS topics, such as less than 50 percent for the "practice of medicine."[23] Interestingly, students appear to have a desire for additional HSS education, as students with more exposure to systems education report a higher satisfaction than students from schools with lower exposure to concepts such as medical economics, health care systems, managed care, and practice management.[23] These data highlight the environment and potential for further integrating HSS into educational programs.

For learners in US medical schools, the HSS educational content to which they are exposed is highly variable and often partial in scope. The inclusion of HSS concepts is generally dependent upon local expertise and resources rather than reflecting a complete HSS "gold standard" curriculum across schools. As a result, medical students are exposed to educational concepts in HSS that are limited in the range of topics and vulnerable to the ebbs and flows of faculty and institutional resources and interest. For example, even if learners are enrolled in a school where they are exposed to educational sessions on "high-value care" and quality improvement, this does not ensure exposure to the entire diverse array of potential HSS concepts that are required for graduates to ably function in the evolving health care system.

The gaps in formal HSS education have been filled to some extent through the hidden or informal curriculum, that is, lessons that are not explicitly taught, but rather learned through the everyday activities and behaviors of the settings in which students are exposed, if it is learned at all.[24,25] This unstructured approach is insufficient for optimal education as the faculty, nursing staff, other health care providers, and the processes of current-day health care may not be conducive to teaching learners the key concepts that are potentially lacking. Worse yet, since the hidden and informal curriculum is rarely evaluated, there is no way of knowing if HSS teaching and role modeling are appropriate, effective, or even correct. Most current-day faculty were not educated within a system that promoted a focus in HSS, and therefore, may view their professional role as one related to more traditional physician-centric knowledge and skills alone (see Chapter 1). This situation may greatly limit the degree of "on the job" education for learners in the HSS, creating an even more emergent need for the HSS in formal curricular activities.

In the literature related to HSS knowledge and skills at the GME level, resident physicians report perceived deficiencies when exposed to the need to apply them in actual clinical settings. In such clinical situations, physician trainees struggle with managing transitions of care, discharge planning, and mitigating medication barriers due to insufficient finances or insurance.[26] Consequently, patients' health improvements are often stymied by lack of health care professionals' understanding of their individual contexts, the determinants of health within the patients' community or social networks, and whether barriers are cultural, financial, educational, or a mixture of all three. In addition to creating potentially unsafe situations for patients, it is hypothesized that these curricular deficiencies may contribute to unnecessary costs within the health care system. Specifically, recent articles highlight the association between learning environment (specifically spending patterns and health care intensity experienced during training) and subsequent trainee knowledge, attitudes, and behaviors related to cost-conscious care.[27–29]

III. DEVELOPMENT OF AN HSS CURRICULAR FRAMEWORK

In 2013, the American Medical Association funded grants to 11 of the 141 eligible US allopathic medical schools to "accelerate change in medical education."[30] This consortium of 11 schools began collaborative work to close gaps and advance critical areas of medical education. One of the early focus areas was Systems-Based Practice (SBP), resulting in the formation of an SBP working group. This group reviewed the literature and brainstormed the major issues and challenges related to needed curricula in medical education beyond the basic and clinical sciences. This iterative process resulted in the sharpened focus, reflected in the group's name changes as the scope became more apparent. The working group chose **Health Systems Science** as the title for the third medical science, embarked on a project to develop a shared definition of HSS, and sought to fulfill the primary need of developing a comprehensive and integrated HSS curricular framework for medical education.

Several conceptual models could have been utilized to pursue the development of an HSS definition and curricular framework. Each potential model and method has its advantages and disadvantages as an overarching HSS framework, and the group was cognizant that the choices would likely result in potential insufficiencies and curricular gaps. Conceptual models considered for the HSS curricular framework included the Social Medicine approach espoused by Virchow, the Systems Management model proposed by Donabedian, and the Systems Thinking and Theory model.[31–33] The group sought to use a comprehensive, broad-based lens that had little likelihood of omitting or neglecting potential curricular topic areas. They selected George Engel's **Bio-Psycho-Social (BPS) model of medicine**, which utilizes a systems thinking approach to all levels beyond the "organism" as the basic theoretical model for HSS.[34]

A. Engel's Bio-Psycho-Social Model

In the 1970s, George Engel described the goals of the patient-physician relationship as including 1) the promotion of healing, 2) the relief of suffering, and 3) encouragement and education regarding behaviors to improve health.[34] He explained the need for physicians to understand his or her patient in several dimensions, both diagnostically and personally, to achieve the goals of this relationship. He emphasized the perspective of illness manifesting at numerous levels of patient- and systems-related factors in addition to disease pathophysiology. His BPS model of medicine proposes that effective physicians in the 21st century cannot isolate and focus on only one component (i.e., pathophysiology) of the organized whole, as doing so will neglect or compromise the object of study (the patient). Physicians must have holistic approaches that integrate the biological, psychological, social, and systems components in order to help patients make the most informed and effective medical decisions, resulting in the greatest impact on the process and outcomes of care. The BPS perspective requires one to consider a human being to be both a biological organism and a person who lives in the context of family and community. Engel believed the following:

> Patients' journeys through health and illness are often not predictable. Clinicians who have the skills and willingness to accompany their patients on these complex journeys will be more effective as healers and more satisfied with their work.

The foundation of Engel's model is based upon general systems theory, as described by Bertalanffy, and later by Senge (Fig. 2.1).[33,35] Systems theory proposes that every level of organization, including molecular, cellular, organic, personal, interpersonal, familial, societal, and biospheric, affects every other level. Systems theory provides a conceptual framework whereby both the organized whole and component parts can be studied and, as such, supplies the basis for HSS. The HSS curricular framework and definition is an expanded view of the "sociological" domain to include sciences related to health care delivery and improvement sciences.

Using Engel's conceptual model and the proposed definition of HSS, in 2014 the American Medical Association's HSS working group initiated a comprehensive analysis of existing and planned curricula within 11 consortium schools to develop an HSS curricular framework based on current

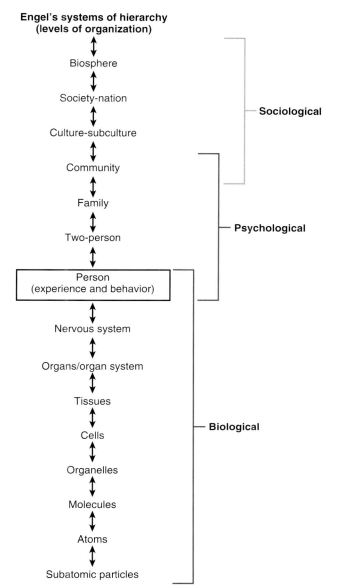

Engel's systems of hierarchy (levels of organization)

- Biosphere
- Society-nation
- Culture-subculture
- Community
- Family
- Two-person
- Person (experience and behavior)
- Nervous system
- Organs/organ system
- Tissues
- Cells
- Organelles
- Molecules
- Atoms
- Subatomic particles

Sociological

Psychological

Biological

Fig. 2.1 Engel's Bio-Psycho-Social conceptual model for medicine used in the identification of a health care delivery science curriculum. The three tiers—biological, psychological, and sociological—are designated on the right side of the figure.

thinking and planning by educators (versus recommended or conceptualized topics). The results of this work have been presented in several forums, and are briefly summarized next.[36,37]

IV. HSS CURRICULAR DOMAINS

Three categories of curricular topics or domains are included in the HSS curricular framework: 1) core, 2) cross-cutting, and 3) linking domains. Fig. 2.2 illustrates the relationship among all three types of domains. Here, all domains are described with a working definition for curricular content; these domains also coincide with subsequent chapters. Subtopics in the core curricular domains are organized using previously published conceptual frameworks, as described later. As with any emerging science, conceptual domains of content will evolve in an iterative manner as new concepts are identified, subcategories

of content expand into individual domains, and relationships across domains are better understood across professional disciplines and in multiple educational settings.

A. Core Domains

There are six core curricular domains, which include content categories that align directly with HSS; for each domain, the 11 schools identified, where possible, an existing theoretical framework to inform the domain's content.

1. Health Care Structures and Processes

Health Care Structures and Processes include all issues related to the organization of individuals, institutions, resources, and processes for delivery of health care to meet the needs of patients or populations of patients, including the processes of collaboration and coordination. Several specific examples of curricular content in this domain include 1) knowledge of clinical settings (e.g., clinics, hospital units) and processes occurring within outpatient and inpatient settings, 2) fragmentation and insufficiencies encountered by patients in the health care continuum, and 3) ability to identify the importance of teamwork within clinical "teams" and "communities" that span diverse settings.

2. Health Care Policy, Economics, and Management

Health Care Policy, Economics, and Management encompasses all issues related to the decisions, plans, and actions undertaken to achieve specific health care goals and the issues related to efficiency, effectiveness, value, and behavior in the production and consumption of health care. These sciences are used to promote health through the study of all components of the health care system and managed care. Specific examples of curricular content in this domain include 1) history and core principles of health care policy, 2) the basics of how health care is financed and the impact of health care policy on insurance and reimbursement, and 3) incentives for providers and hospitals within different US payment models.

3. Clinical Informatics/Health Information Technology

Clinical Informatics/Health Information Technology includes all issues related to the application of informatics and information technology to deliver health care services, including clinical decision support, documentation, electronic medical records, and the utilization of data to improve health. Specific curricular examples in this domain include 1) core principles of informatics sciences, including biomedical informatics, patient security, and rights protection in regard to data; 2) awareness of real-time data viewing and decision support to manage data registries and analyze clinical reports; and 3) awareness of current functionality and challenges in current health information exchange.

4. Population Health

The Population Health domain includes all issues related to traditional public health and preventive medicine, including

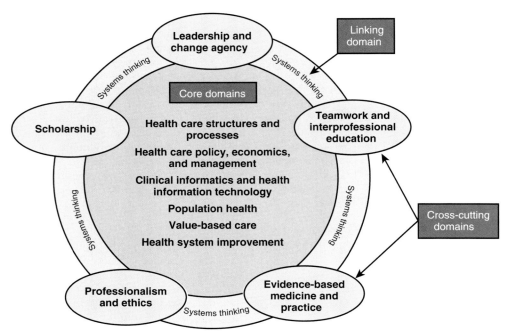

Fig. 2.2 Core, cross-cutting, and linking domains for a Health Systems Science curriculum. The five cross-cutting domains are curricular areas that traditionally may have been included in medical education curriculum, but have a new context in Health Systems Science. The one linking domain, Systems Thinking, unifies or "links" all core and cross-culture domains (depicted in this figure) and other areas of the curriculum (such as the basic and clinical sciences).

the full range of health determinants affecting the entire population rather than sick individuals. The content in this domain also includes the organized assessment, monitoring, or measurement to prevent disease and injury, promote health, prolong life, or improve any other health outcome for a group of individuals (e.g., geographic populations such as nations, communities, ethnic groups, or any other defined group), including the access and distribution of such outcomes within the group, and the dynamic interrelationships among various personal, socioeconomic, and environmental factors that relate to health outcomes or prevention. Specific curricular examples for this domain include 1) ability to build a community asset map to identify local resources that can help address a leading health indicator, 2) definition of patient risk behaviors within the context of health determinants in uninsured populations, and 3) development of cultural skills to work with individuals from diverse cultural backgrounds.

5. Value-Based Care

Value-Based Care broadly includes content related to the performance of a health system in terms of quality of care delivery, cost, and waste. From the quality perspective, the content in this domain maps to one of the six Institute of Medicine dimensions of quality: patient safety, effectiveness, patient-centeredness, timeliness, effectiveness, and equity.[18,38] The content also includes all issues related to the cost of health care, waste components, and service requirements. Finally, the content includes understanding the epidemiology of, as well as seeing and classifying, gaps in care and care delivery. Specific curricular examples for this domain include 1) definition and stakeholder perspectives of value in health care; 2) components of high-value health care systems; 3) key correlations between quality and safety

principles with patient outcomes; 4) the importance of identifying, reporting, and analyzing safety events; and 5) the relationship between quality and cost and efforts by health care professionals and teams to address the costs of care.

6. Health System Improvement

Health System Improvement includes all content related to processes of identifying, analyzing, or implementing changes in policy, health care delivery, or any other function of the health care system to improve the performance of any component of the health care system. Issues herein include quantifying and closing gaps (action), variation/measurement (specifically related to quantifying and closing gaps, not to health care measures in general), analysis of data, and interventions. Specific curricular examples in this domain include 1) selecting a quality indicator and developing an improvement plan, 2) drafting a Plan-Do-Study-Act worksheet that outlines a test of change, and 3) having the ability to adapt to different improvement challenges with different evidence-based methodologies.

B. Cross-Cutting Domains

Topics (knowledge and skills) identified as transcending multiple core curricular domains were clustered into cross-cutting domains. These domains, especially professionalism, teamwork, and evidence-based practice, relate to direct patient-care competencies, and serve to connect and highlight the relationship (and sometimes tensions) between direct patient care priorities and a systems-focused view. As such, many UME curricula traditionally address this content, but these domains must be emphasized within the HSS context.

1. Leadership and Change Agency

Leadership and Change Agency includes all content related to inspiring motivation in others to create goals toward a desirable vision. In the context of UME, leadership pertains to team-based care, quality improvement projects, and so on. Specific curricular examples for this domain include 1) types of leadership in health care (and key competencies required for each type) and key skills physicians must develop to become true leaders, 2) reflection on personal values and synchrony with life goals as well as understanding how successful leaders have alignment between personal and institutional values, and 3) recognition that each health care professional has the power to suggest and implement changes in the health care system.

2. Teamwork and Interprofessional Education

Teamwork and Interprofessional Education includes all issues related to collaboration and team science, specifically through the process of individuals working together on specified tasks to achieved shared goals. Specific curricular examples for this domain include 1) knowledge and awareness of interprofessional providers' roles and skills, 2) communication required to function in teams in an integrated/coordinated system, and 3) skills to function in teams and apply reflective practice in the context of quality improvement and patient safety.

3. Evidence-Based Medicine and Practice

Evidence-Based Medicine and Practice encompasses content related to the conscientious, explicit, and judicious use of current best evidence in making decisions about the care of individual patients, populations of patients, or interventions in health care delivery improvement. Specific curricular examples in this domain include 1) appropriate use of decision support tools in decision-making processes within a virtual health system environment, 2) utilization of evidence-based guidelines and bundled protocols to ensure appropriate care delivery for patient panels, and 3) epidemiology and biostatistical methods required to understand gaps in care and disparities for populations of patients.

4. Professionalism and Ethics

Professionalism and Ethics includes the ethical behavior and professionalism including conduct congruent with generally accepted moral principles and values and with professional guidelines based on those principles and values. This definition includes general leadership ethics, such as honesty and responsibility, as well as ethics and professionalism specific to the HSS domains. Specific curricular examples in this domain include 1) definition of professionalism, its relationship to trust and improving value in health care, and its importance for success as a leader; 2) professionalism involved with collaborative team-based models of care; and 3) awareness of professionalism in the context of social media.

5. Scholarship

Scholarship as a cross-cutting domain includes all content relevant to the conduct and scholarly dissemination of HSS content and/or health services research that investigates any HSS domain. Scholarship is defined as 1) discovery, which is consistent with traditional research; 2) integration, which makes connections across disciplines and places specialties in a larger context; 3) application, which demonstrates the vital interaction between research and practice; and 4) teaching (educational scholarship), which emphasizes the creation of new knowledge about teaching and learning in the presence of learners.[39] Specific curricular examples in this domain include 1) development, completion, and presentation of scholarly quality and patient safety projects; 2) opportunities for population-based research projects; and 3) expertise through advanced application of knowledge and skills in interprofessional team-based care, quality improvement, leadership, and change management, as demonstrated through scholarly projects.

C. Linking Domain: Systems Thinking

Systems Thinking as a linking domain refers to the content that unifies or "links" the core curricular domains or subcategories to other core curricular domains, or core curricular domains or subcategories to contents of the broader medical school curriculum.[33] The knowledge and skills of Systems Thinking allow students to be cognizant of and apply a comprehensive holistic approach to medical care and health care issues. All issues relate to the attention of a complex web of interdependencies, an awareness of the "whole," not just the parts, and the ability to recognize multidirectional cause-effect relationships with all causes emerging as the effect of another system dynamic. For example, Systems Thinking allows a student to understand the influence of the Affordable Care Act on the determinants of health within a community, and as a result, the ability for his or her patient to access health care and adhere to care plans.

As with any emerging science and its inclusion in professional education, the richness and greatest impact lies at the intersection of conceptual content domains, and there is considerable overlap of concepts across the domains described earlier. These domains are not discrete and separate categories but overlap and interrelate as they compose the integrated whole of HSS. For example, discussion of health care processes and microsystems directly relates to specific and detailed discussions regarding teamwork; provider incentives discussed in health policy and economics directly influence value-based care and improvement; and professionalism implications must be included in conversations related to patient data protection concepts in clinical informatics and health information technology.

CASE STUDY 1

Renal Disease and Treatment: Where Basic, Clinical, and Health Systems Sciences Merge

Evolutionary developmental steps whereby concepts are introduced at each stage, but with increasing complexity to match the level of the learner.

FIRST YEAR OF MEDICAL SCHOOL DILEMMA

A first-year student is learning about kidney biochemistry and physiology. The student notes that on the chronic kidney disease equation (CKD-EPI) for estimating glomerular filtration rate (GFR) found on the National Institutes of Health website (http://www.niddk.nih.gov/health-information/health-communication-programs/nkdep/lab-evaluation/gfr/estimating/Pages/estimating.aspx), the formulas are divided between "blacks" and "whites." She asks her renal faculty member who has lectured for decades during the Renal Block about this, and he replies that these are the established formulas, and no one has ever questioned them before. When probing deeper, he suggests that the reason may be due to greater muscle mass among blacks. The student asks further questions:

1. What is the scientific basis for the racial "profiling" of renal function or muscle mass?
2. Is there evidence that blacks have different kidneys than whites?
3. What might be the interwoven social, medical, and economic factors that play into this—from occupational differences, to poverty, to differential access to care and treatment?
4. Who is considered "black," and who is considered "white" in the United States? She herself has a dark brown complexion with parents from Argentina and Brazil, while her anatomy partner is dark skinned, but his parents are from southern India.

INTERN DILEMMA

A family medicine intern prepares to discharge from the hospital to home a 71-year-old male patient following a long hospitalization for new-onset congestive heart failure complicated by acute renal failure. The discharge instructions include six new medications, a low-salt diet, support hose, and exercise and follow-up with a primary care physician in 5 days. The intern orders a visiting home nurse to go to the house and provide guidance, help administer and monitor medication adherence, check home safety, and measure blood pressure and weight. Unfortunately, the medications are administered on different schedules (e.g., once a day in the morning, twice a day, three times a day, once in the evening), and two of the medications are "off-formulary" and are unaffordable for the patient. There are no primary care physicians in the patient's area that accept his insurance. The patient lives in a community that is a "food desert" and is unable to get low-salt food; there are no sidewalks, and the visiting home nurses consider his neighborhood too dangerous to service. The patient quickly deteriorates, and after 4 days he decompensates sufficiently that his family calls 911. An ambulance takes him back to the hospital's emergency room, and he is admitted to the Intensive Care Unit for 1 week.

1. How might the discharge be handled, given the barriers to care?
2. How can rehospitalization be avoided?
3. How might the hospital, residents, staff, and attending physicians help reduce the health disparities in the community?
4. How can the health system assume responsibility for "episodes of care" including follow-up?
5. How might community-wide interventions reduce the rates of disease prevalence and incidence?

RENAL FELLOW DILEMMA

A renal fellow quickly masters the treatments for renal failure including the physiology and chemistry of renal dialysis. While involved in renal consults in a major teaching hospital, he notices that many of the patients who are scheduled to start renal dialysis have other serious comorbidities ranging from advanced Alzheimer's disease to end-stage metastatic cancer. He is pretty certain that neither quality of life nor life expectancy are influenced by the dialysis, but his attending chides him, "Look, who are you to be a one-man death panel" and, "Anyway, there is a special federal law that pays for all of it that was pushed by kidney patients in the 1980s."

1. What are the indications and counter-indications for dialysis for patients at end of life?
2. How might renal dialysis or other expensive medical interventions be judiciously applied to individual patients and populations, and is rationing reasonable?
3. What evidence is required to support the broad utilization of a medical intervention?
4. What health policy and legislative initiatives are reasonable for special interest groups?

V. KEY PRIORITIES IN IMPLEMENTING HEALTH SYSTEMS SCIENCE IN MEDICAL EDUCATION

As the result of a 2-year collaborative effort and deliberative, focused discussions, the AMA ACE Consortium identified the key priority areas and strategies for advancing and integrating HSS in medical education programs.[40] These priorities and strategies highlight several challenges and future directions for HSS in the learning agenda for students and faculty.

A. Develop Comprehensive, Standardized, and Integrated Curricula

As described earlier, medical education does not currently have one unified comprehensive HSS curricular framework that appropriately integrates the basic and clinical sciences at the appropriate time in students' professional development and education. The curricular content across medical schools is highly variable, and not of a unified standard. Increasingly, medical schools are collaborating on steps toward a comprehensive, standardized, and integrated HSS curriculum for health profession schools. Local schools and health systems and national discussion forums and societies can raise awareness of this need and promote discourse around the core content and concepts to be included in such curricula.[36] Efforts to achieve standardization will need to be sufficiently rigorous to ensure that all trainees gain competencies in HSS areas, but not so inflexible that they discourage innovation and ongoing evaluation of topics as health care realities change. Leadership in this area may come from medical education organizations, health care organizations, or trainees; collaborative ventures among all stakeholders will have the greatest chance of success. Students must be aware of this lack of cohesion as they approach their studies in these areas.

B. Develop, Standardize, and Align Assessments

High-quality assessment methods are essential to ensure learner progress in achieving HSS competencies. In addition, assessment drives student learning, and itself facilitates learning through assessment-enhanced information retrieval and workplace-based assessments.[41] There is a relative paucity of validated assessment methods targeting HSS domains, including a robust framework of milestones, competencies, and entrustable professional activities. One challenge to developing and implementing HSS assessment methods is the lack of a clear developmental paradigm for mastery in these domains. Foundational HSS knowledge is currently being defined, and the roles and expected level of student performance in the practice elements of HSS have not been elucidated.[37] Furthermore, it is difficult to construct high-quality, multiple-choice items to assess knowledge in key HSS domains with or without a synthetic HSS curricular framework. Assessments of more practical aspects of HSS will require the development and implementation of observational methods in the "workplace," where approaches to ensuring high-quality, reliable, and valid assessment outcomes are evolving.[42,43] As ongoing work defines the core curriculum, the new types of assessment methods that are needed will become clearer.[36] There are several existing assessment methods that currently could be used for HSS assessment and can provide an initial "toolkit." For example, assessment methods related to teamwork, quality, safety, and evidence-based practice include multiple-choice examinations, knowledge application tests, work-product ratings, simulation-based tools, indirect observation methods (e.g., peer assessment, multisource feedback), and direct observation of clinical activities.[44–58] Unfortunately, most assessment methods involve locally developed tools or modifications of existing "national" tools using small samples of students with variable psychometric characteristics. This forbids the use of existing validity data in informing the use of the tool, prevents comparisons across studies, and hinders rigorous analysis of new tools.[59,60] Future work will increasingly enhance and develop validated tools to ensure that assessments for learners in the HSS are of high quality.

C. Partner with Licensing and Accrediting Bodies to Align Standards and Examinations

One of the leading priority areas for HSS in medical education is aligning assessments with the desired goals of medical education across the continuum of UME, GME, and CME/practice. At present, curricular content, skills, and competencies related to HSS are not significantly integrated into national standards or licensing examinations, and there is scant consistency between accrediting bodies and their assessments. The United States Medical Licensing Examination (USMLE) and the National Board for Medical Examiners (NBME) "shelf examinations" focus primarily on the basic and clinical sciences.

In the current culture, these examination scores are highly valued by students, educators, and residency programs, and often serve as criteria for residency selection.[61] While students realize the importance of learning about health systems and performing authentic systems-based roles, they also feel locked into a pathway that does not assess or reward such an educational agenda. Educators trying to include HSS in a meaningful way face constraints imposed by both students themselves, as they decide what is and what is not important, and by the current educational system, which incentivizes

biomedical learning at the expense of other areas, including HSS. One work-around strategy would be to relegate HSS learning to the "other" category, with content that is at the periphery of the curricular map or that can be learned on the side or at some "later" date. While this approach in the past may have been sufficient for the purposes of accreditation, the expectations of the clinical environment have changed, and health care organizations are increasingly viewing HSS-related experiences as contributing to the development of essential physician skills.[6,62] Students can appreciate this transformation and understand the implications. With increased educational reform that aligns with this transformation, students are seeking additional focus in these areas, and clinical care systems are requesting it. However, as evidenced by student and health systems leaders' opinions regarding the knowledge and skills of current graduates in these areas, change has been slow.[16,23] Research has shown that students seem trapped in an education world, where student focus is dominated by examinations, clerkship performance, and residency vetting that largely ignores the importance of HSS (Fig. 2.3).

The national standards for curricular content in medical schools are developed after widespread acceptance among the education community has occurred. Only then can the standards become an integral part of the standards implemented by the Liaison Committee for Medical Education (LCME) and the Accrediting Council for Graduate Medical Education (ACGME). Similarly, only HSS content that has achieved a level of acceptance and credibility in the educational and regulatory communities will be incorporated into national assessment procedures, such as the USMLE. This process may require years to complete, and in 2016, the HSS curricular content areas have not yet become an integral component of accreditation or licensing standards. It is anticipated that over the next several years, the HSS concepts will be increasingly incorporated into these processes and outcomes. Until HSS is fully aligned with accrediting and licensing standards, students should be encouraged to remain diligent about the need to balance their educational priorities that are most aligned with long-term goals.

D. Improve the Undergraduate-to-Graduate Medical Education Transition

In the current education model, students progress from medical school into residency programs, often in different health systems. This transition between UME and GME creates unique challenges for education programs seeking to enhance learning and assessment in HSS-related competencies.[6,16,62,63] The GME milestones as part of the ACGME Next Accreditation System and the UME AAMC Entrustable Professional Activities (EPAs) outcome goals for graduating medical students are not similar in language or content, limiting the assessment in this transition.[2,64,65] Although EPAs and milestones can be used in a complementary manner, ideal educational "handoffs" are hindered by a lack of consistency in how they are defined and developed.[66] Additionally, variation across GME programs' expectations of graduating medical student competence in HSS, and assessment and prioritization of these areas in the residency selection process further reinforce gaps in the UME-to-GME transition. Medical education initiatives are seeking to achieve a common language to guide learning and assessment, specifically for HSS, to reliably ensure that physicians are prepared to meaningfully

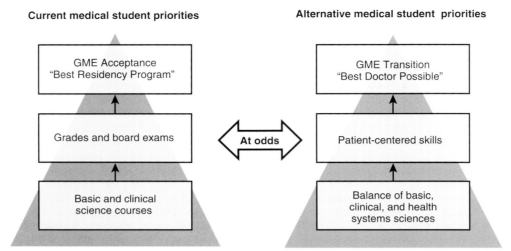

Fig. 2.3 Medical student competing agendas as the primary pedagogical challenge for a Health Systems Science curriculum in undergraduate medical education. The left side of the figure reflects student perspectives of current priority areas for their education. The basic and clinical sciences are viewed as essential components of learning for grades and board examinations, both of which primarily test biomedical concepts. These evaluative measures are perceived as the primary influence on acceptance into the best residency program of their choice. The right side of the figure demonstrates student perspectives on their awareness of the importance to focus on alternative areas. Students identify the importance of balancing basic, clinical, and Health Systems Sciences, which will allow them to develop a skillset for patient-centered care. Students identify these skills as critical for transitioning into graduate medical education training to be able to better care for patients.

participate in complex, evolving, team-based care models. In the coming years, a common "transition" competency and assessment language and system will allow for a more meaningful and seamless transition from UME to GME.

E. Enhance Knowledge, Skills, and Incentives of Faculty

It is critical to identify faculty who understand, practice, and effectively teach HSS content in order to successfully integrate these concepts into existing curricula. Traditionally trained clinical faculty typically need to enhance their own HSS expertise to close these curricular deficiencies.[6,16] This means clinical teachers are challenged to teach HSS while they are learning it and simultaneously working in a continuously changing environment.[67] Competing priorities for time and inadequate resource allocation, coupled with increased emphasis on clinical productivity, make it difficult for faculty to undertake intensive training or integrate newly developed skills into clinical practice and teaching. Currently, little training and support of faculty capabilities in care improvement, educational innovation, and dissemination of HSS scholarship are available to support a sustainable clinical learning environment. Collaboration with the health care system provides the hands-on learning opportunities required to integrate new concepts and practices into the daily work environment. Institutional faculty development programs and learning communities are being created that use a mixture of online, face-to-face, and experiential learning that is supported by a shared repository of educational modules and materials. Institutions can support faculty by facilitating honorific recognition of professional development, structural support for maintenance of certification and CME, streamlined institutional review board processes to encourage quality improvement

interventions, protected time to advance learning and teaching, leadership and career opportunities in related clinical and educational environments, assistance with scholarly productivity, and inclusion in promotion guidelines. National discussions are ongoing around a national certificate program that could promote the dissemination of information to a broad base of medical educators, while allowing institutions to focus on local integration and faculty support for continued learning and improvement.

F. Demonstrate the Potential for Adding Value to the Practice

Traditionally, clinical training experiences in UME link students directly with resident and attending physicians during clinical care duties.[68] This apprenticeship model requires time to mentor and educate students, which often decreases efficiency and negatively impacts physician productivity and profitability of the health system.[69–73] The increasing need for physicians and care delivery models to optimize efficiency and quality while minimizing cost, and the added work in mentoring medical students in today's models needs to be re-examined. Faculty and schools have traditionally presumed that students cannot add value to patient care today. Recommendations have been made for increased education and research into further integrating medical schools with academic health centers and community health programs.[74,75] Recently, educators have recommended an increased focus on identifying and providing value-added roles for medical students to "share the care" of health care delivery.[76,77] The application of HSS competencies in experiential roles within the health care system can often times be "lower stakes" (e.g., health coaching) compared with traditional biomedical decisions (e.g., ordering medications). This key difference opens several opportunities for medical students to engage with the health system by performing authentic systems-based tasks that can add value and improve care processes and patient outcomes, while also promoting learning of HSS content.[9,11,77] Students can add value by serving as patient navigators and health coaches, facilitating effective care transitions, and assisting with medication reconciliation and education. These meaningful roles align with the clinical care needs of the health system, specifically focusing on important quality and efficiency metrics such as reducing re-admissions, improving care transitions, and improving patient satisfaction. These new student roles have the potential to lessen the "burden" on the system and mentors, enhance student education in HSS, and potentially improve health outcomes.

G. Address the Hidden Curriculum

The hidden curriculum is the influence of institutional structure and culture on the learning environment.[24] Policies, the formal curriculum, examinations, and professional development of faculty reflect institutional goals and values, which, in turn, affect the learning environment.[18,25,78] Additionally, the hidden curriculum often reinforces the notions of physician autonomy and authority, influencing trainee's perceptions of patient worth and team member roles as they model faculty behaviors.[79–81] Although trainees have identified gaps in their HSS education, this content is assigned a lower priority because it is not included in licensing and board examinations and residency placement criteria.[23,61,82,83] The environment in which physicians are training may have a lasting effect on their behaviors. Emerging evidence suggests that students who train in clinical environments with lower resource utilization are more likely to practice similar methods in the future, suggesting that role modeling during training years is a critical element to learner development.[27,28] If role models do not demonstrate HSS-informed clinical practice, learners will be less likely to incorporate these behaviors into their own practice. Creating initiatives to introduce HSS curricula will require a change in institutional values and culture. As such, implementation and evaluation of specific curricular changes will model the expected value changes for the rest of the medical education community at each institution.[24] Since perceptions of learning environments vary between institutions, efforts to evaluate the effects of the hidden curriculum must be directed toward each specific locale.[85] Understanding each community's readiness for educational change will assist the institution's leadership in understanding the barriers and tensions of implementing the formal curriculum, and allow them to devise incentive structures for faculty (via resources and promotion) and students (via examinations) accordingly. Increasing students' recognition of the importance of HSS to their careers could be addressed by exposing students to integrated, longitudinal, and meaningful patient-centered experiences. Aligning their HSS education with positive experiences in health systems improvement efforts may reduce gaps in the curriculum and create a "fluid" learning environment. Evolving discourse on HSS education at the national level should include conversations about student, medical school, and physician accountability in espousing HSS tenets in their practice and teaching of medicine.

VI. SUBSEQUENT CHAPTERS IN THE HSS TEXT

Most of the remaining chapters in this book will provide more detail on the HSS content domains represented in Fig. 2.2 (Table 2.1).

Chapter 3 details the dynamic health care delivery system (including the structures and processes) and anticipated changes to the system in the coming years based on external forces in US health care. Chapter 4 is an in-depth look at value in health care. Chapters 5 (Patient Safety) and 6 (Quality Improvement) address the two main components of health care improvement efforts at the health system level (i.e., what is within the control of health care organizations to change). Chapters 7 and 8 highlight teamwork and leadership; Chapter 9 offers in-depth discussions on clinical informatics and technology. Chapter 10 (Population Health) provides an overview of these broad topics; because social determinants of health are a major contributor to health outcomes, Chapter 11 (Socio-Ecologic Determinants of Health) provides a necessary discussion of this subtopic. Chapter 12 discusses health care policy and economics.

Table 2.1 Health Systems Science Curricular Domains and Chapters Addressing Domain

Curriculum Domains	Chapter in Book
Health Care Structures and Processes *World Health Organization*[86] *Donabedian*[32,87]	3
Value-Based Care *Institute of Medicine*[38] *Porter*[88]	4, 5
Health System Improvement *Graban*[89]	5, 6
Teamwork	7
Leadership *Conger*[90]	8
Clinical Informatics and Health Information Technology *American Medical Informatics Association*[91] *Hersh*[92] *and Otero*[93]	9
Population Health *Public Health Foundation*[94,95] *World Health Organization*[96] *Roux*[97] *Young*[98] *Glass*[99] *Kilbourne*[100]	10, 11
Health Care Policy, Economics, and Management[101]	12
Evidence-Based Medicine and Practice *Sackett*[102]	13
Professionalism and Ethics	13
Scholarship *Boyer*[39]	13
Systems Thinking *Senge*[33]	13

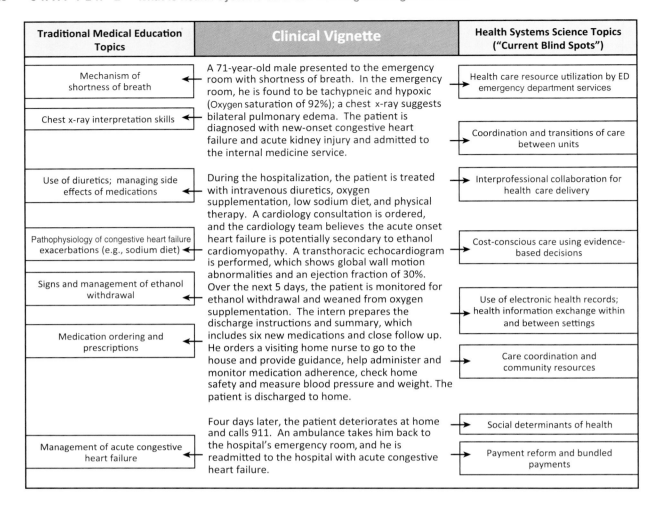

Traditional Medical Education Topics	Clinical Vignette	Health Systems Science Topics ("Current Blind Spots")
Mechanism of shortness of breath	A 71-year-old male presented to the emergency room with shortness of breath. In the emergency room, he is found to be tachypneic and hypoxic (Oxygen saturation of 92%); a chest x-ray suggests bilateral pulmonary edema. The patient is diagnosed with new-onset congestive heart failure and acute kidney injury and admitted to the internal medicine service.	Health care resource utilization by ED emergency department services
Chest x-ray interpretation skills		Coordination and transitions of care between units
Use of diuretics; managing side effects of medications	During the hospitalization, the patient is treated with intravenous diuretics, oxygen supplementation, low sodium diet, and physical therapy. A cardiology consultation is ordered, and the cardiology team believes the acute onset heart failure is potentially secondary to ethanol cardiomyopathy. A transthoracic echocardiogram is performed, which shows global wall motion abnormalities and an ejection fraction of 30%. Over the next 5 days, the patient is monitored for ethanol withdrawal and weaned from oxygen supplementation. The intern prepares the discharge instructions and summary, which includes six new medications and close follow up. He orders a visiting home nurse to go to the house and provide guidance, help administer and monitor medication adherence, check home safety and measure blood pressure and weight. The patient is discharged to home.	Interprofessional collaboration for health care delivery
Pathophysiology of congestive heart failure exacerbations (e.g., sodium diet)		Cost-conscious care using evidence-based decisions
Signs and management of ethanol withdrawal		Use of electronic health records; health information exchange within and between settings
Medication ordering and prescriptions		Care coordination and community resources
	Four days later, the patient deteriorates at home and calls 911. An ambulance takes him back to the hospital's emergency room, and he is readmitted to the hospital with acute congestive heart failure.	Social determinants of health
Management of acute congestive heart failure		Payment reform and bundled payments

Chapter 13 provides selected examples of how some of the foundational skills represented in the cross-cutting domains are applied in HSS. Chapter 14 specifically focuses on how assessments of HSS-related knowledge and skills can be used to provide feedback to learners in this important competency area. Finally, Chapter 15 offers some insight on the future of HSS. Educators, students, and clinical faculty are encouraged to pursue deeper dives in these chapters and to frequently refer back to Fig. 2.2 to see how the broad topic domains interrelate.

VII. CHAPTER SUMMARY

HSS is the third science in medical education, and it must be successfully integrated with the basic and clinical sciences to enable graduates to achieve the Triple Aim. An HSS curricular framework for medical education is needed for students, clinical faculty, and medical educators to ensure that health profession graduates have the necessary competencies to contribute to the Triple Aim. An HSS curricular framework, based in Engel's bio-psycho-social model and informed by existing and planned curricula at 11 schools, was developed to meet this need.

There are three domains of content in this HSS curricular framework: core, cross-cutting, and linking domains. The core domains of content (not traditionally represented in basic and clinical sciences) are Health Care Structures and Processes; Health Care Policy, Economics, and Management; Clinical Informatics/Health Information Technology; Population Health; Value-Based Care; and Health System Improvement. The cross-cutting domains (traditional topics applied with a third science lens) are Leadership and Change Agency; Teamwork and Interprofessional Education; Evidence-Based Medicine and Practice; Professionalism and Ethics; and Scholarship. Systems Thinking is a final "linking" domain that is critical for all other content areas.

There are a number of key priorities for educators and students in order to ensure successful implementation of HSS in medical education. Comprehensive, standardized, and integrated HSS curricula must be developed. Assessment tools must be developed, standardized, and aligned curriculum and learning objectives. Educational groups must partner with licensing and accreditation bodies to align HSS content with regulatory processes and standards. UME and GME educators must improve the transition of trainees across their programs. Schools must enhance the knowledge, skills, and incentives of faculty in HSS. All stakeholders in HSS education must work to demonstrate the ability for HSS-focused education to add value to clinical practices, and schools must address the hidden curricula that may impede successful HSS education efforts.

QUESTIONS FOR FURTHER THOUGHT

1. What are the six Institute of Medicine dimensions of quality, and how do they relate to the elements of value-based care?
2. Why are leadership competencies and professionalism important to effectively manage your patient and patient population in our current health care environment?
3. How does systems thinking help you understand the dynamic relationship between the care of individual patients and the system elements that impact the quality and efficiency of that care?
4. What assessment methods currently used in medical education are useful in providing feedback on HSS-related competencies (teamwork, quality of care, understanding health policy and health systems structure)?
5. What is the hidden curriculum, and how may it have a positive or negative impact on acquiring the skills and internalizing the attitudes intrinsic to HSS?

Annotated Bibliography

American Medical Association: *Accelerating Change in Medical Education Initiative*. 2013. http://changemed.org.
  Includes key information to understanding medical education transformation.
Berwick DM, Nolan TW, Whittington J. The Triple Aim: care, health, and cost. *Health Aff (Millwood)*. 2008;27(3):759–769.
  Sets the stage for the current quality movement.
Gonzalo JD PH, Papp KK, Wolpaw DR, Moser E, Wittenstein RD, Wolpaw T. Educating for the 21st-Century Healthcare System: an Interdependent Framework of Basic, Clinical and Systems Sciences. *Academic Medicine* (ahead of print). 2015.
  Outlines the framework for health systems science and forms the basis for this textbook.
Skochelak SE. A decade of reports calling for change in medical education: what do they say? *Acad Med*. Sep 2010;85(suppl 9):S26–S33.
  Summarizes the modern medical education reform movement.

References

1. Berwick DM, Nolan TW, Whittington J. The triple aim: care, health, and cost. *Health Aff (Millwood)*. 2008;27(3):759–769.
2. *ACGME Outcomes Project*. Accreditation Council for Graduate Medical Education; 1999.
3. Association of American Medical Colleges. *Core Entrustable Professional Activities for Entering Residency: Curriculum Developers' Guide*. 2014.
4. Fink LD. *Creating Significant Learning Experiences: An Integrated Approach to Designing College Courses*. San Francisco, CA: Jossey-Bass; 2003.
5. Kern DE, Thomas PA, Hughes MT. *Curriculum Development for Medical Education: A Six-Step Approach*. 2nd ed. Baltimore, MD: Johns Hopkins University Press; 2009.
6. Crosson FJ, Leu J, Roemer BM, Ross MN. Gaps in residency training should be addressed to better prepare doctors for a twenty-first-century delivery system. *Health Aff (Millwood)*. 2011;30(11):2142–2148.
7. Frenk J, Chen L, Bhutta ZA, et al. Health professionals for a new century: transforming education to strengthen health systems in an interdependent world. *Lancet*. 2010;376(9756):1923–1958.
8. Chang A, Ritchie C. Patient-centered models of care: closing the gaps in physician readiness. *J Gen Intern Med*. 2015;30(7):870–872.
9. Gonzalo JD PH, Papp KK, Wolpaw DR, Moser E, Wittenstein RD, Wolpaw T. Educating for the 21st-century health care system: an interdependent framework of basic, clinical, and systems sciences. *Acad Med*. 2015. [Epub ahead of print].
10. Lucey CR. Medical education: part of the problem and part of the solution. *JAMA Intern Med*. 2013;73(17):1639–1643.
11. Gonzalo JD, Haidet P, Wolpaw DR. Authentic clinical experiences and depth in systems: toward a 21st century curriculum. *Med Educ*. 2014;48:104–105.
12. Pershing S, Fuchs VR. Restructuring medical education to meet current and future health care needs. *Acad Med*. 2013;88(12):1798–1801.
13. Skochelak SE. A decade of reports calling for change in medical education: what do they say? *Acad Med*. 2010;85(suppl 9):S26–S33.
14. Armstrong G, Headrick L, Madigosky W, Ogrinc G. Designing education to improve care. *Jt Comm J Qual Patient Saf*. 2012;38(1):5–14.
15. Core Competencies for Interprofessional Collaborative Practice: Report of an Expert Panel. *Interprofessional Education Collaborative (IPEC)*; 2012. https://www.aamc.org/download/186750/data/core_competencies.pdf. Accessed February 29, 2013.
16. Combes JR, Arespacochaga E. Physician competencies for a 21st century health care system. *J Grad Med Educ*. 2012;4(3):401–405.
17. Wachter RM. *Understanding Patient Safety*. 2nd ed. New York: McGraw Hill Medical; 2012.
18. Moriates C, Arora V, Shah N. *Understanding Value-Based Healthcare*. New York: McGraw-Hill Education; 2015.
19. Askin E. *The Health Care Handbook: A Clear and Concise Guide to the United States Health Care System*. 2nd ed. St Louis, MO: Washington University in St Louis; 2014.
20. Bazell C, Davis H, Glass J, Rodak Jr J, Bastacky SM. The Undergraduate Medical Education for the 21st Century (UME-21) project: the Federal Government perspective. *Fam Med*. 2004;36(suppl):S15–S19.
21. *Strengthening Behavioral and Social Science in Medical School Education (R25)*. National Institutes of Health; 2011.
22. *Behavioral and Social Science Foundations for Future Physicians*. Association of American Medical Colleges; 2011. https://www.aamc.org/download/271020/data/behavioralandsocialsciencefoundationsforfuturephysicians.pdf. Accessed August 21, 2015.
23. Patel MS, Lypson ML, Davis MM. Medical student perceptions of education in health care systems. *Acad Med*. 2009;84(9):1301–1306.
24. Hafferty FW. Beyond curriculum reform: confronting medicine's hidden curriculum. *Acad Med*. 1998;73(4):403–407.
25. Hafferty FW, O'Donnell JF. *The Hidden Curriculum in Health Professional Education*. Hanover, NH: Dartmouth College Press; 2014.
26. Greysen SR, Schiliro D, Curry L, Bradley EH, Horwitz LI. "Learning by doing"—resident perspectives on developing competency in high-quality discharge care. *J Gen Intern Med*. 2012;27(9):1188–1194.
27. Chen C, Petterson S, Phillips R, Bazemore A, Mullan F. Spending patterns in region of residency training and subsequent expenditures for care provided by practicing physicians for Medicare beneficiaries. *JAMA*. 2014;312(22):2385–2393.
28. Sirovich BE, Lipner RS, Johnston M, Holmboe ES. The association between residency training and internists' ability to practice conservatively. *JAMA Intern Med*. 2014;174(10):1640–1648.
29. Ryskina KL, Halpern SD, Minyanou NS, Goold SD, Tilburt JC. The role of training environment care intensity in US physician cost consciousness. *Mayo Clin Proc*. 2015;90(3):313–320.
30. American Medical Association. *Accelerating Change in Medical Education Initiative*. 2013. http://www.ama-assn.org/sub/accelerating-change/index.shtml.
31. Pridan D. Rudolf Virchow and Social Medicine in Historical Perspective. *Med Hist*. 1964;8:274–278.
32. Donabedian A. Evaluating the quality of medical care. *Milbank Q*. 2005;83(4):691–729.
33. Senge PM. *The Fifth Discipline: The Art and Practice of the Learning Organization*. Revised and updated edition. New York: Doubleday/Currency; 2006.
34. Engel GL. The clinical application of the biopsychosocial model. *Am J Psychiatry*. 1980;137(5):535–544.
35. von Bertalanffy L. *Perspectives on General Systems Theory: Scientific and Philosophical Studies*. New York: Braziller; 1975.
36. Gonzalo J, Dekhtyar M, Starr SR, et al. *Identifying and Defining Content Domains for a Science of Healthcare Delivery Curriculum: Results from the American Medical Association Accelerating Change in Medical Education Systems-Based Practice Working Group*. Toronto, Ontario, Canada: Paper presented at: Society of General Internal Medicine National Conference, April 23, 2015; 2015.

37. Gonzalo JD, Starr SR, Borkan J, et al. Healthcare delivery science curricula in undergraduate medical education: identifying and defining a potential curricular framework. *Acad Med.* 2016 Apr 5. [Epub ahead of print].

38. Institute of Medicine (U.S.) Committee on Quality of Health Care in America. *Crossing the Quality Chasm: A New Health System for the 21st Century.* Washington, DC: National Academy Press; 2001.

39. Boyer EL. *Scholarship Reconsidered: Priorities of the Professoriate.* Princeton, NJ: Carnegie Foundation for the Advancement of Teaching; 1990.

40. Gonzalo JD, Baxley E, Borkan J, et al. Priority areas and potential solutions for successful integration and sustainment of health systems science in undergraduate medical education. *Acad Med.* 2016 May 31. [Epub ahead of print].

41. Larsen DP, Butler AC, Roediger 3rd HL. Test-enhanced learning in medical education. *Med Educ.* 2008;42(10):959–966.

42. van der Vleuten CP, Schuwirth LW. Assessing professional competence: from methods to programmes. *Med Educ.* 2005;39(3):309–317.

43. Schuwirth L, Ash J. Assessing tomorrow's learners: in competency-based education only a radically different holistic method of assessment will work. Six things we could forget. *Med Teach.* 2013;35(7):555–559.

44. Aboumatar HJ, Thompson D, Wu A, et al. Development and evaluation of a 3-day patient safety curriculum to advance knowledge, self-efficacy and system thinking among medical students. *BMJ Qual Saf.* 2012;21(5):416–422.

45. Daud-Gallotti RM, Morinaga CV, Arlindo-Rodrigues M, Velasco IT, Martins MA, Tiberio IC. A new method for the assessment of patient safety competencies during a medical school clerkship using an objective structured clinical examination. *Clinics.* 2011;66(7):1209–1215.

46. Dory V, Gagnon R, De Foy T, Duyver C, Leconte S. A novel assessment of an evidence-based practice course using an authentic assignment. *Medical Teach.* 2010;32(2):e65–e70.

47. Hughes C, Toohey S, Velan G. eMed Teamwork: a self-moderating system to gather peer feedback for developing and assessing teamwork skills. *Medical Teach.* 2008;30(1):5–9.

48. Meier AH, Boehler ML, McDowell CM, et al. A surgical simulation curriculum for senior medical students based on TeamSTEPPS. *Arch Surg.* 2012;147(8):761–766.

49. Mookherjee S, Ranji S, Neeman N, Sehgal N. An advanced quality improvement and patient safety elective. *Clin Teach.* 2013;10(6):368–373.

50. Olupeliyawa AM, O'Sullivan AJ, Hughes C, Balasooriya CD. The Teamwork Mini-Clinical Evaluation Exercise (T-MEX): a workplace-based assessment focusing on collaborative competencies in health care. *Acad Med.* 2014;89(2):359–365.

51. Olupeliyawa A, Balasooriya C, Hughes C, O'Sullivan A. Educational impact of an assessment of medical students' collaboration in health care teams. *Med Educ.* 2014;48(2):146–156.

52. Paige JT, Garbee DD, Kozmenko V, et al. Getting a head start: high-fidelity, simulation-based operating room team training of interprofessional students. *J Am Coll Surg.* 2014;218(1):140–149.

53. Sharma N, Cui Y, Leighton JP, White JS. Team-based assessment of medical students in a clinical clerkship is feasible and acceptable. *Medical Teach.* 2012;34(7):555–561.

54. Singh MK, Ogrinc G, Cox KR, et al. The Quality Improvement Knowledge Application Tool Revised (QIKAT-R). *Acad Med.* 2014;89(10):1386–1391.

55. Tartaglia KM, Walker C. Effectiveness of a quality improvement curriculum for medical students. *Med Educ Online.* 2015;20:27133.

56. White JS, Sharma N. "Who writes what?" Using written comments in team-based assessment to better understand medical student performance: a mixed-methods study. *BMC Med Educ.* 2012;12:123.

57. Wright MC, Segall N, Hobbs G, Phillips-Bute B, Maynard L, Taekman JM. Standardized assessment for evaluation of team skills: validity and feasibility. *Simul Healthc.* 2013;8(5):292–303.

58. Havyer RD, Wingo MT, Comfere NI, et al. Teamwork assessment in internal medicine: a systematic review of validity evidence and outcomes. *J Gen Intern Med.* 2014;29(6):894–910.

59. Oates M, Davidson M. A critical appraisal of instruments to measure outcomes of interprofessional education. *Med Educ.* 2015;49(4):386–398.

60. Gillan C, Lovrics E, Halpern E, Wiljer D, Harnett N. The evaluation of learner outcomes in interprofessional continuing education: a literature review and an analysis of survey instruments. *Med Teach.* 2011;33(9):e461–e470.

61. Gonzalo JD, Haidet P, Blatt B, Wolpaw DR. Exploring challenges in implementing a health systems science curriculum: a qualitative analysis of student perceptions. *Med Educ.* 2016;50(5):523–531.

62. Thibault GE. Reforming health professions education will require culture change and closer ties between classroom and practice. *Health Aff (Millwood).* 2013;32(11):1928–1932.

63. Hirsh DA, Ogur B, Thibault GE, Cox M. "Continuity" as an organizing principle for clinical education reform. *New Engl J Med.* 2007;356(8):858–866.

64. *Core Entrustable Professional Activities for Entering Residency Curriculum Developers' Guide.* Washington, DC: American Association of Medical Colleges; 2014.

65. *Accreditation Council for Graduate Medical Education:* Milestones; 2015.

66. Hawkins RECW, Holmboe ES, Kirk LM, Norcini JJ, Simons KB, Skochelak SE. Implementation of competency-based medical education: are we addressing the concerns and challenges? *Med Educ.* 2015;49(11):1086–1102.

67. Clay 2nd MA, Sikon AL, Lypson ML, et al. Teaching while learning while practicing: reframing faculty development for the patient-centered medical home. *Acad Med.* 2013;88(9):1215–1219.

68. Ludmerer KM. *Time to Heal: American Medical Education from the Turn of the Century to the Era of Managed Care.* New York: Oxford University Press; 1999.

69. Jones RF, Korn D. On the cost of educating a medical student. *Acad Med.* 1997;72(3):200–210.

70. Shea S, Nickerson KG, Tenenbaum J, et al. Compensation to a department of medicine and its faculty members for the teaching of medical students and house staff. *New Engl J Med.* 1996;334(3):162–167.

71. Baldor RA, Brooks WB, Warfield ME, O'Shea K. A survey of primary care physicians' perceptions and needs regarding the precepting of medical students in their offices. *Med Educ.* 2001;35(8):789–795.

72. Chandra A, Khullar D, Wilensky GR. The economics of graduate medical education. *New Engl J Med.* 2014;370(25):2357–2360.

73. Wynn B, Smalley R, Cordasco KM. *Does It Cost More to Train Residents or to Replace Them? A Look at the Costs and Benefits of Operating Graduate Medical Education Programs.* 2013.

74. Clancy GP. Good neighbors: shared challenges and solutions toward increasing value at academic medical centers and universities. *Acad Med.* 2015;90(12):1607–1610.

75. Walsh K. *Oxford Textbook of Medical Education.* Oxford: Oxford University Press; 2013.

76. Lin SY, Schillinger E, Irby DM. Value-added medical education: engaging future doctors to transform health care delivery today. *J Gen Intern Med.* 2015;30(2):150–151.

77. Gonzalo J, Thompson B. *Value-Added Student Roles That Align Education and Health System Needs*; 2015. [Internet]. www.iamse.org. Podcast.

78. Hafler JP, Ownby AR, Thompson BM, et al. Decoding the learning environment of medical education: a hidden curriculum perspective for faculty development. *Acad Med.* 2011;86(4):440–444.

79. Michalec B, Hafferty FW. Stunting professionalism: the potency and durability of the hidden curriculum within medical education. *Soc Theor Health.* 2013;11(4):388–406.

80. Karnieli-Miller O, Vu TR, Frankel RM, et al. Which experiences in the hidden curriculum teach students about professionalism? *Acad Med.* 2011;86(3):369–377.

81. Higashi RT, Tillack A, Steinman MA, Johnston CB, Harper GM. The "worthy" patient: rethinking the "hidden curriculum" in medical education. *Anthropol Med.* 2013;20(1):13–23.

82. Brooks KC. A piece of my mind. A silent curriculum. *JAMA.* 2015;313(19):1909–1910.

83. Garvey KC, Kesselheim JC, Herrick DB, Woolf AD, Leichtner AM. Graduate medical education in humanism and professionalism: a needs assessment survey of pediatric gastroenterology fellows. *J Pediatr Gastroenterol Nutr.* 2014;58(1):34–37.

84. Deleted in review.

85. Skochelak SE, Stansfield RB, Dunham L, et al. Medical student perceptions of the learning environment at the end of the first year: a 28–medical school collaborative. *Acad Med.* 2015. [Epub ahead of print].

86. *Strengthening Health Systems to Improve Health Outcomes: WHO's Framework for Action.* Geneva, Switzerland: World Health Organization; 2007.

87. McDonald KM, Sundaram V, Bravata DM, et al. *Closing the Quality Gap: A Critical Analysis of Quality Improvement Strategies (Vol. 7: Care Coordination):* Rockville, MD. 2007.

88. Porter ME. What is value in health care? *New Engl J Med.* 2010;363(26):2477–2481.

89. Graban M. *Lean Hospitals: Improving Quality, Patient Safety, and Employee Engagement.* 2nd ed. New York: Productivity Press/Taylor & Francis; 2012.

90. Conger JA, Kanungo RN. Toward a behavioral theory of charismatic leadership in organizational settings. *Acad Manage Rev.* 1987;12(4):637–647.

91. *Clinical Informatics.* American Medical Informatics Association; 2015. https://www.amia.org/applications-informatics/clinical-informatics. Accessed May 29, 2015.

92. Hersh WR, Gorman PN, Biagioli FE, Mohan V, Gold JA, Mejicano GC. Beyond information retrieval and electronic health record use: competencies in clinical informatics for medical education. *Adv Med Educ Pract.* 2014;5:205–212.

93. Otero P, Hersh W, Jai Ganesh AU. Big Data: are biomedical and health informatics training programs ready? Contribution of the IMIA Working Group for Health and Medical Informatics Education. *Yearb Med Inform.* 2014;9(1):177–181.

94. *Core Competencies for Public Health Professionals.* The Council on Linkages Between Academia and Public Health Practice; 2014. http://www.phf.org/resourcestools/Documents/Core_Competencies_for_Public_Health_Professionals_2014June.pdf. Accessed May 5, 2015.

95. *Population Health Competencies.* Public Health Foundation; 2015. http://www.phf.org/phfpulse/Pages/PHF_ACHI_Exploring_Population_Health_Competencies.aspx. Accessed May 5, 2015.

96. *Health Impact Assessment: the Determinants of Health.* World Health Organization; 2015. http://www.who.int/hia/evidence/doh/en/. Accessed May 5, 2015.

97. Roux AVD. Conceptual approaches to the study of health disparities. *Annu Rev Publ Health.* 2012;33:41–58.

98. Young L. Population health: concepts and methods. *Am J Hum Biol.* 2006;18(1):159–160.

99. Glass TA, McAtee MJ. Behavioral science at the crossroads in public health: extending horizons, envisioning the future. *Soc Sci Med.* 2006;62(7):1650–1671.

100. Kilbourne AM, Switzer G, Hyman K, Crowley-Matoka M, Fine MJ. Advancing health disparities research within the health care system: a conceptual framework. *Am J Public Health.* 2006;96(12):2113–2121.

101. *Health Economics.* Altarum Institute: Systems Research for Better Health; 2015. http://altarum.org/areas-of-expertise/health-economics. Accessed May 29, 2015.

102. Sackett DL, Rosenberg WM, Gray JA, Haynes RB, Richardson WS. Evidence based medicine: what it is and what it isn't. *BMJ.* 1996;312(7023):71–72.

3

The Health Care Delivery System

Stephanie R. Starr, MD, and Robert E. Nesse, MD

LEARNING OBJECTIVES

1. Describe the desired outcomes of health care delivery and the implications of recent changes (Affordable Care Act, accountable care, and payment for value) on health care delivery systems.
2. Understand the objectives (structure and processes), deliverables (outcomes), and limitations of current health care delivery.
3. Review the congruence of current delivery systems with accountable care performance requirements and new population health care models.
4. Summarize the use of improvement strategies, population management, and data analytics to close the gaps in health care delivery.

US health care delivery is evolving rapidly. All health professionals must have a basic understanding of the dynamic and complex delivery system and the challenges posed by anticipated changes. As discussed in Chapter 1, the system is not currently designed to center on outcomes from patients' perspectives and does not align incentives to achieve the Triple Aim. The Affordable Care Act (ACA), accountable care, and payment for value based on outcomes and total cost (versus a fee-for-service model) are demanding and accelerating change in the system. Those who seek to be collaborative members of high-functioning teams must adopt a patient-centered view of the system. They must understand how planned payment reforms will realign this system, and how care teams must leverage health care improvement strategies, data analytics, and population management to close current deficiencies in care delivery and ensure that patients receive care, education, and support to maximize their health.

CHAPTER OUTLINE

I. DESIRED OUTCOMES OF HEALTH CARE DELIVERY

The complex US health care system is not the product of a deliberate, thoughtful, coordinated, and evidence-based approach to maximizing the health of members of society. Individual health professionals and small front-line multidisciplinary teams may be exemplary in their training and practice, but optimal health outcomes do not occur when these professionals and teams are not effectively integrated in a patient's episode of care. In addition, there have been competing priorities, politics, legislation, and a series of accommodations based on the burning issues of health in different eras (infectious diseases, public health, safety, and medical errors) without explicit focus on the "health" of the system itself. The diverse population of patients in the United States (spread across a wide geographic footprint) and the influence of multiple stakeholders with different perspectives contribute to the complexity we see today.

Health professionals and trainees often have personal experiences as patients and family members that serve to highlight the system's flaws. Even as insiders (i.e., members of health care teams directly observing the system), they frequently feel powerless to address the gaps they see. This sense of powerlessness stems in part from the lack of understanding of current health care systems, the factors contributing to gaps in these systems, and the tools to close the gaps. This lack of understanding is not specific to the level of training or profession.

Few participants in the system have even a limited understanding of the network of interactions, competing priorities, resources, and economic pressures that must be factored into the comprehensive new model of health care needed for us to truly heal the sick, ameliorate suffering, and—ideally—achieve health for all. Health professionals often are called to their roles because of a desire to heal, cure, and maintain health for individual patients. In recent years, the health professions have recognized where poorly integrated care models and health care systems have failed the patients they are called to serve. The Institute of Medicine's (IOM) *To Err is Human*[1] and *Crossing the Quality Chasm*[2] reports ignited national conversations about the gaps in health care delivery and health outcomes, and, most concerning, how the system itself has harmed the patients who entrust their care to physicians and other health professionals.

It wasn't until 2008 that the health professions began to share a common mantra for societal health system goals that also considered both the gains and the costs in the ledger: The Triple Aim.[3] Published by the Institute for Healthcare Improvement (IHI), the Triple Aim seeks to ensure 1) health for all individuals (population health), 2) an ideal experience for all patients as they interface with the system (including quality and satisfaction), and 3) achieving both at the lowest possible cost (reducing the per capita cost of health care). Physicians and other health professionals have an opportunity and moral obligation to transform and align the US system to achieve the Triple Aim by closing gaps in all aspects of health care quality. The IOM defines quality as including six dimensions: care that is safe, timely, effective, efficient, equal, and patient-centered[2] (sometimes abbreviated as STEEEP). The system must focus on the needs of the population (society) and the needs of individual patients.

So what do patients need in an ideal system? The immediate goals of active patients are the relief of symptoms and suffering and the preservation of health. All patients deserve interactions with the health care system that incorporate their preferences, their values, and their capacity to complete the recommendations from their care teams. Patients need timely access to and respect from the physicians and other professionals in the system, and for those professionals to share decision making with them to help ensure that they understand the choices they make concerning their care. Patients with certain social determinants of health are at increased risk for disparities in care delivery; Chapter 11 discusses social determinants of health and health inequities in more detail. Patients need to accomplish the goals of care without having to choose food over medications, or worry about financial ruin because of a chronic or life-threatening health condition. Health care organizations, payers, and our society need a system that achieves the Triple Aim, rewards high-value care (as defined later in the chapter[2]), and ensures the recruitment, development, and retention of caring and competent health professionals.[4]

II. CATALYSTS FOR CHANGE IN US HEALTH CARE DELIVERY

The US health care system presently includes a plethora of health care organizations including academic, public, private, not-for-profit multispecialty, community-based, and government institutions, such as the military, the Indian Health Service (IHS), and the Veterans Administration (VA). Historically, hospitals (and by extension, outpatient centers and clinics) and acute care facilities are the central focus of health care delivery. From patients' perspectives, this system exists in name only in that the continuum of care (self-care, primary care within patient-centered medical homes [PCMHs], episodic specialty, and inpatient care) is often not coordinated, and the health care personnel working in these settings do not reliably communicate or share resources in an effective way. Reimbursement has prioritized the relative value of procedures, tests, and other interventions at the relative exclusion of nonvisit care and coordination of care. The **fee-for-service model** has provided a distinct disincentive to analyzing and prioritizing the quality and cost of episodes of care over time or the patient's experience of care and the system over time. In addition to transforming our system to ensure that we truly meet our patients' and society's needs, we recognize the unprecedented misallocation of resources and the waste in our system that must be addressed.[5]

One way of benchmarking the health care system and its historical evolution is to compare it with the airline industry. Both the health care and airline industries have similar origins as "craftsman" systems, in which successful outcomes were determined largely on the capability (intelligence, memory, and other skills) of individual professionals (health care providers and pilots, respectively).[6] It is helpful to reflect on how the two systems have diverged significantly. Pilots are trained and work in a "production" model, whereby they perform "standard work" with frequent data provided to them in real time to allow and support needed changes in the protocol. In contrast, health professional education and care delivery can currently best be described as an "apprentice" model, with a focus on learning at the individual level and not on system performance. In the apprentice model, there is infrequent recognition of "standard work" (Fig. 3.1). Patient outcomes frequently depend on the physician they select, as well as the strengths or weaknesses of the systems and processes that inform and support the delivery of their care.[6] The Dartmouth Institute has documented the variations in quality and use of resources in our current system (including overuse and underuse of care with poorer outcomes associated with higher use of resources).[7] While some variation in care is appropriate based on comorbid conditions and patient preferences and values, there is compelling evidence that we can improve care delivery by developing "standard work" for common conditions where there is strong evidence for best care.

Comparing both industries provides two insights: the opportunity to improve health care by applying a

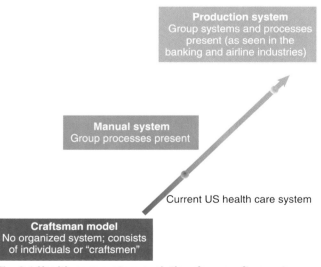

Fig. 3.1 **Health care system evolution, from craftsman to production system.** (Modified with permission from Burton DA. The anatomy of healthcare delivery model: how a systematic approach can transform care delivery. *Health Catalyst.* 2014. https://www.healthcatalyst.com/anatomy-healthcare-delivery-model-transform-care.)

production model where appropriate, but also to recognize the important differences between the health care industry and the airline industry, especially as they relate to patient safety.[8] Pilots operate complex machines doing duplicative work. Physicians and other providers function in a less predictable environment. Health care delivery is complex and requires critical thinking and incorporation of patients' preferences and values (i.e., care that reflects the needs of individual patients), but clinicians often lack systems that inform them and support them to deliver care that is evidence-based and provide quality care (safe, effective, timely, equal, patient-centered, and efficient) for all patients. The practice of health care and the profession of medicine ideally use a hybrid model that combines the effective use of production systems (standard work for the majority of patients and situations for a given condition or in a given setting) in order to create capacity for the artful diagnosis and compassionate treatment of patients as individuals based on trusting relationships. Both approaches are needed to achieve the Triple Aim.

A. Accountable Care Organizations

Several recent developments will accelerate change in health care delivery. **Accountable Care Organizations (ACOs)** are growing with financial and legislative support based on the ACA. ACOs are provider-led organizations charged with management of the entire continuum of care, overall costs, and quality of care for a defined population.[9] ACOs seek to improve coordination of care and provide a "medical home" to coordinate and manage patient care. Traditionally, a small minority of organizations provide truly comprehensive, continuing care for a defined population; the fragmentation of care across organizations and systems has contributed significantly to errors and other gaps in quality while also increasing costs (such as those attributed to redundant care). ACOs can take a variety of forms and functions. Outpatient practice settings, such as primary care clinics, large integrated group practices, government systems such as the Department of Defense and the VA, and hospital practice groups, are all implementing ACOs. ACO financial models include total cost models with "gain-share" models that share the financial rewards of meeting cost and quality targets; other ACO payment models share risk with rewards and penalties for cost and quality performance and partial or fully capitated models in which per-member per-month payments, quality, access, and safety deliverables are determined at the beginning of the contract.

B. Value-Based Payment

The ACA focuses on insurance reform. It provides financial incentives and supports demonstration projects to develop new care and payment models for a more integrated, less fragmented system focused on high value (highest quality at the lowest cost). In April 2015, Congress repealed the sustainable growth rate formula for Medicare payments and empowered the Secretary of Health and Human Services to replace that system with the Medicare Incentive Payment System (MIPS). The MIPS will support value-based incentive payments along with alternate payment models. In 2019 and beyond, alternate payment models (such as episodes of care and ACOs) will be eligible for a lump sum annual bonus based on their Medicare expenditures. In 2016, the Centers for Medicare and Medicaid Services (CMS) mandated bundled payments for hip and knee replacements in 67 US markets. In addition to this specific payment model change, Health and Human Services Secretary Sylvia Burwell stated that 90 percent of Medicare fee-for-service payments will be tied to quality or value, and 50 percent of Medicare payments will be delivered using alternate payment models by 2019.[10]

Value in health care can be expressed as the quality of care (the sum of outcomes, safety, and service) divided by the cost of care over time.[11,12] Many stakeholders are now using an expanded definition that reflects the IOM STEEEP dimensions of quality mentioned earlier. The value equation relates directly to the Triple Aim as it encompasses the overarching goal of best experience of care and best health (outcomes) for the population at the lowest cost, but its components allow stakeholders in the system to more easily measure quality and value gaps in order to improve care. Chapters 4 and 6 provide more detail on the concepts of value, quality, and measurement.

The shift from a fee-for-service model to a value-based model is complex and faces many challenges. Value-based models are dependent on reporting of quality, safety, and patient experience measures. In a value-based model, providers need sophisticated analytics to enable ongoing monitoring of financial and quality performance for each population of patients. The ACA includes a number of provisions designed to positively affect the Triple Aim, including expanded use of PCMHs, bundled payments, value-based purchasing, and payment reform. All of these initiatives depend on sharing of clinical information and improved feedback regarding performance that is actionable and available in a timely manner. In addition, the shared responsibility for resource use and performance over an episode of care or over time requires system integration and shared systems for effective implementation.[13]

III. COMPONENTS OF HEALTH CARE DELIVERY SYSTEMS

A. Structures, Processes, and Clinical Microsystems

In order to build the system patients and society need, we must understand the common current flow or "steps" in care delivery that currently exist. It is important to understand the difference among structures, processes, and outcomes to ensure a shared understanding of the vocabulary as we consider steps in care delivery and in varying levels by which we can define or "view" the system. It is also important to remember that the US system cannot be viewed as static at any given time; it is dynamic and constantly changing.

In 1988, Donabedian described an approach to assessing health care quality based on using three categories or components: structures, processes, and outcomes.[14] These categories enable health professionals to use a common language across the system; you will learn more about these in Chapter 6. Structures are the characteristics of

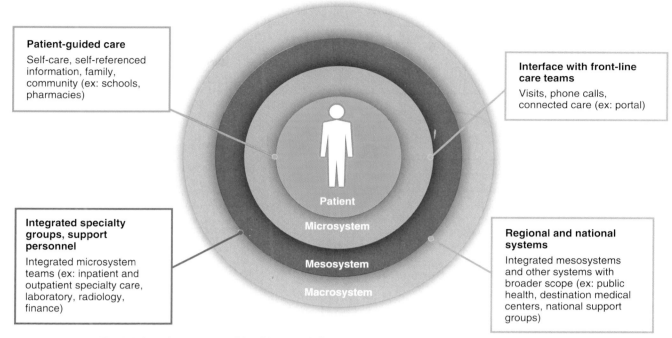

Patient-guided care

Self-care, self-referenced information, family, community (ex: schools, pharmacies)

Interface with front-line care teams

Visits, phone calls, connected care (ex: portal)

Integrated specialty groups, support personnel

Integrated microsystem teams (ex: inpatient and outpatient specialty care, laboratory, radiology, finance)

Regional and national systems

Integrated mesosystems and other systems with broader scope (ex: public health, destination medical centers, national support groups)

Patient

Microsystem

Mesosystem

Macrosystem

Fig. 3.2 **A patient-centered health care delivery system.** (Modified from Nelson EC, Godfrey MM, Batalden PB, et al. Clinical microsystems, part 1. The building blocks of health systems. *Jt Comm J Qual Patient Saf.* 2008;34(7):367–378.)

the settings in which care occurs (e.g., hospitals, clinics) and include material resources (e.g., facilities, equipment, and money), human resources (personnel), and organizational structures (e.g., medical staff organization, peer review, and revenue cycle). Processes are the actions taken by care teams and staff as they deliver care to patients, and the processes that support the needs of the business. Outcomes are what patients experience as a result of the care that is provided.

In addition to the basic structures and processes of care, it is helpful to also visualize the delivery system at four levels or as four concentric circles. Patients (the population for whom the system is responsible) and their families are appropriately in the center of this model. The subsequent levels (larger circles beyond the center) are clinical microsystems, mesosystems, and macrosystems[4] (Fig. 3.2). The clinical microsystem most familiar to patients is the team of providers that provide care and support for patients in a clinic or during a hospitalization. This "microsystem" or care team typically consists of physicians, nurses, therapists, and other professionals who directly contact patients. These microsystems also include administrative support (desk staff, secretaries) as well as the processes (e.g., ensuring that results of laboratory tests are provided to patients) needed to ensure good care. Mesosystems are the collection of microsystems; they include the clinical programs and centers that are often part of larger organizations. For example, there are often many individual microsystems or care teams within one hallway of a larger mesosystem (e.g., a family medicine clinic, a sports medicine center). Macrosystems (such as hospitals, multispecialty group practices, and integrated health systems) are the larger collection of mesosystems.

The ideal is for patients to interact with each level seamlessly as they engage the system from start to finish.

Consider this common example as a way to better understand one of many processes in health care and the different levels of the system. A woman decides to contact her primary care clinic because she has a new symptom and wants to schedule a visit with her physician. She starts by calling the desk staff (or sends an internet-based portal message) to schedule an appointment. On the day of the appointment, she is greeted by a receptionist and escorted to a room by another team member, who often obtains vital signs and clarifies the reason for the visit. Next, the physician conducts the office visit and, if needed, orders additional tests and images and/or a consultation to make an accurate diagnosis and appropriate treatment plan. If a prescription is written, the patient next encounters the pharmacy team (another microsystem) to get information regarding the drug and have the prescription filled. If the patient's symptoms resolve, she may not reconnect with the system until the next time she has a health concern or preventive services are due. If tests are ordered, she needs to learn the results of the tests, and how to best manage her condition and (if necessary) schedule follow up care. If the patient requires hospitalization, her physician may transfer her immediate care to an inpatient care team (another new microsystem involved in her episode of care).

The many steps in the process represented in this example appear to many patients as being relatively straightforward. Fig. 3.3 is one representation of our patients' view of processes across our current health care system. However, health care professionals and the nonclinical teams that constitute the mesosystems and macrosystems of care delivery must

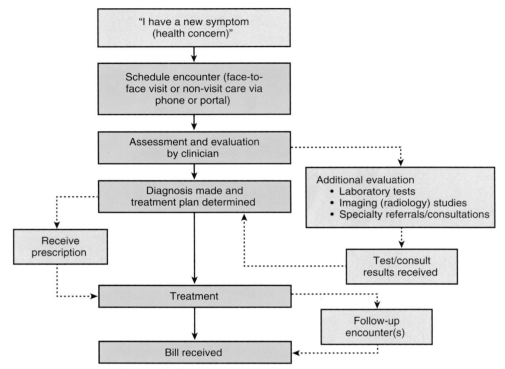

Fig. 3.3 **Patient's view of the health care encounter.**

cope with the complexity of the current system in a way most patients do not see. Fig. 3.4 is one representation of the current health care delivery system as seen by many working within the system.[6] This chaotic flow diagram is representative of most current systems, which were not deliberately designed and do not align with patient priorities or the Triple Aim. It is important to contrast this representation of the system with the representation in Fig. 3.2, which places patients and families in the center. It is understandable that the complex "system" represented by Fig. 3.4 often frustrates and baffles professionals as they deliver care. As mentioned earlier, even where exemplary health professionals or microsystems exist, they often are not optimally integrated with other microsystems. One common example is poor integration across microsystems during times of **patient handoffs** (such as dismissal from the hospital team to the outpatient team, or from the emergency department to the intensive care unit). Those who receive care must be supported as they navigate this system, or their care will suffer. While health care will remain complex, those within the system can only improve it if the system is oriented around the patients. Health professionals must work in multidisciplinary teams to modify the processes exemplified in Fig. 3.4 to center on patients and their quality of care. Chapter 6 will provide more detail regarding methods used in process improvement.

Health professionals must understand where and how often patients actually encounter the health care system in order to ensure that the system is truly patient-centered and designed to address the Triple Aim. Fig. 3.5 represents the percentage of US health care system encounters by one segment of patients (adults 55 to 64 years of age) over 12 months, by visit type.[15] Approximately 12 percent of adults (55 to 64 years of age) had no physician visits whatsoever. This should not surprise us as we maintain our focus on ensuring a

patient-centered health care system (see Fig. 3.2); efforts at achieving and maintaining health start at home by patients and families themselves. Patients and families are more likely to interact next to address health with community-based components of the system (e.g., schools and pharmacies) outside of traditional clinics and hospitals. Traditionally, the greatest focus on costs and poor outcomes has been for those patients admitted to the hospital; this makes sense given the greater cost and acuity if hospitalized. It is critically important to note that for this age cohort, approximately 10 percent of all individuals in this age group were hospitalized. To achieve the Triple Aim, our system structures and processes must include all individuals, whether or not they directly interface with the medical portion of the system.

B. New Structures for Health Care Delivery

As noted earlier, structures include both the materials and personnel needed to provide care. Within these material structures, clinical settings are commonly represented as being inpatient or outpatient. In the future system, connected care (supporting nonvisit health needs of patients) and clinical models aligned with delivery and continuing care will grow. PCMHs are medical groups that have achieved recognition and in many cases certification for their ability to provide coordinated ongoing care to include health maintenance and wellness, acute care needs, and chronic care needs.[16] PCMHs may be primary care clinics within a variety of practice models, such as multispecialty group practices, integrated health care systems, or community health centers, but also can be care teams dedicated to patients with specific complex needs. An increasing number of integrated community care practices have begun to provide team-based care and coordinated nonvisit patient care support.

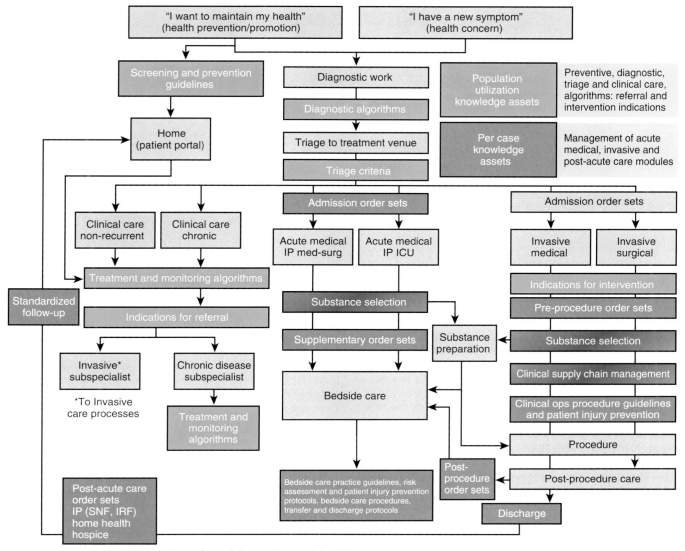

Fig. 3.4 **A system view of the anatomy of health care.** (Modified with permission from Burton DA. The anatomy of healthcare delivery model: how a systematic approach can transform care delivery. *Health Catalyst.* 2014. https://www.healthcatalyst.com/anatomy-healthcare-delivery-model-transform-care.)

In addition to the changes in "typical" practices, new models of outpatient care have developed. Retail clinics, often located in pharmacies and grocery stores, compete for patients that require routine care and vaccination. Concierge practices compete for patients who value personal high-service care delivery that is supported by extra fees for access and service. Hospitals are now delivering more complex care in an outpatient environment. For example, while inpatient admissions have fallen in recent years, the use of outpatient observation for patients with acute medical needs has increased. Sophisticated imaging such as magnetic resonance imaging has increased the precision of diagnoses prior to admission. And outpatient surgery has grown. It is critical to note that whether the structures of the system are existing models of care (e.g., nursing homes) or new models of care (e.g., PCMHs and retail clinics), they are not executed uniformly and frequently are not effectively integrated with other portions of the system.

The personnel that provide care and support our care delivery system are varied. In an integrated system, all personnel engaged in health care delivery are part of a team, and over time the emerging models of high-value care and responsibility for the well-being of a population of patients have highlighted the importance of high-performance teams in the delivery and outcomes of patients. The success of high-functioning teams hinges on the skill and reliability of all team members to work together.[17] Team-based health care is the provision of health services to individuals, families, and/or their communities by at least two health providers who work collaboratively with patients and their caregivers—to the extent preferred by each patient—to accomplish shared goals within and across settings to achieve coordinated, high-quality care.[18]

In the past, training and practice has focused on the physician as the center of the team; we now recognize the patient as the central member of any high-functioning care team, and that all members of the team play a critical role to optimize patient health outcomes. The roles necessary for a high-functioning team at the clinical microsystem level will depend on the setting. For example, the operating room

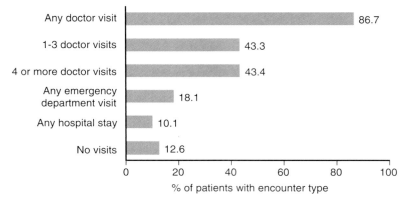

Fig. 3.5 Patient-reported (55 to 64 years of age) encounters with the US health care system in the previous 12 months (2012–2013). Respondents were asked about their health care contacts in the past 12 months. Less than 1% had an emergency department visit or a hospitalization, but no doctor visits, in 2012–2013. No visit is no doctor visit, emergency department visit, or hospital stay, in the past 12 months. (Modified from CDC/NCHS, National Health Interview Survey, United States, 2014. Centers for Disease Control and Prevention Web site. http://www.cdc.gov/nchs/data/hus/hus14.pdf. Published May 2015. Accessed February 13, 2016.)

teams include operating room nurses and technicians, anesthesiologists and nurse anesthetists, and surgeons. Neonatal intensive care units include pediatric pharmacists and dieticians, neonatal nurses, neonatologists, neonatal nurse practitioners, social workers, respiratory therapists, as well as chaplains and unit secretaries.

Given the growth of accountable care models, the composition of primary care delivery teams is changing dramatically to reflect their role as the "core" population health teams. The roles and professions represented on traditional primary care teams (physicians, RNs, LPNs, desk staff, administrative assistants) have expanded to include nurse practitioners, physician assistants, RNs in care manager roles, social workers, and other integrated behavioral health professionals such as psychologists. Many other roles may be selectively represented on expanded teams, including pharmacists, therapists, audiologists, dieticians, podiatrists, optometrists, oral health providers, and community health workers. A primary goal of these population health teams is to implement processes of care delivery that enable every member to perform at the maximum of his or her licensure.

There are many other health professionals and members of health care teams not listed specifically in this chapter; it is impossible to accurately summarize each of their roles, as even with the same professional training and licensure, a health professional may function in a myriad of roles depending on the setting, context, and state licensure rules. For further reading, *The Health Care Handbook* has an expanded list of health care professionals, their training, and their common roles in the system.[19] The concept of teamwork is addressed in Chapter 7.

C. Process Example: Care Transitions Across Clinical Microsystems

Each microsystem has numerous processes or flow of work that are part of daily work and routines. Health care improvement projects (discussed in detail in Chapter 6) often focus on these processes of care, especially when decreased variation in the process has been linked with better patient outcomes. Processes regarding transitions of

care across clinical microsystems are particularly important to address to improve the patient experience and identify and close gaps in care delivery. Many providers and patients have experienced and understand typical transitions such as the transition from hospital care to home care. These transitions often occur within an established health care setting (e.g., from an emergency department to an intensive care unit). Transitions also occur across health care settings (e.g., from a hospital inpatient unit to the outpatient setting, or from a provider visit to ongoing nonvisit care conducted between patients and population health teams). PCMH models also generate transitions between traditional health care, individual care locations, and community partners (such as public health departments, schools, and health clubs). Patients often are more vulnerable to errors and unsafe care by the system during these times of transition due to poor exchange of information and the complexity of transitions that accompany an integrated high-value health care system; diligent attention is needed to deliver seamless care. New information systems, such as an electronic medical record that can share information simultaneously in multiple settings, are increasingly essential to share the information generated in different settings to prevent errors and duplication of work.

IV. CONGRUENCE OF CURRENT DELIVERY SYSTEMS WITH ACCOUNTABLE CARE AND POPULATION HEALTH

To succeed in the new health care system, provider groups must develop a network of providers with aligned purpose that considers all contacts individuals may have with the health care system, as demonstrated earlier via one patient segment (adults 55 to 64 years of age) in Fig. 3.5. They can then use interdisciplinary teams to coordinate the care delivery supported by timely actionable analytics and an aligned financial model. The overriding goal of the system is to maximize value.[20] The Centers for Medicare and Medicaid Services (CMS) accountable care performance requirements are designed to foster a high-value system that meets the goals of patients and of the Triple Aim. New population health models, based on the premise that the foundation of the ideal health system lies in PCMHs, seek to operationalize this system.[9]

Accountable care requirements rely on timely performance measurement to evaluate the quality of care that is provided. Alignment between the metrics for financial success and performance incentives can make provider teams aware of both potential overuse (i.e., in disintegrated systems) and underuse (e.g., in organizations that lack awareness of patient needs for preventive care).[9] The existing culture in many organizations and communities is entrenched in a narrow view of each "service line" (such as cardiovascular surgery) or the structures, processes, and outcomes associated within or across microsystems, when evaluating value and cost. Significant change (with strong leadership) is required to transform these silos within the system into a coordinated and cohesive mesosystem or macrosystem, with a focus on aligning incentives for high-value care models based on patient outcomes and costs of care over time.

The presence of a coordinated system of care for primary care needs (a "medical home" such as the PCMH model) is critically important to health system reform.[9] A PCMH model can help increase value by providing higher-quality care at a lower cost over time in a coordinated way. It combines attention to the ongoing and acute care needs of patients in a patient-centered manner that is supported by practice innovations, including population health approaches to chronic disease, effective uses of information technology, and new models of health care delivery and health care improvement.[9] This model focuses on the preferences and values of patients and their families as well as payment reform that rewards value over finite interventions and provisions of care.

The transformation to accountable care and the PCMH model is challenged by the current state of many health care systems. Current information technology systems (discussed in more detail in Chapter 9) are often insufficient to measure and provide real-time feedback to front-line teams and to help leaders anticipate whether the mesosystem or macrosystem is on track to meet ACO requirements. Clinical revenue systems have traditionally used production-based work flow and compensation models that do not align the systems to support collaborative discussions regarding transitions in care, much less high-value care or the Triple Aim.

CASE STUDY 1
Health Improvement at the Macrosystem Level

A team responsible for the health of a large population of Native Americans identified multiple gaps in care delivery and health outcomes. How did they use health care improvement strategies at the organizational (macrosystem) level to help close the gaps they identified?

The Chinle Service Unit (CSU) serves 31 Navajo communities in the central region of the Navajo Nation as part of the Indian Health Service (IHS). The IHS is a federal agency in the US Department of Health and Human Services. After developing a patient-centered culturally influenced improvement model in 2005 and engaging in primary care transformation via a collaborative in 2007, the CSU committed to further pursue the Triple Aim to provide higher-value care for their population of over 35,000 primarily Native American patients. They created

and implemented a portfolio of projects to include a medical home model (including childhood immunizations, emergency department visits, and access to care), inpatient safety, diabetes, inpatient satisfaction, and collaboration of the IHS's Community Health Improvement Councils.

The CSU organized the projects based on the Triple Aim. Their project outcome measures included emergency department and urgent care visits, childhood immunization rates (medical home care), diabetes outcome bundle control (hemoglobin $A1_C$, low-density lipoprotein, blood pressure), hospitalization rates (diabetes), and coalition development scores (community health improvement council collaboration). The teams also followed population outcome measures for each dimension of the Triple Aim: population health (self-reported health status, childhood healthy weight, diabetes incidence and prevalence), experience of care (ambulatory care patient satisfaction, 30-day re-admission rate, and diabetes outcome bundle and per capita cost, estimated based on emergency department and urgent care utilization and hospital bed days). The teams made significant and sustained improvement in many of their measures; participation in the projects has positively impacted the long-term culture of quality improvement across their unit.[36]

V. CLOSING GAPS IN THE HEALTH CARE DELIVERY SYSTEM

Chapter 1 provided a high-level view of the US health care system and its transition from a physician-centered to a patient-centered system as a foundation for the Third Science. The first part of this chapter provides detail regarding the dynamic milieu of the health care system and the direction in which the system is heading. The breadth and speed of changes and the rapid emergence of high-value care models to meet the Triple Aim of care requires physicians and other health professionals to re-envision and execute on specific opportunities to advance the system forward for patients and society. The remainder of the chapter provides a broad look at several approaches used to close gaps at the macrosystem level (i.e., health care organizations, regionally and nationally): population management, health care improvement, and data analytics.

How can the health care system define and capture the promise of population health, and how does this differ from public health? Many authors have offered definitions of population health, including "the health outcomes of a group of individuals, including the distribution of such outcomes within the group."[21] Chapter 10 provides a detailed review of population health and its intersection with public health. Public health typically assumes a direct relationship with government health departments, whereas population health is a broader topic that includes the health care delivery system in total.[22] Currently, most consider population health as a spectrum, where the population in any given context may be patients defined by specific characteristics such as their residence, their provider group, their disease, or their insurer.

Health professionals must improve population health one patient at a time; professionals in teams at all levels of the system (microsystems, mesosystems, and macrosystems) must proactively provide high-value care and promote health for individual patients as well as the group of patients they are responsible for. The system must include the structures (personnel, training, team composition, settings, means of communication) and processes that ensure the care provided is truly patient-centered. Health professionals must be facile in effective shared decision-making and incorporate patients' preferences, values, context, and capacity for completing care recommendations with advanced information systems and analytics.[23] Any viable future for population health requires production, display, understanding, and implementation of practice changes using data analytics.

There are three fundamental prerequisites for an information system designed to support the Triple Aim: content, analytics, and deployment.[24] Content broadly includes "What should we be doing?" such as applying evidence-based decision making regarding diagnosis, treatment, and prevention, as well as the best practices (including care models) needed to provide optimal care to patients. Analytics refers to the system that answers "How are we doing?" What is the system's performance on measures of importance? For example, what percentage of children in a particular population is fully vaccinated at 2 years of age (process measure)? What is the inpatient mortality rate for patients admitted with a diagnosis of myocardial infarction (outcome measure)? Analytics that connect the processes of care to patient outcomes are particularly important and require a data source that transcends any particular structure in the system. Content includes extant evidence (knowledge, including practice guidelines) as well as the implementation of the evidence (via health care improvement strategies) to minimize delays between identifying what physicians and other health care professionals should do and actually ensuring that it happens consistently in practice. Deployment ensures that improvements become part of routine care delivery through changes in culture, dissemination, leadership, and accountability.[24] Effectiveness depends upon how improvements are adapted or adopted by microsystems of care.

A. Health Care Improvement Strategies

Health care improvement is a broad term that encompasses traditional process and quality improvement and patient safety efforts to close gaps aligned with the six IOM dimensions of quality. Batalden and Davidoff defined it as "the combined and unceasing efforts of everyone—health care professionals, patients and their families, researchers, payers, planners, and educators—to make the changes that will lead to better patient outcomes (health), better system performance (care), and better professional development."[25] Chapters 5 and 6 provide detailed explanations of patient safety and quality improvement strategies and tools that are used up to the macrosystem (health care organization) level. Health care improvement empowers every member of the health care team to close gaps and hold gains in quality and value within the system. It also adds the challenge of change management and the work necessary to disseminate, adapt, and operationalize improvements across a system. Health care improvement is fundamental to both content ("What should we be doing?") and deployment ("How do we transform?").

Five types of knowledge must be applied in concert to drive system improvement: scientific evidence, context awareness, performance measurement, plans for change, and execution of planned changes. Scientific evidence informs plans for change (or interventions aimed to make the desired improvement) within a particular context (microsystem setting); knowledge related to system improvement (change

management, leadership) is required to ensure that the needle successfully "moves" from baseline performance measure to desired performance measure. Quality improvement efforts occur at the microsystem, mesosystem, and macrosystem levels; successful initiatives include representatives from all roles in the process or "work" that is being improved.

Every health professional should understand early in their education and training that they have two jobs: delivering high-value care to patients and improving the process and outcomes of care.[25] Although health professionals (even within a single discipline) will have varying levels of expertise in planning and executing quality improvement projects, it is important for all team members to visualize health care delivery as a series of processes that become "standard work" (see Fig. 3.1); systematizing care will ensure better outcomes and provide capacity for individualizing care when needed. Chapter 6 describes rapid cycle changes; Lean, Six Sigma, and change management by leaders; and the importance of measurement. Related chapters include Chapter 8 (a broad overview of leadership) and Chapter 12 (discusses health policy, a means for improving the system at a level higher than the macrosystem or health care organization level).

CASE STUDY 2
Clinical Use of Patient Registry to Improve Pediatric Asthma Care

A patient-centered medical home in the upper Midwest sought to improve the quality of life and outcomes for their pediatric asthma patients. They used a population health model approach. What structures and processes might be needed to implement such an approach?

This practice started by building a registry of chronic asthma patients 5 to 18 years of age within their practice in order to identify which group of children they would target to optimize care. The database was populated using billing codes from the electronic medical record. They used registered nurses as care managers, who then applied standard processes (e.g., frequency of phone calls or portal messages to parents to assess asthma control) to the patients in the database (without the need for additional provider visits in most cases) to improve outcomes (missed school days, asthma control, amount of medication needed for asthma control). They collaborated with patients' parents to help ensure an improved quality of life for these children.[35]

B. Population Management

The IHI defines **population management** as management of and payment for health care services for a discrete or defined population. Contrast this with **population medicine,** which the IHI defines as the design, delivery, coordination, and payment of high-quality health care services to manage the Triple Aim using the best resources available.[26]

Effective population management requires the stratification or segmentation of patients based on level of risk of poorer health outcomes. Roughly one half of patients in a primary care population are healthy (bottom of the pyramid) and constitute 10 percent to 20 percent of total health care dollars spent. Thirty to 45 percent of the population has limited and/or stable chronic disease; the cost of caring for this group is roughly 30 percent to 40 percent of total costs. The sickest patients are in the smallest percentage (5 percent) of the population and are often described as "super-utilizers." They often are elderly, frail, disadvantaged socioeconomically, have psychosocial barriers to care, and have multiple health issues and/or many emergency department visits and hospitalizations. They account for 45 percent to 50 percent of health care costs in the population.[27]

Health organizations seeking to meet the Triple Aim and improve outcomes while minimizing cost must target high-risk, high-cost "sub-populations" proactively and differently than those with lower risk. At the outset, this requires organizations to correctly identify these patients. For example, ACOs must be able to determine which patients are at high risk for re-admission, with a focus on patients with a rising risk index such as congestive heart failure patients with sudden weight gain or diabetic patients with worsening hemoglobin $A1_C$ values.[28] Current risk prediction models lack precision and are difficult to generalize across a broad diverse population. Ongoing study of internal performance and benchmarking to similar groups will allow a broader understanding of risk. Emerging systems are collecting and sharing de-identified data from electronic medical records and other sources to better characterize and predict risk to help ACOs with projections of patient outcomes and financial performance.[29]

Patient registries are organized systems that use observational study methods to collect uniform data (including clinical data) to evaluate specific outcomes (predetermined for scientific, clinical, or policy purposes) for a population of patients.[30] The population of patients may be defined by a particular disease, condition, or exposure. The file or files derived from the registry is called the **registry database.** Registries are designed according to their purpose, as different levels of rigor are required for registries used to support decision making as compared to those used for descriptive purposes. Registries may be used for determining clinical, cost, or comparative effectiveness of a test or treatment. They may be used to monitor or measure the safety of specific products and treatments; to measure or improve quality of care within a health care improvement initiative at the microsystem, mesosystem, or macrosystem level; or to assess the natural history, magnitude, incidence, prevalence, and/or trend of a disease over time.[30] In the context of population management, patient registries are important tools not only for quality and process improvement efforts, but for active management or care of patients with specific diseases or conditions by front-line (microsystem) teams.

C. Data Analytics

Data analytics that collate and display observational data from national and international billing data and de-identified clinical data is another critical tool for closing the knowledge gap between the current health care system and the system of the future. These "big data" collections consist of large integrated data sources accessed with alternate techniques such as machine learning. Data are often displayed as graphic analytics and "heat maps" of data that can link diagnoses and use of resources. The complexity and breadth of the data plus the need to access multiple databases simultaneously to develop a comprehensive observational data set requires the use of resources and software that is beyond the capacity or purpose of commonly available data management software that is used for internal process and outcomes analytics.

While "big data" are a potential resource to better understand national care patterns and the natural history of diseases, it presents several limitations. Big data are generally limited to administrative or observational data, and decisions regarding specific clinical interventions may often require more detailed clinical studies. In addition, most providers are primarily interested in discovering and benchmarking the performance of their front-line team. This type of data analysis includes three phases: data collection, data sharing, and data analytics. Data analytics is the discovery and communication of meaningful patterns in data.[31] Institutions across the health care system have or are moving toward electronic health records (EHRs), but this intervention alone is not enough to significantly close system gaps, since they typically benchmark past performance. The return on investment for EHRs will primarily occur once we have a data-driven health care culture aligned with rapid cycle improvement where data is analyzed, exploited, and benchmarked to other providers to improve outcomes and align financial incentives in a value-based model to the work of clinical teams.[31]

It is helpful to consider how organizations might improve their awareness of unexpected practice variation and improvement of their performance through adoption of analytics. Many start by collecting and integrating data through the use of standardized vocabulary to allow collation of information and develop patient registries. Analysis of internal data benchmarked to other providers can improve understanding of performance gaps and drive a response to waste and unexpected variation in care. Eventually the system will evolve to a higher level, allowing population health management and predictive analytics. Predictive modeling is a statistical process that analyzes historical data in order to create an algorithm that can be used to determine the likelihood of a future event. Predictive modeling helps to identify the risk of an outcome, based on an in-depth understanding and analysis of what has happened in the past.[32] At this more advanced level, organizations may seek to use clinical risk intervention and analytics to tailor patient care based on population outcomes and genetic data.[31]

Organizations that have achieved an evidence-based, patient-centered, data-driven culture with a consistent analytic feedback loop for understanding clinical outcomes can effectively execute population health management and likely move closer to the Triple Aim. These organizations are aligned with the goals of accountable care, sharing the financial risk and reward of clinical outcomes, with more than one half of acute care cases managed under bundled payments (payments based on an entire episode of care, not on a fee-for-service for each health care intervention or encounter).[31]

D. Displays of Population Data

To become successful in providing high-value care to a population of patients, provider groups must structure their practice to analyze data and intervene when needed to support the health and well-being of the population that they serve. The emerging model of team-based care is well-aligned with this care model. Good intentions must be supported by sophisticated analytics that display the current status of the population with enough granularity and timeliness to support action, move forward, and proactively manage and predict risk for the population. With this in place, medical groups must develop data-based learning communities to accelerate the adoption of new care models and adapt the system when confronted with unexpected outcomes or evidence of low-value care. Electronic medical records will provide evidence and focus caregiver attention based on formal problem lists, reconciled medication lists, tests, and imaging. However, the clinical profile of patients at present is not fully captured by available risk scoring or formal documentation and coding.[33] Large databases that selectively navigate provider and payer databases are often supported by natural language processing and have large patient cohorts with the power to reach statistical significance for subsets of the population that cannot be profiled by many groups. These systems offer health care providers the potential to use integrated data for detailed predictive care modeling and comparison with a national database of matched de-identified patients.[34]

VI. CHAPTER SUMMARY

US health care is undergoing unprecedented and exponential change. The complexity of the current system and the magnitude of change the system will undergo in the next decade present enormous challenges to health professionals and trainees. Patients and society need the health care system to maximize the health of all individuals (population health) and ensure a patient-centered experience of care while minimizing unnecessary costs (i.e., the Triple Aim).

All health professionals must have a basic understanding of this dynamic system and its anticipated changes by catalysts such as the ACA, accountable care, and value-based (versus fee-for-service) payment reform. A more detailed discussion of value in health care, defined as quality of care divided by total cost of care over time, is provided in Chapter 4. Health professionals must see the components of the health care system as structures, processes, and outcomes. They must conceptualize the levels of a patient-centered system (defined as microsystems, mesosystems, and macrosystems), how these levels are related, and how they as professionals must both deliver and improve care for both individual patients and populations of patients.

Physicians and other health professionals must appreciate the dissonance between what the patients perceive as the system of care, what currently exists as an unorganized patchwork of processes that are not patient-centered, and how the present system is not congruent with accountable care performance requirements and new population health models. They should understand how health care improvement strategies (patient safety and quality improvement efforts), population management, and data analytics are used to close current gaps in the health system. Population health models and data analytics will be required to effectively segment patient populations so that health care improvement interventions can be designed, deployed, and adapted to meet the particular needs of these patient groups. Concepts regarding social determinants of health, a key consideration in population management, are discussed in Chapter 11. Clinical informatics is discussed in Chapter 12.

Systemic health care improvement efforts must target how best to achieve and maintain health outcomes for all individuals by closing gaps in each of the six IOM domains of quality. Together, these evolving efforts must be integrated with compassionate care that reflects the preferences and values of individual patients. More details regarding patient safety, quality improvement, and population management are discussed in Chapters 5, 6, and 10, respectively.

QUESTIONS FOR FURTHER THOUGHT

1. How do the financial models utilized by Accountable Care Organizations (ACOs) facilitate achievement of the Triple Aim for the patient populations covered by those organizations?
2. What are the elements that make up the value equation for health care?
3. What processes and structural elements of our current health care systems need to change to enable delivery of accountable or value-based care?
4. Why does stratification or segmentation of patients based on level of risk of poorer health outcomes lead to more effective population management?
5. What are the advantages and disadvantages of using "big data" in data analytics to guide population management approaches?

Annotated Bibliography

Burton DA. The anatomy of healthcare delivery model: how a systematic approach can transform care delivery. *Health Catalyst*. 2014. https://www .healthcatalyst.com/anatomy-healthcare-delivery-model-transform-care.
This white paper provides a high-level overview of how US health organizations can transform to close gaps in value (quality and cost) in the evolving environment.
Burton DA. Guide to successful outcomes using population health analytics. *Health Catalyst*. 2014. https://www.healthcatalyst.com/wp-content/uploads/2015/05/A-Guide-to-Successful-Outcomes-using-Population-Health-Analytics.pdf.
This white paper gives a high-level overview of how population health and data analytics can be successfully used to improve health and health outcomes.
Nelson EC, Godfrey MM, Batalden PB, et al. Clinical microsystems, Part 1. The building blocks of health systems. *Jt Comm J Qual Patient Saf.* 2008;34(7):367–378.
This journal article provides a commonly used nomenclature for understanding and communicating the different levels of the health care system (microsystems, mesosystems, and macrosystems).
Rittenhouse DR, Shortell SM, Fisher ES. Primary care and accountable care—two essential elements of delivery-system reform. *N Engl J Med.* 2009;361(24):2301–2303.
This commentary article nicely summarizes the importance of primary care and accountable care as two necessary ingredients for US health care delivery reform.

References

1. To err is human: building a safer health system. Institute of Medicine. http://www.qu.edu.qa/pharmacy/development/documents/14ay/To_Err_is_Human_1999__report_brief.pdf. Published November 1999. Accessed January 22, 2016.
2. Crossing the quality chasm: a new health system for the 21st century. Institute of Medicine. http://www.nationalacademies.org/hmd/Reports/2001/Crossing-the-Quality-Chasm-A-New-Health-System-for-the-21st-Century.aspx. Published March 1, 2001. Accessed January 22, 2016.
3. Berwick DM, Nolan TW, Whittington J. The triple aim: care, health, and cost. *Health Aff*. 2008;27(3):759–769.
4. Nelson EC, Godfrey MM, Batalden PB, et al. Clinical microsystems, Part 1. The building blocks of health systems. *Jt Comm J Qual Patient Saf*. 2008;34(7):367–378.

5. Berwick DM, Hackbarth AD. Eliminating waste in US health care. *JAMA*. 2012;307(14):1513–1516.

6. Burton DA. The anatomy of healthcare delivery model: how a systematic approach can transform care delivery. *Health Catalyst*. 2014. https://www.healthcatalyst.com/anatomy-healthcare-delivery-model-transform-care.

7. A Dartmouth Atlas Project Topic Brief. Effective care: there is unwarranted variation in the practice of medicine and the use of medical resources in the United States. The Dartmouth Atlas Web site. http://www.dartmouthatlas.org/downloads/reports/effective_care.pdf. Published January 15, 2007. Accessed February 13, 2016.

8. Kapur N, Parand A, Soukup T, Reader T, Sevdalis N. Aviation and healthcare: a comparative review with implications for patient safety. *JRSM Open*. 2015;7(1):205427041561654.

9. Rittenhouse DR, Shortell SM, Fisher ES. Primary care and accountable care—two essential elements of delivery-system reform. *N Engl J Med*. 2009;361(24):2301–2303.

10. Burwell S. Setting value-based payment goals—HHS efforts to improve US health care. *N Engl J Med*. 2015;372(10):897–899.

11. Smoldt RK, Cortese DA. Pay-for-performance or pay for value? *Mayo Clin Proc*. 2007;82(2):210–213.

12. Porter M. What is value in health care? *N Engl J Med*. 2010;363(26): 2477–2481.

13. Berwick DM. Launching accountable care organizations—the proposed rule for the Medicare shared savings program. *N Engl J Med*. 2011; 364e32.

14. Donabedian A. The quality of care: how should it be assessed? *JAMA*. 1988;260(12):1743–1748.

15. Health, United States, 2014. Centers for Disease Control and Prevention Web site. http://www.cdc.gov/nchs/data/hus/hus14.pdf. Published May 2015. Accessed February 13, 2016.

16. Joint Principles of the Primary Care Medical Home: Patient-Centered Primary Care Collaborative. https://www.pcpcc.org/about/medical-home; 2015.

17. Mitchell P, Wynia M, Golden R, et al. Core principles & values of effective team-based health care. Institute of Medicine; October 2012. https://www.nationalahec.org/pdfs/VSRT-Team-Based-Care-Principles-Values.pdf.

18. Naylor MD, Coburn KD, Kurtzman ET, et al. *Inter-Professional Team-Based Primary Care for Chronically Ill Adults: State of the Science.* Philadelphia, PA: Unpublished white paper presented at the ABIM Foundation meeting to Advance Team-Based Care for the Chronically Ill in Ambulatory Settings; March 24–25, 2010.

19. Askin E, Moore N, Shankar V. Chapter 6: Health Care Providers. In: *The Health Care Handbook: A Clear and Concise Guide to the United States Health Care System.* Washington University in St. Louis Press; 2014.

20. Rouse WB, Cortese DA. Chapter 1: Introduction. In: *Engineering the System of Healthcare Delivery.* IOS Press; 2010.

21. Kindig DA, Stoddart G. What is population health? *Am J Public Health*. 2003;93:3669.

22. Stoto MA. Population health in the Affordable Care Act era. *Acad Health*. February 21, 2013.

23. May C, Montori V, Mair FS. We need minimally disruptive medicine. *Br Med J*. 2009;339(7719):485–487.

24. Burton DA. Guide to successful outcomes using population health analytics. *Health Catalyst*. 2014. https://www.healthcatalyst.com/wp-content/uploads/2015/05/A-Guide-to-Successful-Outcomes-using-Population-Health-Analytics.pdf.

25. Batalden P, Davidoff F. What is "quality improvement" and how can it transform healthcare? *Qual Saf Health Care*. 2007;16:2–3.

26. Lewis N. Populations, population health, and the evolution of population management: making sense of the terminology in US health care today. Institute for Healthcare Improvement. Published March 19, 2014. http://www.ihi.org/communities/blogs/_layouts/ihi/community/blog/itemview.aspx?List=81ca4a47-4ccd-4e9e-89d9-14-d88ec59e8d&ID=50.

27. CliftonLarsonAllen. Moving from traditional care delivery models to population health management. http://www.claconnect.com/Health-Care/Transition-From-Traditional-Care-Delivery-Models-to-Population-Health-Management.aspx. Accessed January 24, 2016.

28. Just E. Understanding risk stratification, comorbidities, and the future of healthcare. *Health Catalyst*. 2014. https://www.healthcatalyst.com/wp-content/uploads/2014/11/Understanding-Risk-Stratification-Comorbidities-and-the-Future-of-Healthcare.pdf.

29. Furukawa MF, Patel V, Charles D, Swain M, Mostashari F. Hospital electronic health information exchange grew substantially in 2008–12. *Health Aff (Millwood)*. 2013;32(8):1346–1354.

30. Gliklich RE, Dreyer NA, eds. *Registries for Evaluating Patient Outcomes: A User's Guide.* April 2007. (Prepared by Outcome DEcIDE Center [Outcome Sciences, Inc. dba Outcome] under Contract No. HHSA29020050035I TO1.) AHRQ Publication No. 07-EHC001-1. Rockville, MD: Agency for Healthcare Research and Quality. http://effectivehealthcare.ahrq.gov/ehc/products/21/12/PatOutExecSumm.pdf.

31. Sanders D, Burton DA, Protti D. The healthcare analytics adoption model: a framework and roadmap. *Health Catalyst*. 2013. https://www.healthcatalyst.com/wp-content/uploads/2013/11/analytics-adoption-model-Nov-2013.pdf.

32. Predictive Modeling—To Improve Outcomes in Patients and Home Care. OCS. 2008. http://docplayer.net/11574556-Predictive-modeling-to-improve-outcomes-in-patients-and-home-care.html.

33. Mechanic RE. Mandatory Medicare bundled payment—is it ready for prime time? *N Engl J Med*. 2015;373:1291–1293.

34. Providers convert health information to health intelligence. Optum One Web site. http://www.humedica.com/solutions/providers/optum-one/. Published 2013.

35. Rank MA, Branda ME, McWilliams DB, et al. Outcomes of stepping down asthma medications in a guideline-based pediatric asthma management program. *Ann Allergy Asthma Immunol*. 2013;110(5):354–358.

36. Whittington JW, Nolan K, Lewis N, Torres T. *Indian Health Service Chinle Service Unit: A Triple Aim Improvement Story.* Cambridge, MA: Institute for Healthcare Improvement; November 2015. Institute for Healthcare Improvement Web site. http://www.ihi.org/resources/Pages/Publications/IndianHealthServiceChinleTripleAim.aspx.

4

Value in Health Care

Neera Agrwal, MD, Donna Williams, MD, Timothy Dempsey, MD, MPH, and Natalie Landman, PhD

LEARNING OBJECTIVES

1. Explain the concept of value and how it applies to health care.
2. Review the essential components of a high-value health care system.
3. Summarize the current state of value in US health care.
4. Discuss key barriers to patient-centered, high-value health care.
5. Understand key strategies physicians can use to promote high-value care.

Value in health care is a strategic priority in the United States. All members of society want to have a health system that provides care that is highly effective, safe, patient-centered, and affordable. In this chapter, the reader is introduced to the definition of value in health care, followed by an exploration of what value means to all the stakeholders in society, and a discussion of the barriers to high-value health care. While on average, the US health care system falls short on value, many institutions and health care systems in the United States are championing high-value initiatives. This chapter will highlight some of these high-value systems that are providing much needed innovations in the field of health care delivery.

CHAPTER OUTLINE

"Making systems work in health care—shifting from corralling cowboys to producing pit crews—is the great task of your and my generation of clinicians and scientists."

—Dr. Atul Gawande

"Quality is the match between work and need. It has to do with how close what we are doing is to what people need, or what society needs."

—Dr. Don Berwick

I. INTRODUCTION TO VALUE IN HEALTH CARE

Payment for health care is moving from the traditional fee-for-service and volume-based reimbursement to one that is value-based, in part, because of recent mandates from the Department of Health and Human Services (HHS), which houses the Centers for Medicare and Medicaid Services (CMS).[1] HHS has indicated the desire to tie Medicare fee-for-service payments to quality and value, through programs such as Hospital Value Based Purchasing and the Hospital Readmissions Reduction Programs, with the goal of 85 percent of payments meeting these goals in 2016, and 90 percent in 2018.[2] Commercial payers are making this shift as well, and a number of major health care organizations, such as members of the recently formed Health Care Transformation Task Force, have pledged that 75 percent of their overall payments will be linked to value-based reimbursement.[3]

"Achieving high value for patients must become the overarching goal of health care delivery. This goal is what matters for patients and unites the interests of all actors in the system. If value improves, patients, payers, providers, and suppliers can all benefit while the economic sustainability of the health care system increases," wrote Porter.[4] The Institute of Medicine (IOM) has defined high-value care (HVC) as the "best care for the patient, with optimal results for the circumstances, delivered at the right price."[5] HVC is becoming a strategic priority of all major health care institutions. HVC needs to span the full health care continuum from the macrosystem (national and local health care systems) to the microsystem (the team providing care at the individual patient level) (see Chapter 3).

All stakeholders in health care want HVC, whether they are patients, health care professionals, health care delivery institutions, or payers. Historically, much of medical training and practice focused on, and was limited to, acquiring medical knowledge, ordering and interpreting tests, and prescribing medications. With these imminent changes in the health care delivery environment, there is a growing call for HVC educational models and competencies for health care professions training.

II. KNOWLEDGE AND EDUCATION GAPS IN HIGH-VALUE CARE

It has been argued that in order to improve value in health care delivery, we must also improve the education for those providing health care. Gaps in this knowledge base exist throughout the spectrum of health care professionals and across the continuum of physician training. The gaps in undergraduate medical education (UME) and graduate medical education (GME) have been widely recognized, and are described by Skochelak and others.[6] Fifteen US and Canadian reports published over a decade uniformly called for a significant change in education practice to align with the goals of high-value health care delivery. The gaps in HVC education have become wider over time, as the pace of change in medicine becomes steeper each year, and education programs struggle to modernize their curricula.

Ryskina and colleagues conducted a survey of US internal medicine residents' knowledge of HVC. While the residents felt they were aware of the principles of HVC, only one in four reported knowledge of cost information, and less than one half discussed costs of care with patients.[7] A study from Kaiser Permanente surveyed leaders regarding the ability of newly graduated physicians within their divisions to practice within a highly organized care delivery system. The survey included competence in care coordination, continuity of care, familiarity with clinical information technology (IT), leadership and management skills, and systems thinking. Thirty percent to 50 percent of those surveyed felt that this cohort of physicians showed significant deficiencies in these core competencies, indicating a lack of training in health systems science in GME.[8]

The training environment appears to be critical in the development of physicians who can practice HVC. Sirovich and colleagues assessed the ability of first-time test takers of the American Board of Internal Medicine certifying exam to recognize HVC practices. They noted that internists trained in lower-intensity medical practice regions were more likely to recognize when conservative management was appropriate, although they remained capable of choosing appropriate aggressive therapies when indicated.[9] A similar analysis by Chen and coworkers demonstrated that physician training location and local practice patterns determined how they spent resources throughout their careers. Those who trained in lower-spending regions continued to spend up to 7 percent less during the first 15 years of their practice, compared to their counterparts who trained in higher-spending regions. This difference did decrease with time, and by 16 to 19 years of practice, there appeared to be no spending differential.[10] These studies serve as examples for the importance of training health care professionals about how health care costs, health care financing, and health care policy affect HVC.

Another key message in health professions training is that HVC is not simply a formula for cost containment, but is a recipe for improved health care outcomes.[11,12] The Accreditation Council for Graduate Medical Education (ACGME) has defined six general competency domains for physician education: medical knowledge, patient care, professionalism, interpersonal and communication skills, practice-based learning and improvement, and systems-based practice. Weinberger proposed that providing high-value cost-conscious care should be a critical seventh general competency for physician training.[13]

Educating health professionals to provide high-value health care is not a simple task, in part because it requires mastery of many competencies. The University of California, San Francisco Center for Healthcare Value Training Initiative has proposed 21 competencies in health care value that should be considered in the education of all health care professionals. These are defined by learner levels and include the core principles of health care delivery, financing, and organizations.[14] The American Hospital Association (AHA) notes "that to work in a reformed health care environment, physicians need to develop skills to both lead and facilitate a care team, understand and use systems theory and information technology to improve quality and patient safety."[15] In order to meet these goals, the AHA recommended lifelong learning in HVC, starting at the medical school curriculum, and continuing through residency and postgraduate practice.[15] One such curriculum that spans the entire educational and practice career has been developed as a collaborative effort by The Alliance for Academic Internal Medicine (AAIM), the American Board of Internal Medicine (ABIM), and the American College of Physicians (ACP).[16] The AAIM-ACP HVC curriculum was launched in 2012, and although initially intended for internal medicine residents and fellows, it has now been adapted for medical students and practicing physicians and could serve as a model for additional health care professionals.

III. DEFINING VALUE

Individuals expect value in their lives, whether buying consumer goods, such as a car, or purchasing a service from an airline or hospital. While some have argued that it is impossible to measure value in health care, there is increasing recognition that it can be measured and improved.

What constitutes high-value health care, and how is it defined? A widely accepted approach was proposed by the IOM in 2001 and includes six health system goals. Health care should be Safe, Timely, Effective, Efficient, Equitable, and Patient-centered (STEEEP).[17]

- *Safe:* Medical errors account for between 44,000 and 98,000 deaths per year,[18] and there is much room for improvement. Avoiding injuries to patients and eliminating medical errors is a crucial component of any high-value system.

- *Timely:* Care should be provided as expeditiously as possible with a premium set on reducing potentially harmful delays in both evaluation and treatment.
- *Effective:* Health care organizations should provide the most up-to-date services following established guidelines and best practices. These services should be evidence-based, and care that does not provide a clear benefit should be withheld to avoid unintended harm.
- *Efficient:* Waste in US health care is an important issue, with some estimates ranging between $500 billion to $900 billion of wasteful care provided each year.[19] Avoiding duplication, ineffective treatments, and other sources of wasteful use of resources is crucial to improving quality.
- *Equitable:* Care should be provided without prejudice to all patients regardless of individual characteristics such as gender, ethnicity, socioeconomic status, or sexual orientation.
- *Patient-centered:* Patients should be at the center of decisions affecting their health and well-being. Care should be taken to ensure individual patient preferences, and values are accounted for at each step in the decision-making process. Consumer-directed values of accessibility, service, effectiveness, and costs should be upheld whenever possible.

A system that is able to improve care in all of these domains will go a long way toward achieving HVC. As the IOM states: "A health care system that achieves major gains in these six areas would be far better at meeting patient needs. Patients would experience care that is safer, more reliable, more responsive to their needs, more integrated, and more available, and they could count on receiving the full array of preventive, acute, and chronic services that are likely to prove beneficial. Health care professionals would also benefit through increased satisfaction from being better able to do their jobs and thereby bring improved health, greater longevity, less pain and suffering, and increased personal productivity to those who receive their care."[17]

The formidable goals put forth by the IOM have since been distilled into an actionable framework known as the Triple Aim, by the Institute for Healthcare Improvement (IHI)[20]:

1. Improve the health of a defined population.
2. Enhance the patient care experience, including quality, access, and reliability.
3. Control and reduce the per capita cost of care.

The Triple Aim in practice would support a defined population, with a system optimized to do so. The system would provide coordinated care for individuals in the population, with access to up-to-date knowledge and evidence on effective care. The costs of doing so should be transparent, especially the costs over time for both the individual and for the population.

After establishing what kind of health care is desired by all members in society and stakeholders in the health care system and the high-level tactics to get there (Triple Aim), a common framework is needed 1) to determine the size of the gap between the current and desired state and 2) to monitor the progress on the path toward a high-value health care system for all. This is where the concept of a value equation becomes particularly useful. While the specific metrics to measure value will vary depending on whose perspective is considered (e.g., patient, payer, provider) and the exact population of patients in question (e.g., asthma vs. diabetes patients), in the simplest terms, value can be defined as *quality relative to costs.*

Fig. 4.1 shows an example of the components of a value equation. Quality, which forms the numerator of the equation, has at least three key elements: *outcomes, safety,* and *service.* Each of these elements is a multidimensional term that can include a variety of specific metrics that reflect stakeholder perspectives and the population of patients being addressed. Outcomes may include patient mortality, complications, functional status, and workplace productivity or consistent school attendance. Safety, one of the most important determinants of HVC, may include metrics such as infection rates, accidental falls, and medication errors. Finally, service may include patient satisfaction, waiting times to be seen by a given health care provider, access to a given treatment or procedure, and access to affordable insurance.[21]

The denominator of the value equation, "total cost," can also be defined in various ways, for example, per line item of service, per visit, per episode, per disease, or per year. However, to determine greatest value, cost must be defined as the total amount spent per patient over the length of the condition being treated. This long-term view is essential, as in some instances higher costs in the short term actually lead to lower overall costs of treatment. Thus, *value in health care is defined as quality achieved per dollar spent for the entire course of the disease over time.*

The following are examples of high-value care that have initial higher costs, but lead to higher quality and, thus, lower overall costs.[22]

- At the Intermountain Medical Group, outpatient mental health care is combined with primary care. Primary care physicians are empowered to provide treatment for more common mental health conditions such as mild or moderate depression, and several types of mental health professionals are integrated into primary care practices. Patients receive coordinated behavioral care, leading to improved outcomes. Although costs are higher upfront, overall costs are lower due to reductions in emergency department visits and other care.
- The Mayo Clinic studied surgeons who, while performing breast cancer surgery, obtain pathology evaluations of frozen specimens in the operating room to see if all surgical margins are cancer free. This adds time in the operating room initially but may prevent a second surgery. In a study of breast cancer lumpectomy surgery at 5 years after procedure, the 30-day reoperation rate was 3.6 percent at Mayo Clinic, compared with 13.2 percent nationally. Thus, the initial costs are higher, but overall costs are lower, promoting HVC.

IV. VALUE FROM STAKEHOLDERS' PERSPECTIVES

Physicians and other health professionals who strive to provide HVC must consider the perspectives of the various stakeholders in the health care system. The health care system is a large ecosystem, ranging from the macrosystem to

$$\text{Value} = \frac{\overset{\text{Quality}}{(\text{Outcomes} + \text{Safety} + \text{Service})}}{\text{Total cost}}$$

Fig. 4.1 The value equation. (Included with permission from Dr. Denis Cortese, Mayo Clinic Health Policy Center.)

the local microsystem (discussed in Chapter 3). An action by a specific entity in the system, whether a provider, a payer, or the patient, may lead to outcomes affecting quality and cost, and have an effect on other stakeholders. Given the currently fragmented nature of the US health care system, the integration across components of the system is not optimized. The lack of synergy across systems means the definition of health care value can vary widely depending on whose perspective is being considered.

Who are the players in our health care system, and what do they value? The health care system can be defined as a complex, intertwined organism comprising five key domains (Table 4.1).

The knowledge domain includes research and education. Stakeholders include a variety of institutions: universities,

Table 4.1 The Five Domains of the US Health Care System

	Care Delivery Domain	Knowledge Domain	Payer Domain	Medical-Legal Domain	Regulatory Domain
Current roles played by each domain	Diagnosis Treatment Rehabilitation Prevention	Medical-related education Clinical training Medical technologies Data collection Measurement	Reimbursement Patient coverage	Confidential and undiscoverable malpractice procedures Compensation for patients and families State-specific policies	Numerous policy and regulations related to the following: • Health • Medical documentation • Billing codes • Payments • Use of information technology • Clinical certification and licenses • State specific scope of practice for providers • State specific insurance rules
Roles for each domain in a future high-value, continuously learning, health care system focused on the patient	• Create high value care on a continuously improving basis. • Develop a continuously learning organization as an output of the health care delivery system.	• Discover and generate new knowledge, novel diagnostics, novel therapeutics that improve value.	• Pay for value.	• Compensate injured patients and families. • Generate safety data and information for continuous improvement by the care domain.	• Develop policies and regulations that foster the self-organization of a high value, continuously learning health care delivery system.
Stakeholders	• Patients • Physicians • Non-physician providers (pharmacists; nurses; social workers; registered dieticians/nutritionists; community health workers; physical, occupational, speech therapists; public health workers) • Health care administrators • Public health departments • Community health centers • Sub-acute care facilities • Ambulatory surgery centers • Hospitals • Home health agencies • Rehabilitation centers • Skilled nursing facilities • Nursing homes • Hospices • Integrated networks • Diagnostic clinics • Imaging units • Laboratory services • Health information technology • Nonprofit/special-interest organizations	• Medical schools • Dental schools • Nursing schools • Physician assistant programs • Physical, occupational, speech therapy programs • Researchers • Universities • US Public Health Services (AHRQ, ATSOR, CDC, FDA, HRSA, HIS, NIH, SAMHSA) • State Departments of Health • Professional associations • Trade associations • Medical equipment manufacturers • Biomedical suppliers • Pharmaceutical companies • Biotechnology companies • Nonprofit/special-interest organizations	• Commercial insurers • Self-insured employers • Government payers (Medicare/Medicaid, Veterans Affairs, Tri-care, Indian Health Services, Federal Employees Health Benefits, State Children's Health Insurance Program) • Individual/Consumers/Patient	• Lawyers • State Government • Justice system	• Congress • The White House • Federal government agencies • State government agencies • State legislatures • State medical licensing bodies • Accreditation agencies including professional specialty boards for providers

Reprinted with permission from Dr. Natalie Landman and Dr. Denis Cortese.

research institutes, academic medical centers, pharmaceutical and medical device manufacturers, as well as the agencies that fund their activities, such as the National Institutes of Health.[21] Maximizing return on investment by these organizations can contribute to increasing health system costs.

The care delivery domain is the primary place where patients "reside." It includes the broad range of health care professionals and institutions across the patient care continuum, from primary care to postacute and long-term care. In defining value, the patient's perspective includes outcomes of mortality, survival, complications, return to normal activity, and access to care. The health care professional is concerned with mortality, survival, complications, and patient satisfaction. Neither group has historically focused on the cost of care, although awareness of costs of care is changing as patients share an increasingly higher proportion of out of pocket payments for health care.

The primary function of the *payer domain* is to pay for health care services provided and includes individuals, private insurance companies, employers, and state and federal government agencies. Private payers want to keep the bottom line solvent, as many must report to stockholders, while self-insured employers look for satisfied employees and their rapid return to work, as well as a healthy bottom line.

The medical-legal domain, which includes the malpractice system, often exists in an adversarial relationship with the care delivery domain. Although, this domain often may serve a watchdog function, under the current structure it also has the ability to profit from the health system's mistakes.

Finally, *the regulatory domain,* the domain of legislative enactment and associated administrative interpretation, derived from national, state, and local actions exerts as a powerful influence across the other domains. Regulatory efforts may increase or decrease costs, sometimes through unintended or anticipated consequences.

Although understanding the value from the perspective of all stakeholders in the health care system is important, the most important perspective to be considered is that of the patient. Thus, defining value (and paying for value) requires measuring what actually matters to patients.[23] Ideally, a high-value health care system would identify each individual's priorities and measure the extent to which these priorities are met.

Despite the need for a patient-centric definition of HVC, the vast majority of current quality metrics reflect professional standards. For example, outcomes of interest to people living with frailty or advanced illnesses may not be well represented in the current set of quality metrics used by CMS. Among the elderly, priorities include maximizing physical comfort, avoiding delirium, receiving care at home, maintaining independence, and maintaining relationships with family and friends. Younger disabled persons may have a different set of priorities: restoring function, returning to work, earning a living, supporting a family, and being in control of one's own life. Thus, high-value care may be a moving target and must be defined for each patient in a manner that meets their needs.

CASE STUDY 1

Virginia Mason Medical Center Marketplace Collaborative Low Back Pain Value Maps

Given that the definition of value can vary widely among health care ecosystem participants, and may at times conflict, how can payers and care delivery organizations find common ground to provide the highest value to the patient? What potential challenges will delivery organizations face as they embark on the road of providing high-value care?

In 2004, Virginia Mason Medical Center (VMMC) an integrated, not-for-profit health care delivery system was approached by self-insured employers in the Seattle, Washington, area seeking a solution to rising health care costs. VMMC prides itself as an organization that prioritizes patients' interests, but they also realized that the employers were paying the bills for patient care. To better meet the needs of its customers, VMMC invited the employers to collaborate on identifying and solving perceived quality and cost issues. The overall vision was to improve patient care, while making it more affordable to those who purchase care, the patients' employers.[24]

A series of discussions between VMMC and self-insured employers followed. A set of key principles to drive the development of the new models of care was agreed upon, including: 1) focus on highest costs, 2) adopt employers' definition of value: better, faster, and more affordable, 3) create evidence-based clinical value streams, 4) employ systems engineering tools to remove waste, and 5) use a cost-reduction business model.

In accordance with these principles, VMMC began identifying cost and quality concerns of employers. One employer identified low back pain as a significant problem for the workforce that resulted in high health care costs and loss of employee productivity. By analyzing claims data, the VMMC team discovered that 80 percent to 85 percent of patients with back pain suffered from uncomplicated conditions best treated by physical therapy. Following this finding, the team proceeded to develop a value stream map for back pain care at VMMC. Value stream maps are a Lean quality improvement tool (read more about Lean in Chapter 6). The map identified each step in the process of back pain care, revealing that the current state of treatment was far from ideal. VMMC determined that 90 percent of the existing evaluation and treatment process was not helpful in improving patient outcomes. Armed with these observations, evidence-based protocols, and the customer definition of value, the VMMC team set off on a radical redesign of the treatment plan for patients with uncomplicated back pain.

The back pain collaborative has resulted in substantial improvements in patient outcomes (94 percent of patients returned to work the same day, or the day after) and in access to care (the waiting period for an appointment went from 31 days to same-day access), while reducing overall treatment costs (from 5 percent above the national average to 9 percent below).[25] In turn, VMMC was able to recoup the loss of revenue from unnecessary procedures by freeing up capacity so staff could see and treat other patients. Employers also increased reimbursement rates to VMMC for physical therapy for uncomplicated back pain. Building on the success of the back pain collaboration, VMMC has expanded marketplace collaborations to address a total of 15 high-cost diagnoses, including headache, large joint pain, breast masses, and acute respiratory infection all with improved results, better access, and lower costs.

V. ASSESSING THE CURRENT VALUE OF US HEALTH CARE

Much has been written about the rapidly rising costs, uneven access to health care services, and patient outcomes that consistently place the United States at the bottom of the developed world when ranked against other nations' health care systems.[26] However, beneath the surface there is a more complex story—perhaps not surprisingly, given the sheer size and heterogeneity of the US population. A deeper look at US health care data suggests that value is variable and often falls short on basic dimensions of quality and cost.[5] As the IOM says in its 2012 report, *Best Care at Lower Cost: The Path to Continuously Learning Health Care in America,*

> If banking were like health care, automated teller machine (ATM) transactions would take days or longer as a result of unavailable or misplaced records… If home building were like health care, carpenters, electricians, and plumbers each would work with different blueprints, with very little coordination… If shopping were like health care, product prices would not be posted, and the price charged would vary widely within the same store, depending on the source of payment… If airline travel were like health care, each pilot would be free to design his or her own preflight safety check, or not to perform one at all… If automobile manufacturing were like health care, warranties for cars that would require manufacturers to pay for defects would not exist. As a result, few factories would seek to monitor and improve production line performance and product quality.

So where does the United States stand in terms of achieving high-value health care for all? Let's examine each of the components of the value equation individually.

A. Outcomes

The US health care system produces some of the best and some of the worst patient outcomes in the world, as measured by mortality amenable to health care. The measure of "deaths… before age 75 potentially preventable with timely and effective health care" is often used to assess the performance of health systems.[27] Data collected by the Commonwealth Fund show that the United States consistently ranks last in mortality amenable to health care among developed nations. However, a more detailed review highlights a more than twofold variation in this measure across the United States, ranging from 56 deaths per 100,000 people in Minnesota (the best performing state) to 137 in Mississippi (the worst performing state).[28] This variation within the United States is more extensive than what has been observed across Organization for Economic Cooperation and Development (OECD) member nations. Moreover, the top five states in the United States consistently rank among the best OECD nations, while the bottom five states trail all of OECD.

The variability in mortality outcomes holds true, even when we look at a smaller subset of health care providers (e.g., teaching hospitals). We might expect that teaching hospitals would consistently show the best patient outcomes in the country given their access to the latest in medical technology and use of best practices. However, analysis of Medicare Provider Analysis and Review (MEDPAR) data showed that in 2009, mortality outcomes in teaching hospitals varied approximately 3-fold between the best and the worst facilities.[29]

B. Safety

Safety is a major factor contributing to the poor quality care. The IOM's landmark 1999 report, *To Err is Human: Building a Safer Health System* estimated that avoidable medical errors contribute between 44,000 and 98,000 annual deaths in the United States. Despite numerous initiatives over the past 10+ years, medical errors remain a major system issue. A 2010 HHS report showed that nearly one in seven (or 13.5 percent) hospitalized Medicare beneficiaries experienced an adverse medical event, while an additional 13.5 percent experienced temporary harm. The same study determined that nearly one half of these events were clearly or likely preventable.[30] A 2011 study of a broader patient population by Classen and colleagues found that one in three patients in the United States experiences an adverse event during a hospital stay.[31] Medical errors also increase health care costs. Van Den Bos and colleagues estimated that medical errors cost the United States approximately $17.1 billion in 2008.[32]

The Hospital Safety Score, published by the Leapfrog Group, is quickly becoming a key measure of patient safety. A single score is calculated based on 28 approved performance measures and represents a hospital's overall performance around preventable harm and medical errors. The 2015 Hospital Safety Score report showed that only 31 percent of over 2500 hospitals across the nation received an A grade. The data also showed significant variability in hospital safety scores across the nation. For example, the percent of hospitals that received grade A scores in a given state ranged from 68.8 percent in Maine to 0 percent in New Mexico.[33]

Variability in patient safety is also found when examining specific individual procedures. For example, a 2012 study of total joint procedures by the High-Value Healthcare Collaborative (a consortium of 17 health care delivery systems and The Dartmouth Institute) showed "substantial variations across the participating health care organizations in… in-hospital complication rates."[34]

C. Service

Patient satisfaction, one metric of service, varies greatly across the nation. The Hospital Consumer Assessment of Healthcare Providers and Systems (HCAHPS) survey is a national, standardized, publicly reported survey of patients' perspectives of hospital care. The July 2015 HCAHPS release showed that 86 percent of patients were highly satisfied with their experience at the best ranked hospitals, while only 56 percent reported the same level of satisfaction in facilities ranked in the bottom 5 percent.[35] At the state level, percent of patients who "would definitely recommend the hospital" ranged from 78 percent in South Dakota (the best performing state) to 63 percent in New Mexico (the worst performing state).[36]

It should be noted that while patient satisfaction continues to play a role in Medicare's Value-Based Purchasing Program, a growing number of quality experts and health services researchers are moving away from patient satisfaction to patient experience of care metrics. In contrast to patient satisfaction surveys, which focus on patient "opinion" of care received, patient experience surveys are designed to collect information on what patients actually did or did not experience in their interactions with the health care system.[33] For example, instead of asking whether the patient would recommend a given facility (a measure of patient satisfaction), a patient experience of care survey may inquire about ease of scheduling appointments or transparency regarding the costs of care. Thus, surveys of patient experience are presumed to not only provide more accurate, but also more actionable information toward understanding and improving the value of health care.

D. Cost of Care

"Price is what you pay, value is what you get." —Warren Buffet

The United States spends significantly more per capita and a higher percentage of its gross domestic product (GDP) on health care than other countries spend (Fig. 4.2).[37] In 2013, the United States spent 17.1 percent of its GDP on health care. In contrast, the next highest spender, France, saw 11.6 percent of its GDP go to health care, while the United Kingdom spent 8.8 percent of its GDP on financing the health of its citizens. Per capita spending in the United States stands at $8713, more than double that of France ($4124) and the United Kingdom ($3235).[38] Private health care spending, which includes both insurance premiums and out-of-pocket spending, is also highest in the United States. All of these observations are sources of concern in assessing value in US health care.

Due to high (and rising) costs, health care in the United States is becoming increasingly unaffordable for the average citizen[39] and, as one of the major contributors to US debt, may be putting the financial health of the nation at risk.[40] Federal spending on health care has grown from 5 percent of the federal budget in 1970 to nearly one fourth of the federal budget in 2013. Some have estimated that if the current trends continue, the federal spending on Social Security and health care plus payment for interest on the national debt, may exceed total US revenue by 2025. Thus, no federal funding would be available for other government initiatives, including education, infrastructure, social services, and defense.

Does higher US spending on health care translate to higher-quality care? Unfortunately, many studies demonstrate that the higher spending does not necessarily translate into better quality of care (and thus higher value). For example, when compared with other developed nations, the Commonwealth Fund reports show that in 2013 Americans had fewer physician visits (4 vs. 6.5 average for member nations); fewer practicing physicians (2.6 per 1000 population vs. an average of 3.3 across OECD countries); and poor population health despite the high level of health care spending. In 2013, the US life expectancy at birth was 78.8 years, whereas the average life expectancy of OECD member nations was 80.5 years.[37] One explanation for why higher health care spending in the United States does not lead to higher life expectancy is that the majority of health care dollars in the United States are spent on a relatively small population of highly sick patients[41] and on acute interventions that have limited impact on life expectancy of the overall population. Comparatively little funding goes to primary prevention and health promotion, addressing lifestyle, environmental, and social circumstances that might have much greater impact on overall population health than health care delivery.

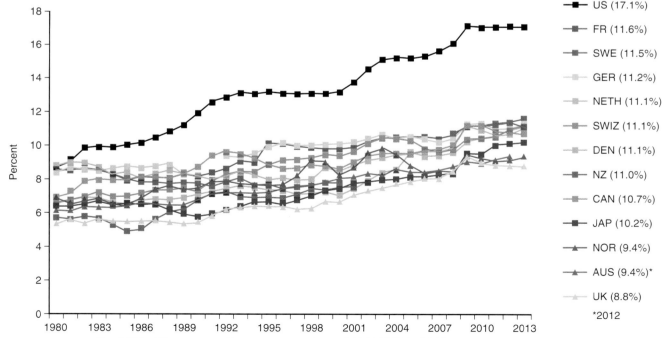

Fig. 4.2 Health care spending as a percentage of GDP, 1980 to 2013. Notes: GDP refers to gross domestic product. Dutch and Swiss data are for current spending only, and exclude spending on capital formation of health care providers. (Source: OECD health data 2015. Reprinted with permission from Squires D, the Commonwealth Fund. *US health care from a global perspective: spending, use of services, prices, and health in 13 countries.* October 2015.)

The limited correlation between quality and cost of care also holds true when we examine specific patient populations or conditions. Fig. 4.3 provides an illustration of quality of care and costs of care for a subset of Medicare beneficiaries.[42] The near-zero correlation between the dollars spent and patient mortality suggests significant waste and room for improvement. Analysis of coronary artery bypass grafting (arterial grafts for blocked coronary arteries) outcomes and costs in California hospitals have resulted in similar observations and set of conclusions.[43]

An estimated 15 to 30 percent of all health care spending is either low-value or of no value at all to the patient. To put this degree of waste into perspective, the 30 percent estimate (approximately $750 billion in 2010) is greater "than our nation's entire budget for K-12 education."[44] The IOM defines six categories of health care waste, two of which—unnecessary services and inefficient care—are the influence of health care providers and account for nearly one half of the estimated health care waste.

Geographic variation in the cost of care for Medicare beneficiaries has been well documented over the past 20 years by the Dartmouth Atlas Project *(www.dartmouthatlas.org)*. In 2011, the IOM released its own set of standardized and risk-adjusted Medicare data that corroborated Dartmouth's findings. While on average, Medicare spent $7500 per beneficiary (in 2008), there was a 40 percent difference in spending between the geographic areas with the 10 percent lowest cost providers and those with the 10 percent highest cost providers.[45] In the much discussed article in *The New Yorker*, "The Cost Conundrum," Atul Gawande examined two Texas towns, McAllen and El Paso, which despite similarities in location and demographics, cost Medicare vastly different amounts of money. In 2006, McAllen cost $14,946 per Medicare enrollee, essentially double the cost of $7504 per enrollee in El Paso.[46] Data from the Dartmouth Atlas Project suggest that the difference is due to the amount of care ordered for patients—a difference driven foremost by physician practice style and in response to system incentives.

VI. KEY ATTRIBUTES OF A HIGH-VALUE HEALTH CARE SYSTEM

The experience of select health care organizations such as Advocate Health Care and Kaiser Permanente, discussed in detail later, suggests that high-value health care in the United States is both feasible and occurring in some parts of the country. What health care system features need to be in place to support the STEEEP aims put forth by the IOM and create high-value health care for all? The key components of a high-value health care system include the following:[21,21a]

1. A clear, shared vision, with the patient at the center, to deliver the highest-value care possible
2. Leadership and professionalism on the part of health care professionals, with corresponding training that emphasizes teamwork, systems engineering, and process improvement
3. A robust IT infrastructure that supports the development and maintenance of a learning health care system, one characterized by seamless information exchanges, stringent peer review and use of best practices, and evidence-based medicine
4. Insurance for all, where individuals own their insurance and have the means to choose and access appropriate medical care
5. Reimbursement models that remove incentives for volume-based care, and instead promote integration and coordination, prevention, and health promotion

In the absence of a carefully designed national system that supports HVC, it is not surprising that the focus

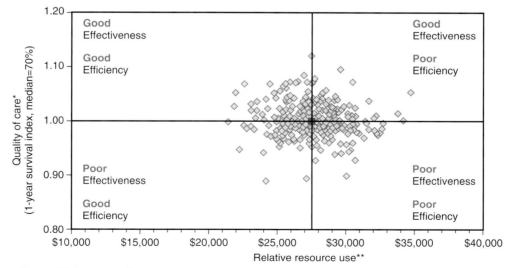

Fig. 4.3 Higher spending does not correlate with better outcomes, suggesting system waste and room for improvement. Quality and costs of care for Medicare patients hospitalized with heart attacks, hip fractures, or colon cancer by hospital referral region (2004). *Indexed to risk-adjusted 1-year survival rate (median = 0.70). **Risk-adjusted spending on hospital and physician services using standardized national prices. (Data from Fisher E, Sutherland J, Radley D. Dartmouth Medical School analysis of data from a 20% national sample of Medicare beneficiaries. Source: *Commonwealth Fund national scorecard on U.S. health system performance,* 2011. Adapted from the Commonwealth Fund. Reprinted with permission from the Commonwealth Fund, Dr. Natalie Landman, and Dr. Denis Cortese.)

on HVC often falls to organizations under the umbrella of "integrated" systems. An **integrated health care system** is one that aligns the incentives of health care professionals to deliver value-based care for its patient population. A 2009 survey of health care leaders performed by the Commonwealth Fund revealed that promoting the growth of integrated delivery systems was viewed as the best way to reduce the growth in US health care costs.[47]

Case Study 2
Advocate Health Care/Physician Partners Asthma Outcomes Initiative

Advocate Health Care/Physician Partners (based in Oak Brook, Illinois) is the largest integrated health care system in Illinois with 12 hospitals, more than 250 outpatient care sites, and over 4800 physicians on staff.[48] The idea of integration began in the early 2000s as an attempt to coordinate care between the organization's hospital-based physicians with doctors working within the surrounding community. They accomplished this through the Clinical Integration Program, which "focuses on five broad improvement categories: enhancing clinical outcomes, improving patient safety, adopting clinical technology, improving patient satisfaction, and increasing efficiency"[49] Progress in each category is tracked via performance metrics, which are quality measures derived from industry standards that provide goals for each provider and the system as a whole to achieve. In order to better accomplish this mission, Advocate implemented cutting-edge technology as well as evidence-based protocols and guidelines.

Advocate's Asthma Outcomes Initiative provides one specific example of how they improved outcomes across an integrated system.[48] After realizing that asthma was a major burden for their patients (as of 2011, 13.5 percent of the Illinois population carries a diagnosis of asthma)[50] and payers (costs for hospitalizations due to asthma totaled more than $380 million per year in Illinois in 2011),[51] Advocate set out to develop a multidisciplinary plan to improve value for all components of its system. Standardized protocols and tools are used by physicians and care providers. These include asthma action plans—individualized management and education tools for each patient to use at home to help guide asthma treatment and discussed with every asthma patient at every visit. In addition to asthma action plans, asthma coordinators are available to patients in the inpatient setting to ensure coordination upon discharge. A community outreach program is currently being tested as is an interactive mobile application for patients and providers. Through the implementation of these collaborative tools and protocols, Advocate has achieved an asthma control rate 24 percent above the national average, and has saved payers more than $17 million annually when compared with national asthma costs.[48]

Compare the strategies of the Clinical Integration Program adopted by Advocate with the components for a high-value system discussed in the beginning of this section. Advocate used care coordination, evidence-based tools, and innovative technology that allowed for individualized treatment plans and promotion of preventive care and attended to patient needs. By following the components for HVC outlined by the IOM, health care systems can improve quality

(the numerator of the value equation) while decreasing costs (the denominator), thus producing higher value associated with better patient outcomes.

VII. BARRIERS TO HIGH-VALUE CARE

The previous sections have described ways to achieve high-value health care delivery in the United States and, as highlighted in Fig. 4.2, each of the domains of the health care system plays a role in promoting HVC. This begs the question, "What are the key barriers that stand in the way of high-value health care delivery being the norm in the United States?"

A. Conflicting Stakeholder Incentives

One barrier that precludes full adoption of HVC practice is conflicting incentives across various stakeholder groups including health care professionals, patients, private payers, industry, and policymakers. Health care professionals play a pivotal role in determining health care spending because of their responsibility for ordering services, medications, and treatments. It has been estimated that physicians are responsible for more than 80 percent of health care costs, based on the decisions made about patient treatment plans.[51] Certainly much of this spending is necessary to provide appropriate care; however, the amount of overuse is substantial. Health care in the United States has historically been permeated by the idea that more care is better care, and this concept has been reinforced over generations of training.[52] More recently, physicians and other health care professionals have started to actively combat the challenge of health care waste through initiatives such as Choosing Wisely[53] and The Do No Harm Project.[54]

Patients also sometimes assume that more medical care is better, despite the potential harm of unnecessary testing. Direct-to-consumer advertising by pharmaceutical, medical device, and other health care companies may lead patients to request specific tests, drugs, and procedures that may be unnecessary. Direct-to-consumer advertising in the form of television and magazine advertisements may be used to promote the sale of newer, more expensive medications that may not necessarily increase value or safety over other, lower-priced medications.[55] It has been suggested that advertisements for medications should include cost information or a notation that generics may be cheaper; however, this is not current practice.[56] In past decades, patients with health insurance have become increasingly insulated from the true costs of care and thus may have few incentives to be prudent consumers of health care services. Insurers have recently employed strategies such as copays and deductibles, bringing at least a portion of health care costs to light for patients.

In contrast, the payers (i.e., insurance companies) are interested in decreasing the use of health care services and the corresponding cost of health care, sometimes with different motivation. Over the past few decades, insurance companies have tried a variety of ways to contain costs and spending, including setting prices (government payers), negotiating discounts (the success of which frequently depends on relative market clout between the two parties), aggressive gatekeeping of services, bundled payments to hospitals based on the patient's specific diagnosis, and financial incentives to physicians for their ordering habits.[57]

Porter wrote, "In any field, improving performance and accountability depends on having a shared goal.… In health care, however, stakeholders have myriad, often conflicting goals.… Lack of clarity about goals has led to divergent approaches, gaming of the system, and slow progress in performance improvement."[4]

B. Lack of Shared Reality

In order to improve health care value, all stakeholders need to openly and honestly appraise the current state of US health care. This shared reality is pivotal to dispelling deeply ingrained assumptions and generalizations, and helps drive actions and prioritization of opportunities. Yet, the fragmented nature of the health care system and the current state of health care IT systems make it difficult to measure and improve health care value. Ideally health professions would make assumptions on reliable, relevant, and meaningful data. However, lack of a national health data infrastructure and poor health IT interoperability, even within the same organization, limit the ability to collate data, study outcomes, and publish results. IT is vital in providing safe and effective ongoing care for all patients and mandatory if we are to generate new strategies for HVC. In an ideal state of health care IT, all information about an individual's health care would be immediately available to both physician and patient, anywhere in the world, with the simple click of a computer key. Currently, this ideal is far from realized.

These inherent challenges in measurement have encouraged an explosion of quality metrics and quality measuring agencies, and focus on what is easy to measure (process) instead of what is meaningful (outcomes). As stated by Porter, "Since value depends on results, not inputs, value in health care is measured by the outcomes achieved, not the volume of services delivered… Nor is value measured by the process of care used; process measurement and improvement are important tactics but are no substitutes for measuring outcomes and costs."[4] The future of quality measurement may lie in harnessing the big data available in electronic medical records across systems to identify areas where better value can be achieved. A recent article by Bates and colleagues suggests that there are six practical areas where big data can be used to reduce costs of health care: high-cost patients, re-admissions, triage, decompensation, adverse events, and treatment optimization for diseases affecting multiple organ systems.[58] Through this approach, organizations may have an opportunity to increase the quality of care while decreasing costs. A more in-depth discussion of quality improvement and measurement is included in Chapter 6.

C. Poor Integration and Coordination

Increasing specialization and the growing number of health care professionals involved in a given patient's care, combined with insufficient communication among them (in some cases even within the confines of the same organization), have resulted in a health care system that may be complex, highly fragmented, and characterized by lack of care continuity and coordination. This current system is discussed in additional detail in Chapter 3. In the worst examples, this can be a system of duplicated tests, confusion about care plans, and not surprisingly, poor patient outcomes at higher costs.[39] Improvement is possible; the integrated delivery systems discussed earlier show both higher quality and better cost containment than the status quo.[21] On average, integrated delivery systems engage in more prevention and health promotion than nonintegrated groups and score better on a variety of Healthcare Effectiveness Data and Information Set (HEDIS) measures.[59] These organizations provide "a coordinated continuum of services to a defined population … and [are] held clinically and fiscally accountable for the outcomes … of the population served."[60] They are the precursors of **Accountable Care Organizations (ACOs)** and accomplish their results through a combination of aligned incentives, robust IT infrastructure, and the greater use of team-based care.

D. Inadequate Education of Health Care Professionals

Currently, most health care professions training programs lack formal education on methods to systematically improve care delivery. Health care professionals may have some exposure to these concepts as part of their training, but often it is not at the level of rigor that includes how value is measured and monitored, and how data can be used for continuous improvement. Despite the growing recognition that team-based care results in higher value for patients and the health care system overall, health professions training programs continue to struggle to develop meaningful interprofessional training.

It is important to understand the role of physicians (and, increasingly, other independent health professionals) in contributing to wasteful spending in health care; it starts with the development of ordering habits in medical school and residency and leads to the formation of practice patterns following training. Indeed, on traditional rounds in a hospital medicine ward, errors of omission (e.g., missing tests that could have been ordered but were not) are more likely to beget the criticism of attending physicians rather than errors of commission (e.g., ordering too many tests that were not necessary). This problem is compounded by the lack of easily accessible costs of laboratory tests and images. It has been shown that making fee information available to providers at the time the order is placed results in decreased ordering.[61] Even so, fee information remains difficult to access at most institutions.

VIII. WHAT CAN HEALTH CARE PROFESSIONALS DO TO PROMOTE HIGH-VALUE CARE?

Professionals can increase value by improving outcomes, decreasing cost, increasing safety, and increasing patient satisfaction through application of principals presented in this chapter. Thus, increasing the numerator and decreasing the denominator raises value (Fig. 4.4).

A. Identify and Classify Value Gaps

In order to avoid the unabated growth in health care spending, health care professionals must serve as leaders in identifying and minimizing care that is inappropriate and focus on delivering care that is appropriate and necessary.[62] An important first step is to identify and understand gaps in

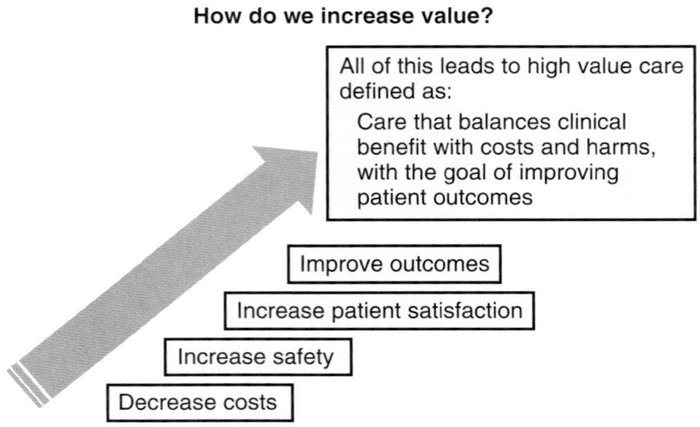

How do we increase value?

All of this leads to high value care defined as:

Care that balances clinical benefit with costs and harms, with the goal of improving patient outcomes

Improve outcomes

Increase patient satisfaction

Increase safety

Decrease costs

Fig. 4.4 **How do we increase value?** (Reprinted with permission from Dr. Neera Agrwal and Dr. Stephanie Starr, Arizona State University and Mayo Medical School Science of Healthcare Delivery, 2015.)

HVC. The most common value gaps include overuse, misuse, underuse, and overdiagnosis. *Overuse* and *misuse* refer to the waste that occurs when care is provided that cannot help patients, such as ordering advanced imaging to evaluate acute low back pain without concerning findings.[19] *Underuse* occurs when screening opportunities are missed, such as early detection of colorectal or cervical cancer in at-risk individuals. On the other end of the spectrum, *overdiagnosis* refers to detection of cancers that will not become symptomatic in a patient's lifetime.[63]

Increasingly, physicians and health care professionals are leading the charge to decrease health care waste and increase value. One example is the Choosing Wisely campaign, which launched in 2012 as a collaboration between the American Board of Internal Medicine and Consumer Reports. In this forum, societies of medical specialists developed lists of tests, treatments, and services that often are used but should be questioned by both health care providers and patients.[64] As of late 2015, over 70 professional societies are represented in the Choosing Wisely campaign. The overarching goal of the Choosing Wisely campaign (www.choosingwisely.org) is to decrease the utilization of services that provide harm or little benefit; next steps include evaluating the effect of the campaign on ordering practices of providers.[65]

Education of future professionals is a key focus in the drive toward high-value health care. It has been shown that internal medicine residents demonstrate inconsistent stewardship practices in hypothetical situations.[66] One way to combat inconsistent education in HVC is to provide a national curriculum in this area. In 2012, the American College of Physicians collaborated with the Alliance for Academic Internal Medicine to launch a national curriculum for internal medicine residents that introduces a framework for HVC delivery and promotes evidence-based, thoughtful, patient-centered care that adds value.[52] The curriculum was updated in 2014 and again in 2016; materials are available at https://hvc.acponline.org/.

B. Understand the Benefits, Harms, and Relative Costs of Interventions

It is critical that all health care professionals understand the benefits and harms of any test, procedure, or medication that they order. Although it is tempting to consider each test we order as a yes or no answer to assist with a specific complaint or diagnosis, this is not often the case. Each test has its own sensitivity and specificity that help increase or decrease our pretest probability of disease. All health professionals must do their best to practice **evidence-based medicine**, which refers to the thoughtful consideration of scientific evidence in application to patient care. With this framework in mind, understanding the characteristics of a test and thinking ahead provides high value. When ordering a test, professionals should be able to answer the following questions:

- What will I do with the results of this test?
- Will these results change the diagnosis, management, or prognosis for my patient?
- If this test is positive, how will the care plan change?
- What if the test is negative?

If the test results will not change the care of the patient, the test should be reconsidered.[67] Similarly, the cost of the test must be taken into consideration. The cost of the test does not only include the financial costs, which may be substantial, but also downstream effects such as radiation exposure, contrast reactions, implications of false-positive or false-negative tests, anxiety or worry for the patient, and incidental findings. When considering downstream costs, downstream savings must also be considered. Sometimes a medication that is more costly per pill (such as certain oral anticoagulants) may cost less in the long run due to greater effectiveness and fewer complications.[68] **Comparative effectiveness research** can assist professionals in making such determinations; this exciting body of literature continues to grow and gain momentum.

C. Decrease or Eliminate the Use of Interventions That Provide No Benefit and/or May Be Harmful

Once the benefits, harms, and costs of the intervention have been considered, it becomes simpler to eliminate those that do not provide benefit to the patient. The concept of eliminating interventions that provide no benefit can be extrapolated beyond the clinical question at hand and applied to routine cancer screening. The prostate cancer screening story should be a cautionary tale. In 2012, the US Preventive Services Task Force (USPSTF) recommended against routine screening for prostate cancer with prostate-specific antigen (PSA) testing, as two large trials reported an overdiagnosis rate of 17 percent to 50 percent.[69] To quote the report, "There is convincing evidence that PSA-based screening programs result in the detection of many cases of asymptomatic prostate cancer, and that a substantial percentage of men who have asymptomatic cancer detected by PSA screening have a tumor that will not progress or will progress so slowly that it would have remained asymptomatic for the man's lifetime." In 2015, the ACP published a value framework for cancer screening, which aims to balance the benefits of screening with the harms and costs introduced.[63] In this framework, one key concept is to consider the "screening cascade," that is, the domino effect that has the potential to lead to diagnosis of important diseases or to increase harm. Classic teaching has recommended against screening patients who are suspected to live less than 10 years due to known comorbidities; it has been suggested that we consider screening only those patients expected to live 15 to 20 years or more.[70] Again, providers of high-quality health care are challenged to practice evidence-based medicine and to thoughtfully, deliberately provide care that helps patients while eliminating interventions that provide no positive benefit.

D. Choose Interventions and Care Settings That Maximize Benefits, Minimize Harms, and Reduce Costs

The setting of care is important in the value equation. Hospital-based care is necessary in many cases and adds value due to concrete benefits from specific treatments not available outside the hospital. However, there is a growing body of literature regarding certain conditions for which inpatient care does not add value, and may in fact increase harm. One such example is treatment of uncomplicated deep vein thrombosis (DVT). Traditionally, patients with DVT were admitted to the hospital for intravenous heparin administration while bridging to oral warfarin for anticoagulation therapy. Since the advent of low–molecular-weight heparin and other agents, outpatient treatment is safe and cost-saving compared to inpatient treatment in selected patients with uncomplicated DVT.[71] Harms of unnecessary hospitalizations include not only financial harm, but exposure to hospital-associated infections such as *Clostridium difficile,* methicillin-resistant *Staphylococcus aureus* (MRSA), and others. Hospital-acquired infections such as MRSA have been associated with higher costs as well as increased utilization of care.[72] With this in mind, it is reasonable to aim to reserve hospital care for only those patients who truly require it in order to avoid unnecessary complications and cost, both short term and long term. It is critical to use shared decision making as a tool for considering the best interventions and care settings for individual patients given their own values and concerns.

E. Customize Care Plans with Patients That Incorporate Their Values and Address Their Concerns

Open and honest communication with patients is critical to achieving HVC. Obtaining a clear vision of each patient's individual goals and values can assist health care professionals in delivering care that is both medically appropriate and consistent with patients' wishes. For example, consider a chronically ill 85-year-old female smoker presenting to the emergency room with fever, shortness of breath, and cough. An initial chest radiograph reveals pneumonia, but also reveals a mass concerning for lung cancer. Should she have a lung biopsy? Should she receive chemotherapy if she has cancer? Should she be referred to hospice to focus on quality of life? Thoughtful discussion with this patient and her family will help her clinical team choose interventions that are appropriate for her ongoing care. Patients with underlying medical conditions who are found to have cancer may choose not to pursue aggressive treatment such as surgery or chemotherapy. If an open and honest discussion is not undertaken regarding the risks and benefits of aggressive

treatment, patients may start down a road of high cost, highly morbid care that may not provide benefit. The 2016 High Value Care curriculum from the ACP/AAIM presents the "High Value Care Conversation Guide" (https://hvc.acponline.org) as a tool to assist in clear conversations aimed at customizing care. This tool includes tips on specific phrases to use to elicit patient values, customize the plan, and confirm patient understanding, among others.

On the other side of the coin, some patients may request care that is unnecessary due to underlying fears of cancer, disability, or other concerns. For example, consider a young man who presents to your clinic complaining of low back pain after helping his friend move to a new apartment 1 week ago. He read on the Internet that he could have a "slipped disc," so he wants you to order magnetic resonance imaging (MRI) to be sure. You perform a complete history and physical, and find no alarming signs or symptoms. In this case, skilled communication is necessary to reassure the patient that his concern (slipped disc) is highly unlikely or at least unlikely to cause disability and that the MRI is unnecessary and potentially harmful. Resources such as Choosing Wisely (www.choosingwisely.org) offer patient handouts on challenging topics such as these to encourage thoughtful communication in the provision of patient care when patients request tests or studies.

F. Identify System-Level Opportunities to Improve Outcomes, Minimize Harms, and Reduce Health Care Waste

Institutional leaders have the responsibility to harness the culture of their organizations and use it to forward the mission of HVC.[73] This mission is often accomplished through quality improvement initiatives driven by those who are on the ground seeing patients and working in the health care system directly. Quality improvement efforts are critical in the quest to provide health care with increased quality at decreased cost, therefore decreasing the denominator of the value equation. One example of a quality improvement success story is found at The Everett Clinic, a physician group practice in Snohomish County, Washington, that employs 500 providers and cares for 300,000 patients. A multidisciplinary team recognized the high expense and minimal benefit of advanced imaging studies (such as computed tomography or CT, MRI, and positron emission tomography or PET scans) when they are not clinically indicated and developed a set of criteria that health care providers must use to order such studies. As a result, unnecessary imaging was reduced by 39 percent in 2 years, saving the system $3.2 million annually.[74] Chapter 6 provides more details about the role of quality improvement in institutional change.

Patient safety efforts, as addressed in Chapter 5, play a key role in both individual and system-level efforts to minimize harms and therefore increase both quality and value. The IOM report "To Err is Human" brought patient safety initiatives to the forefront of medical care. Most institutions have patient safety reporting systems in which any individual who has patient contact may anonymously report witnessed patient safety events. These observations are then investigated in a nonjudgmental fashion, and, in many cases, lead to patient safety improvement efforts throughout the system. The goal of safety reporting systems is to encourage a culture of safety throughout the system.

IX. CHAPTER SUMMARY

Over recent years, health care reimbursement in the United States is shifting from a system based on volume to one based on providing value. Despite this important change, gaps remain in teaching value-based care to health care professionals at all points in training. Encouragingly, there are multiple new initiatives currently under way to combat these deficiencies in the education of HVC, and excellent resources are readily available.

HVC is best defined by the value equation, which states that value is equal to quality over cost. Other ways to understand value-based care include analyzing various domains in the health care ecosystem and determining value from the perspective of these stakeholders. Finally, the IOM's STEEEP model, which says that health care should be safe, timely, effective, efficient, equitable, and patient-centered, provides another way of defining value. This model has been crafted into a framework for action by the Institute of Healthcare Improvement's Triple Aim, which aspires to improve the health of a defined population, enhance the patient care experience, and reduce the per capita costs of care.

Despite the efforts of organizations such as the IHI and IOM, the United States as a whole continues to struggle to provide HVC as evidenced by the variation throughout the country regarding patient outcomes, safety, satisfaction, and costs of care. This may be due to barriers such as poor integration and coordination of services, fragmented and volume-based provider reimbursement, and conflicting stakeholder incentives. Despite the variability in health care quality and value across the United States as a whole, examples of HVC systems, including some integrated systems highlighted in this chapter, have demonstrated the ability to produce high-quality care at low costs.

What can health care professionals do to promote HVC? Health care professionals should understand the relative benefit, harm, and cost of every intervention undertaken. An evidence-based approach should be used to assess options, and if an intervention provides no benefit or is shown to be harmful, it should not be used. Care plans should be customized to each patient's values and address all concerns, placing the patient and his or her family in the center of the decisions made with the care team. Finally, as health care professionals are uniquely positioned to affect change on a systemic level, they should provide leadership in identifying opportunities to improve outcomes, minimize harms, and reduce health care waste.

QUESTIONS FOR FURTHER THOUGHT

1. Among the six IOM goals for quality health care, what are specifically meant by "effective" and "equitable"?
2. Within the health care system, what are the knowledge domain and the payer domain, and how do their value goals differ?
3. How do health care quality outcomes and costs in the United States compare to quality and cost outcomes in other developed countries?
4. What are the key components of a high-value health care system?
5. What are the key barriers to delivery of high-quality care? What can you do to improve the value of the care provided to patients?

Annotated Bibliography

Berwick DM, Hackbarth AD. Eliminating waste in US health care. *JAMA.* 2012;307(14):1513–1516.
This short article identifies the six categories of waste that account for more than 20 percent of total health care expenditures and suggests a model to reduce health care spending.

Institute of Medicine. *Crossing the Quality Chasm: A New Health System for the 21st Century.* Washington, DC: National Academies Press; 2011.
A key publication that outlines the framework that medicine must use to provide high-value care in the 21st century.

Owens DK, Qaseem A, Chou R, Shekelle P. Clinical Guidelines Committee of the American College of Physicians. High-value, cost-conscious health care: concepts for clinicians to evaluate the benefits, harms, and costs of medical interventions. *Ann Intern Med.* 2011;154(3):174–180.
This key article discusses key concepts for understanding how to assess the value of health care services. These concepts serve as the basis for the framework outlined in the ACP High-Value Care Curriculum.

Porter ME. What is value in health care? *New Engl J Med.* 2010;363(26):2477–2481.
This article is an excellent and key synopsis of the framework of value in health care.

Squires D, Anderson CUS. Health care from a global perspective: spending, use of services, prices, and health in 13 countries. http://www.commonwealthfund.org/publications/issue-briefs/2015/oct/us-health-care-from-a-global-perspective. The Commonwealth Fund; October 2015.
This online article discusses data published by the Organization for Economic Cooperation and Development, in which US health care spending is compared to 13 other high-income countries.

References

1. Burwell S. Setting value-based payment goals. HHS efforts to improve US healthcare. *New Engl J Med.* 2015;372(10):897–899.
2. US Department of Health & Human Services. Better, smarter, healthier: in historic announcement, HHS sets clear goals and timeline for shifting Medicare reimbursements from volume to value. 2015. http://hhs.gov/about/news/2015/01/26/better-smarter-healthier-in-historic-announcement-hhs-sets-clear-goals-and-timeline-for-shifting-medicare-reimbursements-from-volume-to-value.html; 2015. Accessed February 18, 2016.
3. Health Care Transformation Task Force. *Major Health Care Players Unite to Accelerate Transformation of U.S. Health Care System.* January 28, 2015. www.hcttf.org/releases/2015/1/28/major-health-care-players-unite-to-accelerate-transformation-of-us-health-care-system.
4. Porter ME. What is value in health care? *New Engl J Med.* 2010;363(26):2477–2481.
5. Smith M, Saunders R, Stuckhardt L, McGinnis JM. *Best Care at Lower Cost: The Path to Continuously Learning Health Care in America.* Washington, DC: National Academies Press; 2013.
6. Skochelak SE. A decade of reports calling for change in medical education: what do they say? *Acad Med.* 2010;85(suppl 9):S26–S33.
7. Ryskina KL, Smith CD, Weissman A, et al. U.S. internal medicine residents' knowledge and practice of high-value care: a national survey. *Acad Med.* 2015;90(10):1–7.
8. Crosson FJ, Leu J, Roemer BM, Ross MN. Gaps in residency training should be addressed to better prepare doctors for a twenty-first-century delivery system. *Health Aff.* 2011;30(11):2142–2148.
9. Sirovich BE, Lipner RS, Johnston M, Holmboe ES. The association between residency training and internists' ability to practice conservatively. *Jama Intern Med.* 2014;174(10):1640–1648.
10. Chen C, Petterson S, Phillips R, Bazemore A, Mullan F. Spending patterns in region of residency training and subsequent expenditures for care provided by practicing physicians for Medicare beneficiaries. *JAMA.* 2014;312(22):2385–2393.

11. Cooke M. Cost consciousness in patient care—what is medical education's responsibility? *New Engl J Med*. 2010;362(14):3.

12. Korenstein D. Charting the route to high-value care: the role of medical education. *JAMA*. 2015;314(22):2359–2361.

13. Weinberger SE. Providing high-value, cost-conscious care: a critical seventh general competency for physicians. *Ann Intern Med*. 2011;155(6):386–388.

14. Moriates C, Dohan D, Spetz J, Sawaya GF. Defining competencies for education in health care value: recommendations from the University of California, San Francisco Center for Healthcare Value Training Initiative. *Acad Med*. 2015;90(4):421–424.

15. Combes JR, Arespacochaga E. Lifelong learning: physician competency development. www.ahaphysicianforum.org/files/pdf/physician-competency-development.pdf; 2012.

16. Smith CD, Levinson WS, Internal Medicine HVCAB. A commitment to high-value care education from the internal medicine community. *Ann Intern Med*. 2015;162(9):639–640.

17. Institute of Medicine. *Crossing the Quality Chasm: A New Health System for the 21st Century*. Washington, DC: National Academies Press; 2011.

18. Institute of Medicine. *To Err Is Human*. Washington, DC: National Academies Press; 1999.

19. Berwick DM, Hackbarth AD. Eliminating waste in US health care. *JAMA*. 2012;307(14):1513–1516.

20. Beasley C. The Triple Aim: optimizing health, care, and cost. *Healthcare Executive*. 2009;24:64–65.

21. Rouse WB, Cortese DA. *Engineering the System of Healthcare Delivery*. Amsterdam: IOS Press; 2010.

21a. McCarthy D, Mueller K, Jennifer Wrenn Issues Research, Inc. *Kaiser Permanente: bridging the quality divide with integrated practice, group accountability, and health information technology*. The Commonwealth Fund; 2009.

22. Kaiser LS, Lee TH. Turning value-based health care into a real business model. *Harvard Business Review*. October 8, 2015.

23. Lynn J, McKethan A, Jha AK. Value-based payments require valuing what matters to patients. *JAMA*. 2015;314(14):1445–1446.

24. Blackmore CC, Mecklenburg RS, Kaplan GS. At Virginia Mason, collaboration among providers, employers, and health plans to transform care cut costs and improved quality. *Health Aff*. 2011;30(9):1680–1687.

25. Kenny C. Better, faster, more affordable: how Virginia Mason Medical Center took a common complaint and delivered uncommon health care. *Seattle Business Magazine*. 2011. http://www.seattlebusinessmag.com/article/better-faster-more-affordable.

26. Davis K, Stremikis K, Squires D, Schoen C. *Mirror, mirror on the wall: how the performance of the U.S. health care system compares internationally*. http://www.commonwealthfund.org/~/media/files/publications/fund-report/2014/jun/1755_davis_mirror_mirror_2014.pdf. The Commonwealth Fund; June 2014.

27. Schoenbaum SC, Schoen C, Nicholson JL, Cantor JC. Mortality amenable to health care in the United States: the roles of demographics and health systems performance. *J Public Health Policy*. 2011;32(4):407–429.

28. Health System Data Center. http://datacenter.commonwealthfund.org/#ind=1/sc=1; 2015. Accessed February 10, 2016.

29. Cortese D, Smoldt R. *A Roadmap to High-Value Healthcare Delivery*. Tempe, AZ: Arizona State University; 2012.

30. Levinson D. *Adverse events in hospitals: national incidence among medicare beneficiaries*. http://www.hospitalsafetyscore.org/state-rankings. Department of Health and Human Services; 2010. Accessed December 5, 2015.

31. Classen DC, Resar R, Griffin F, et al. Global trigger tool shows that adverse events in hospitals may be ten times greater than previously measured. *Health Aff (Millwood)*. 2011;30(4):581–589.

32. Van Den Bos J, Rustagi K, Gray T, Halford M, Ziemkiewicz E, Shreve J. The $17.1 billion problem: the annual cost of measurable medical errors. *Health Aff (Millwood)*. 2011;30(4):596–603.

33. How safe is your hospital? http://www.hospitalsafetyscore.org/state-rankings; 2015. Accessed December 5, 2015.

34. Tomek IM, Sabel AL, Froimson MI, et al. A collaborative of leading health systems finds wide variations in total knee replacement delivery and takes steps to improve value. *Health Aff (Millwood)*. 2012;31(6):1329–1338.

35. HCAHPS hospital survey. www.hcahpsonline.org. Accessed September 24, 2015.

36. Hospital Compare datasets. https://data.medicare.gov/data/hospital-compare; 2015. Accessed February 10, 2016.

37. Squires D, Anderson C. *U.S. health care from a global perspective: spending, use of services, prices, and health in 13 countries*. http://www.commonwealthfund.org/publications/issue-briefs/2015/oct/us-health-care-from-a-global-perspective. The Commonwealth Fund; October 2015.

38. OECD Health Statistics 2015. http://www.oecd.org/els/health-systems/health-data.htm; 2015. Accessed February 10, 2016.

39. Moriates C, Arora V, Shah N. *Understanding Value-Based Healthcare*. New York: McGraw Hill Education; 2015.

40. Meeker MG. *USA Inc.: A Basic Summary of America's Financial Statements*. Menlo Park, CA: Kleiner Perkins Caufield & Byers; 2011.

41. Concentration of health care spending in the US population. http://kff.org/health-costs/slide/concentration-of-health-care-spending-in-the-u-s-population-2010/; 2010. Accessed February 5, 2016.

42. Why Not the Best? Results from the National Scorecard on US Health System Performance, 2011. http://www.commonwealthfund.org/publications/fund-reports/2011/oct/why-not-the-best-2011. The Commonwealth Fund; 2011.

43. Smoldt R, Landman L. *Healthcare Integration: Organizational and Cultural Issues Keynote Session: MGMA Health Systems Forum*; 2014.

44. Gawande A. Overkill. *The New Yorker*. http://www.newyorker.com/magazine/2015/05/11/overkill-atul-gawande; 2015. Accessed November 1, 2016.

45. Newhouse JP, Garber AM, Graham RP et al. *Variations in Health Care Spending*. Washington, DC: National Academies Press; 2013.

46. Gawande A. The cost conundrum. *The New Yorker*. http://www.newyorker.com/magazine/2009/06/01/the-cost-conundrum; 2009. Accessed November 1, 2016.

47. Commonwealth Fund/Modern Healthcare Health Care Opinion Leaders Survey: views on slowing the growth of health care costs. http://www.commonwealthfund.org/interactives-and-data/surveys/2009/april/health-care-opinion-leaders-survey-on-slowing-the-growth-of-health-care-costs. The Commonwealth Fund; 2009.

48. *The 2015 Value Report*. https://www.advocatehealth.com/documents/app/vrweb2015.pdf; 2015. Accessed January 13, 2016.

49. Pizzo J, Grube ME. Getting to there from here: evolving to ACOs through clinical integration programs. http://www.advocatehealth.com/documents/app/ci_to_aco.pdf; 2011. Accessed February 1, 2015.

50. Crosson FJ. Change the microenvironment: delivery system reform essential to controlling costs. http://www.commonwealthfund.org/publications/commentaries/2009/apr/change-the-microenvironment. The Commonwealth Fund; 2009. Accessed December 2, 2015.

51. Illinois Department of Public Health. The burden of asthma in Illinois, 2000–2011; August 2013.

52. Smith CD. Alliance for Academic Internal Medicine–American College of Physicians High Value; Cost-Conscious Care Curriculum Development Committee. Teaching high-value, cost-conscious care to residents: the Alliance for Academic Internal Medicine–American College of Physicians Curriculum. *Ann Intern Med*. 2012;157(4):284–286; 2015.

53. Choosing Wisely: an initiative of the ABIM Foundation. www.choosingwisely.org; 2015.

54. Welcome to The Do No Harm Project. http://www.ucdenver.edu/academics/colleges/medicalschool/departments/medicine/GIM/education/DoNoHarmProject/Pages/Welcome.aspx; 2016. Accessed February 8, 2016.

55. Ventola CL. Direct-to-consumer pharmaceutical advertising: therapeutic or toxic? *PT*. 2011;36(10):669–684.

56. Frosch DL, Grande D, Tarn DM, Kravitz RL. A decade of controversy: balancing policy with evidence in the regulation of prescription drug advertising. *Health Policy and Ethics*. 2010;100(1):9.

57. Riggs KR, Alexander GC. Cost containment and patient well-being. *J Gen Intern Med*. 2015;30(6):701–702.

58. Bates DW, Saria S, Ohno-Machado L, Shah A, Escobar G. Big data in health care: using analytics to identify and manage high-risk and high-cost patients. *Health Aff (Millwood)*. 2014;33(7):1123–1131.

59. Shortell S, McCurdy RK. Integrated health systems. In: Rouse WB, Cortese DA, eds. *Engineering the System of Healthcare Delivery*. Amsterdam: IOS Press BV; 2009:369–382.

60. Shortell S. *Remaking Health Care in America: Building Organized Delivery Systems*. San Francisco: Jossey-Bass; 1996.

61. Feldman L. Impact of providing fee data on laboratory test ordering. *JAMA Intern Med*. 2013;173(10):6.

62. Brook RH. The role of physicians in controlling medical care costs and reducing waste. *JAMA*. 2011;306(6):650–651.

63. Harris RP, Wilt TJ, Qaseem A. High Value Care Task Force of the American College of Physicians. A value framework for cancer screening: advice for high-value care from the American College of Physicians. *Ann Intern Med*. 2015;162(10):712–717.

64. Cassel CK, Guest JA. Choosing Wisely: helping physicians and patients make smart decisions about their care. *JAMA*. 2012;307(17):1801–1802.

65. Bhatia RS, Levinson W, Shortt S, et al. Measuring the effect of Choosing Wisely: an integrated framework to assess campaign impact on low-value care. *BMJ Qual Saf*. 2015;24(8):523–531.

66. Green J, Bell DS, Wenger NS. Stewardship decisions among internal medicine residents: responses to common challenges using vignettes. *Teach Learn Med*. 2013;25(2):141–147.

67. Qaseem A, Alguire P, Dallas P, et al. Appropriate use of screening and diagnostic tests to foster high-value, cost-conscious care. *Ann Intern Med*. 2012;156(2):147–149.

68. Owens DK, Qaseem A, Chou R, Shekelle P. Clinical Guidelines Committee of the American College of Physicians. High-value, cost-conscious health care: concepts for clinicians to evaluate the benefits, harms, and costs of medical interventions. *Ann Intern Med*. Feb 1 2011;154(3):174–180.

69. Moyer VA. U.S. Preventive Services Task Force. Screening for prostate cancer: U.S. Preventive Services Task Force recommendation statement. *Ann Intern Med*. 2012;157(2):120–134.

70. Wilt TJ, Harris RP, Qaseem A. High Value Care Task Force of the American College of Physicians. Screening for cancer: advice for high-value care from the American College of Physicians. *Ann Intern Med*. 2015;162(10):718–725.

71. Segal JB, Streiff MB, Hofmann LV, Thornton K, Bass EB. Management of venous thromboembolism: a systematic review for a practice guideline. *Ann Intern Med*. 2007;146(3):211–222.

72. Nelson RE, Jones M, Liu CF, et al. The impact of healthcare-associated methicillin-resistant *Staphylococcus aureus* infections on post-discharge healthcare costs and utilization. *Infect Control Hosp Epidemiol*. 2015;36(5):534–542.

73. Gabow P, Halvorson G, Kaplan G. Marshaling leadership for high-value health care: an Institute of Medicine discussion paper. *JAMA*. 2012;308(3):239–240.

74. Managing the use of diagnostic imaging. http://www.everettclinic.com/about-us/our-core-values/adding-value-healthcare/managing-use-diagnostic-imaging; 2016. Accessed February 8, 2016.

5

Patient Safety

Luan E. Lawson, MD, MAEd, Jesse M. Ehrenfeld, MD, MPH, and
Danielle Walsh, MD

LEARNING OBJECTIVES

1. Understand the history of the patient safety movement as it has evolved into a priority for high-value care.
2. Understand the classification of medical errors, and analyze the epidemiology of common errors.
3. Understand the elements of full disclosure and apology when dealing with the victims of medical errors.
4. Understand the importance of human factors, systems thinking, Just Culture, and other components that can contribute to improved patient safety.

Patient safety rose to the attention of patients, physicians, payers, and the public after the **Institute of Medicine's (IOM's)** landmark report *To Err is Human: Building a Safer Healthcare System* was released in 1999. Despite significant technological and clinical advances, understanding how to deliver safe care in a complex, rapidly changing environment with tremendous time constraints is one of the greatest challenges in health care today. Too often, errors have been attributed to the mistakes of individuals, instead of focusing on how the health care system can contribute to making health care error prone. This chapter aims to teach the key principles of patient safety and provide foundational learning for health professionals to effectively change the culture and systems in which they care for patients. Understanding the epidemiology and types of errors is essential to investigating solutions. Clinical examples are utilized to demonstrate the types and etiologies of medical errors. This chapter also discusses the importance of error disclosure and care of "second victims," both of which are essential in promoting a **"Just Culture."** Finally, reporting systems and analysis of errors and near misses are described as an opportunity to prevent and correct system failures in a nonpunitive manner. Understanding these concepts will provide health professionals with the requisite knowledge and skills needed to change the future of health care and patient safety.

CHAPTER OUTLINE

I. INTRODUCTION

Patient safety has received increasing focus over the past several decades as the impact of medical errors on health care has drawn increasing attention from the public and medical community. The World Health Organization (WHO) defines patient safety as "the reduction of risk of unnecessary harm associated with health care to an acceptable minimum."[1] Others have described patient safety as "a discipline in the health care sector that applies safety science methods toward the goal of achieving a trustworthy system of health care delivery. Patient safety is also an attribute of health care systems; it minimizes the incidence and impact of, and maximizes recovery from, adverse events."[2] The importance of patient safety came to the forefront of attention in 1999 after the **Institute of Medicine (IOM)** published the landmark report *To Err is Human: Building a Safer Healthcare System,* which estimated that between 44,000 and 98,000 people die each year in US hospitals from medical errors and that over one half of these deaths are preventable.[3] Until this report was released, the inherent high-risk environment of medicine that includes complex patient conditions and required tasks coupled with time and flow pressures was largely unrecognized by the general public. Most importantly, the significant challenges of health care delivery were made transparent to the public in their role as potential patients and advocates for their own health and hastened the systematic evaluation of the problem.

While there is clear evidence that adverse events and medical errors in our health care system are compromising the safety of patients, there remains inconsistency from study to study and ambiguity in terminology as to what constitutes a medical error. This has created significant debate as to the most reliable estimates of errors, near misses, and patient harm. The death estimates reported by the IOM were drawn from over 45,000 discharge records in New York, Colorado, and Utah in the mid-1980s to the early 1990s.[4–6] Another study indicated that 142,000 people die globally each year from medical errors.[7] Using more broad definitions, yet another study suggested that over 400,000 patients die prematurely each year due to preventable medical errors, and patients experience harm 10 to 20 times more frequently than death, making medical errors the third leading cause of death in the United States.[8] Staggering accounts of wrong-site surgeries, missed diagnoses, poor discharge processes, retained surgical sponges, incorrect patient procedures, transfusion and transplant mishaps, and medication errors have been reported. Yet medical errors continue to impact patients and health care providers regularly and represent a leading cause of injury and mortality in the United States. In addition to the impact on patients, families, and health care providers, medical errors and preventable deaths cost approximately $20 billion annually in lost income and health care expenditures.[9] Health care professionals who pursued a career in medicine to help others can find their lives and careers emotionally burdened and potentially derailed by untoward events. Patients and health care professionals alike are united in the call to improve the safety of health care through a non-punitive culture aimed at creating systems less prone to error.

II. BASIC PRINCIPLES OF PATIENT SAFETY

While many patients experience adverse outcomes relative to their underlying medical condition, an **adverse event** is defined as "harm caused by medical treatment," whether it is associated with an error or considered preventable.[4] An **error** is defined as "the failure of a planned action to be completed as intended or the use of a wrong plan to achieve an aim."[10] A **preventable adverse event** is "an adverse event that is attributable to error."[4] Preventable adverse events that satisfy the legal criteria for negligence, where the care provided to the patient did not meet the standard of care an average physician would provide, are known as **negligent adverse events.**[4] A negligent adverse event is one criteria that must be met for **malpractice** (other criteria include demonstration of a doctor-patient relationship, negligence contributed to the injury, and the injury led to specific damages). Moreover, not all errors result in adverse events or harm to the patient. Even **near misses,** in which the unplanned event or close call did not reach the patient or cause an injury or damage to the patient, can impact the patient-provider interaction and serve as valuable learning opportunities to evaluate potential safety risks within the health care system. Historically, the majority of serious, recognized adverse events occurred in hospital-based settings, with the operating room, hospital room, emergency department, intensive care unit, and labor and delivery unit being most commonly involved locations for error, though increasing focus is being shifted to the ambulatory setting.[5]

Understanding patient safety nomenclature is critical to interpreting and applying evidence-based patient safety literature to clinical scenarios. Consider the following patient scenarios to illustrate the subtle differences in patient safety nomenclature. Mr. Jones is a 56-year-old male patient with a history of coronary artery disease who was prescribed daily aspirin to decrease the risk for vascular complications. Unfortunately, Mr. Jones developed a gastrointestinal hemorrhage requiring transfusion, though he did not have a history of peptic ulcer disease. Mr. Jones experienced an **adverse event** as a result of taking aspirin despite receiving standard of care treatment. The gastrointestinal hemorrhage was not considered preventable. If Mr. Jones had a history of remote gastrointestinal bleeding and was prescribed aspirin, this scenario may be described as a **preventable adverse event.** After a thorough risk-to-benefit ratio of the intervention is considered, it may be determined that the potential benefit of the treatment outweighs the risk for side effects. If Mr. Jones had a documented history of anaphylaxis to aspirin and multiple gastrointestinal hemorrhages 2 weeks prior and required a blood transfusion, then prescribing aspirin to this patient could be considered a **negligent adverse event.**

A. Slips, Lapses, Mistakes, and Violations

Another way of looking at errors relates to the level of intent that underlies the action of a physician or other health care professional. Understanding the intent can be useful when trying to understand the nature of an error. One can ask three questions to further understand the nature of an error:
1. Was the action intentional?
2. Did the action occur as planned?
3. Did the action bring about the expected outcome?

A **slip** occurs when an action does not occur as planned. For example, a resident breaks a suture when she is tying it because she pulls too hard on the material. A **lapse** occurs when an action is missed or a person forgets to do something. For example, a nurse forgets to turn on a patient's intermittent pneumatic compression device as indicated to prevent a venous thromboembolism during surgery. A **mistake** occurs when someone does something he or she thought to be correct but was not. For example, a physician writes an electronic order on the wrong patient. A **violation** occurs when a deliberate, illegal, or otherwise unsanctioned action is undertaken.[11] An example would be knowingly skipping a mandatory surgical time out that is both a hospital and **Joint Commission** (accrediting body for health care organizations) requirement.

Not all harms are the result of error. Multiple harms exist in health care related to the underlying condition of a patient, including complications of surgery, postoperative infections, adverse drug reactions, pressure ulcers, or health care–associated infections. Assessing harm in health care is more difficult than in many other industries. Patients frequently present to physicians and other health care professionals in a poor state of health, and it is difficult to separate the impact of an error from the consequences related to the underlying medical condition. Further complicating this separation is that some treatments, such as chemotherapy or radiation, are understood to cause some harm in the process of treating an underlying illness. In a patient-centered approach, providers must weigh the risks and benefits of various testing and treatment options to determine the best approach for each individual patient. Many medical errors may not have immediate obvious negative outcomes, and it may be difficult to attribute the later injury to a specific error.

Despite health care providers' intention to deliver excellent care to every patient, adverse events due to medical errors occur in every hospital on a daily basis. When an error occurs, it is human nature to try and identify "the fall guy," the person who will be individually held responsible for the event. It is tempting to simply say the caregiver most culpable should be fired or reprimanded to prevent further errors. At the same time, health care providers do not come to work intending to do harm. Well-trained, well-meaning professionals still make mistakes and can inadvertently cause patient injury simply because humans are imperfect. In fact, a good mindset is to assume mistakes will be made and go about finding systems and processes to prevent them or minimize their impact. Human errors are frequently a sign that the systems around the person are broken and require further evaluation. In fact, a study of medication errors and near misses found that at least 78 percent of the issues were attributable to system issues, not human errors.[12]

Case Study 1

A patient is discharged from the hospital and goes home with a prescription intended for a different patient. The patient takes the medication, but it cross-reacts with one the patient is already taking and causes an anaphylactic reaction requiring re-admission to the intensive care unit. What happened in this case? Should the physician be reprimanded or fired?

A systems review of this case reveals that an administrator on the floor had called the physician shortly before the event asking that as many patients as possible be discharged right away as there were patients coming out of surgery needing the beds. The physician, who had been up all night with critically ill patients, was trying to discharge three patients simultaneously, but the electronic health record had "gone down." The prescriptions were handwritten instead, and the nurse of one of the patients was helping the physician by putting labels on the prescriptions. The label for an incorrect patient went onto the prescription. Can you identify both the latent and active errors in this case? Do you still think the physician should be reprimanded or fired?

B. Systems Approach to Error

Because defective systems have been identified as the most predominant source of error, health care must adopt a **systems approach** to eliminate preventable errors.[13] A systems approach, focused on improving and redesigning the environment and care processes, provides a comprehensive approach to anticipate and evaluate errors instead of focusing on the behavior of a few individuals. Other industries such as aviation, nuclear power, and the military have made significant improvements in safety, and their containment of errors can serve as a conceptual framework for reducing medical errors. These high-reliability industries emphasize safety by maintaining an environment of collective mindfulness in which all workers identify and report small problems before they pose a significant risk to the organization and result in harm.[14] The traditional health care culture that emphasizes "error-free practice" tends to create an environment that precludes open discussions of error and organizational learning, limiting the ability to improve care.

Dr. James Reason, a British psychologist and leader in the study of accidents and unintended events, described errors as circumstances in which planned actions fail to achieve the desired outcome.[13] He explained that human error can be viewed in either a **persons approach** or **systems approach.** The persons approach focuses on the errors of individuals at the bedside or "sharp end" of the system, such as the physician, nurse, or other caregiver in contact with the patient.[13] The **"sharp end"** refers to any personnel or components of the health care system that directly contact the patient in the provision of care. Such human errors are often attributed to forgetfulness, lack of knowledge, and carelessness. Methods such as poster campaigns, training, and disciplinary measures are utilized to counteract these errors viewed as the responsibility of individuals. In contrast, the **"blunt end"** refers to the many layers of the health care organization removed from direct patient contact, but directly influencing what happens to the patient.[13] Organizational leaders and managers, biomedical engineers, policymakers, and software developers all reside at the "blunt end" away from the patient's bedside. In a **systems approach** to error, one assumes that humans are fallible and human error is likely to occur, even in the best organizations, and that the system of care surrounding the caregivers must be assessed and improved.[15] Using a systems approach, countermeasures to prevent error focus on system defenses, barriers, and safeguards to error.

Reason performed an analysis of errors and determined that most accidents occur as the result of multiple, small errors occurring in an organization with system flaws instead of the singular errors of individuals.[13,15] He went on to describe the **Swiss Cheese model** of system failure (Fig. 5.1) that recognizes error is inevitable, and every step in a process (such as health care delivery) has the potential for failure, with each layer of the system serving as a defensive layer to identify and catch the error before harm reaches the patient.[13] Envision the medical system as a stack of slices of Swiss cheese with the slices representing the system defenses and the holes representing a process failure or system error. In order for harm to reach the patient, the error must pass through holes in multiple defense mechanisms represented by layers of the cheese. Ideally, errors will be prevented through the application of multiple defenses and safeguards (additional layers of cheese) that will function as a safety net to prevent error from reaching the patient.

These holes are the result of both latent and active failures. **Latent failures** (or **latent errors**) occur at the "blunt end" as the result of system or design flaws occurring away from the patient's bedside that allow active errors to occur and result in harm.[13] Latent failures are less obvious than active failures and may include equipment design flaws, decreased staffing for fiscal reasons, and software interface issues. Addressing latent flaws requires an understanding of how the complex system interacts with individuals and may identify flaws in leadership, work environment, or institutional policies as the source of error. **Active failures** (or **active errors**) involve front-line personnel at the "sharp end," and occur as the result of an individual's failure.[13] These types of errors normally occur as the result of mental lapses, errors in judgment, or procedural violations. Examples of active errors include administering the incorrect medication, performing surgery on the wrong site, or ignoring an alarm.

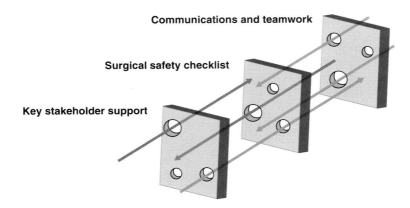

Communications and teamwork

Surgical safety checklist

Key stakeholder support

Latent failures ➡
The organization's information technology does not function.
The pharmacy and the OR do not interface.
The pharmacy does not retrieve medications in time for administration.
A procedure is not in place for changing or verifying gases.
Different types of gases are stored in one holder and location.
Preoperative orders are not formally written.
The RN circulator does not have access to the patient's preoperative order.
The surgical team does not address anticipation of blood loss before the procedure.
The perioperative team does not address the need for special equipment before the procedure.
Members of the nursing team are under pressure to be efficient and quick.
Confirmation of patient identity, procedure, incision site, and informed consent do not occur.
A knowledge deficit potentially exists among members of the surgical team.
Routine verification of patient allergies does not occur.
Regular testing of equipment does not occur.

Active failures ➡
The surgeon performs the surgery on the incorrect limb (i.e., wrong-site surgery).
The surgical team identifies the wrong patient.
A member of the surgical team administers the wrong medication to the patient.
Blood is not available during the procedure when the patient needs it.
A nurse programs a piece of equipment incorrectly during the procedure.
The preoperative RN does not review the surgical schedule.
A team member places the incorrect medical gas on the laparoscopy cart.

Fig. 5.1 The Swiss Cheese model of system failure. (Reproduced with permission from Collins SJ, Newhouse R, Porter J, et al. Effectiveness of the surgical safety checklist in correcting errors: a literature review applying Reason's Swiss cheese model. *AORN J.* 2014;100[1]:65–79.)

Multiple factors can contribute to errors in health care. Reason's Swiss Cheese model of organizational accidents emphasizes that the "root causes" allowing an error to occur should be investigated and identified.[13] Using this as a foundation, Charles Vincent developed a framework for classifying error-prone conditions and organizational factors affecting clinical practice in health care. Contributory factors and influences on safety are divided into seven broad categories including patient factors, task factors, individual factors, team factors, work environment, organization and management factors, and institutional context.[16,17]

Patient factors, such as personality, language, culture, and illness complexity have a direct impact on communication and bias. While the patient's condition has the most direct impact on care, individual patient factors including language, cultural expectations, or psychological factors may impact the way in which the patient interacts with the health care provider. Provider knowledge, skills, experience, and other **individual factors** affect clinical practice and outcomes, especially in stressful conditions requiring high levels of skill. Provider fatigue, stress, or lack of familiarity of procedures can negatively impact the ability to safely perform the procedure and additionally impair the ability to deal with complications. Availability and use of clear protocols and the accessibility of accurate test results are examples of **task factors.** For example, institutions that have protocols where the laboratory technician immediately contacts the physician or nurse with abnormal results are much more likely to address these abnormalities that can lead to increased morbidity and mortality compared to institutions that routinely report these results in the electronic health record without any notification procedures. **Workplace factors** (staffing, physical environment, light, heat, and interruptions) contribute to the provider's ability to carry out a task without being distracted. Heavy workloads without administrative support create a stressful environment that makes communication difficult, limits time at the bedside with patients, and increases the likelihood of an error. Each person is a member of multiple teams contributing to patient care. The respect, mutual support, and communication skills among team members directly

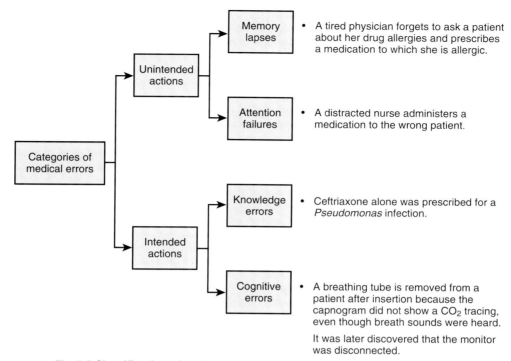

Fig. 5.2 Classification of medical errors and common types of medical errors.

impact the patient and the care provided. It is important to remember that all members of the team, from environmental engineering personnel to leadership executives, are critical team members. Poor communication is most likely to contribute to poor teamwork leading to medical errors, but poor supervision and unwillingness to ask for assistance by less experienced team members have deleterious consequences.

Organizational factors impact care through policies and processes related to leadership, education, supervision, and availability of equipment or supplies. Organizations have the capacity to impact patient safety through engagement by senior management through policy standards and goals that support an organizational safety of culture that is valued above purely financial metrics. External regulatory agencies, medicolegal environment, and financial constraints affect the **institutional context.**

III. SPECIFIC TYPES OF MEDICAL ERRORS

A medical error may be defined as an adverse event in the health care process that was preventable—regardless of whether harm occurred to the patient or patient's family. These errors can occur when physicians and other health care professionals fail to recognize something (often leading to a diagnostic error) or improperly provide care. Common types of medical errors include medication, surgical and diagnostic errors, and errors related to transitions of care, teamwork, and communication. There are a number of classification systems and taxonomies for categorizing medical errors. Fig. 5.2 shows one approach to classification, and Table 5.1 lists examples of common medical errors.

Case Study 2

A 72-year-old veteran with memory loss, diabetes, and hypertension is admitted to the emergency department at his local Veterans Affairs (VA) facility after he developed difficulty breathing, tongue swelling, and facial numbness. He was diagnosed with angiotensin-converting enzyme (ACE) inhibitor angioedema. The patient was stabilized, admitted to the intensive care unit for monitoring, and discharged 48 hours later. Upon discharge, the patient's record was updated to indicate that he had an allergy to ACE inhibitors, and he was prescribed a new antihypertensive medication from a different drug class.

One month later, the patient presented again to the emergency department with signs of angioedema. Upon review, it was determined that the patient had started taking his ACE inhibitor again. The patient was stabilized, admitted for observation, and the internist on call spoke to the patient's wife regarding how this occurred a second time.

The internist discovered that the patient had a local non-VA primary care physician whom he also saw from time to time. After his hospital discharge 1 month earlier, the patient did well until he ran out of his medications. His wife, who is the patient's primary caregiver, called his local doctor to obtain refills. However, the other physician did not have access to the VA records and was unaware that the patient had been recently hospitalized. The local physician refilled all of the patient's medications—including the ACE inhibitor that had been discontinued.

What can be done to prevent this type of error from occurring in the future? How common is it for patients to move among health care systems?

Table 5.1 Examples of Common Medical Errors

Type of Medical Error	Examples
Medication	• A nurse practitioner writes a prescription for 5.0 mg of lisinopril, and the order is misread as 50 mg. • A resident orders Zyban for a patient, not realizing the patient is already taking the drug Wellbutrin—which contains the same active ingredient bupropion. • A pharmacist mistakes a prescription for eribulin for epirubicin (both are drugs used to treat breast cancer).
Surgical	• An elderly patient's left kidney is removed instead of the right kidney. • A surgeon performs a thyroid nodule biopsy on a sedated patient in the intensive care unit. However, it was the wrong patient. • During an emergency laparotomy procedure for a teenager involved in a motor vehicle crash, a surgical towel is left hidden behind the spleen.
Diagnostic	• A 19-year-old patient with abdominal pain, vomiting, and loss of appetite is diagnosed with acute gastroenteritis rather than appendicitis. • A lung nodule on chest radiograph is not recognized by a radiologist. • A 63-year-old woman arrives in the emergency department with shoulder pain and palpitations after lifting a set of heavy boxes. She is diagnosed with a shoulder strain, rather than a myocardial infarction.
Transitions of care	• A 72-year-old woman was re-admitted to a hospital for heart failure 2 weeks after being discharged for treatment of the same condition. Upon reviewing her medication list, the admitting physician discovered the patient's diuretic and ACE inhibitor were not prescribed at discharge. • A 63-year-old man was transferred from a long-term care facility to an emergency department with an acute decline in mental status and shortness of breath. Laboratory analysis revealed that the patient was in acute renal failure. The patient was enrolled in an assisted living facility, and medication reconciliation was completed between a nurse practitioner and a pharmacy technician at a local pharmacy. The patient was restarted on digoxin, a medication stopped by the patient's internist 1 year prior. The patient was subsequently diagnosed with digoxin toxicity.
Teamwork / communication	• A medical intern decides not to wake up her attending physician at 2:00 AM for a patient who has taken a turn for the worse, exposing the patient to unnecessary risk. • A patient is started on a new antihypertensive medication that can increase a patient's potassium level as a side effect. The prescribing physician orders a potassium laboratory test 2 weeks after the medication is started, but forgets to notify the physician assistant who will be seeing the patient in follow-up. One month later, the patient is hospitalized for 3 days with hyperkalemia.

A. Medication Errors

The exponential increase in prescription and over-the-counter drugs has led to a tremendous increase in complexity of prescribing and administering medications. An **adverse drug event,** experienced by at least 5 percent of hospitalized patients, is harm that is experienced by a patient, either from a side effect or as the result of a medication error.[18] It is estimated that over 7000 patients die each year due to preventable medication errors.[19] The costs of medication errors have been estimated to waste over $21 billion annually.[19,20] While many discussions have focused on illegible handwriting as the cause of medication errors, errors can occur in the ordering, transcribing, dispensing, and administration stages.[21] Errors can occur with the prescription or ordering of medications that include the wrong medicine, wrong dose, or failure to consider interactions or contraindications. The wrong medication may be administered either by the pharmacy or a health care provider. In addition, medications may be inappropriately monitored, such as in a patient with mild hepatic insufficiency prescribed glyburide for diabetes in hopes of avoiding insulin injections, or inappropriately taken by the patients themselves.

Medication errors continue to be a surprisingly common and costly source of error across all clinical settings, and were the focus of a 2007 IOM report, *Preventing Medication Errors: Quality Chasm Series.*[20] In this report, authors estimated that 1.5 million preventable adverse drug errors occur in the United States each year, representing $3.5 billion in unnecessary cost to the health care system.[20] To reduce the likelihood of certain types of medication errors, it is recommended to avoid the use of abbreviations or dose designations, which are often misinterpreted.[22] Examples include the abbreviation "µg" for microgram, which is often mistaken as "mg." Instead one should use "mcg." The use of a "naked" decimal point (e.g., .25 mg) can be easily mistaken as 25 mg if the decimal point is not recognized. Instead, one should always write a zero before a decimal point (0.25 mg). Finally, drug abbreviations such as "HCTZ 50 mg" for hydrochlorothiazide can be mistaken as hydrocortisone by someone who reads "HCT250 mg." The Joint Commission has developed a "Do Not Use" list of problematic abbreviations (Table 5.2)[22]

In addition, there are specific medications that are referred to as *high-alert* or *high-hazard* agents because they are thought to be the most likely to cause harm to patients, even when used as directed. The Institute for Safe Medication Practices has published a list of high-alert medications, with insulin, opioids, potassium chloride, albuterol, heparin, vancomycin, cefazolin, acetaminophen, warfarin, and furosemide being the some of the most common drugs associated with medical errors.[23] Special consideration should be given to implementing safeguards to reduce risks and minimize harm when using these medications. These strategies may include mandatory patient education, improving access to drug information, using automated alerts, standardizing prescribing practices, implementing bar code and administration, and standardizing prescribing, dispensing, and administration practices. Geriatric patients are particularly predisposed to adverse drug effects, with the most common drugs causing harm being heparin, insulin, morphine, potassium chloride, and warfarin.[24] Finally, it should be noted that all forms of insulin, subcutaneous and IV, are considered a class of high-alert medications and insulin U-500 (a highly concentrated form of insulin) has been singled out for special emphasis to bring attention to the

Table 5.2　The Joint Commission's "Do Not Use" List

Do Not Use	Potential Problem	Recommended
U, u (unit)	Mistaken for "0" (zero), the number "4" (four), or "cc"	Write "unit"
IU (International Unit)	Mistaken for IV (intravenous) or the number "10" (ten)	Write "International Unit"
Q.D., QD, q.d., qd (daily) Q.O.D., QOD, q.o.d, qod (every other day)	Mistaken for each other Period after the Q mistaken for "I" and the "O" mistaken for "I"	Write "daily" Write "every other day"
Trailing zero (X.0 mg) Lack of leading zero (.X mg)	Decimal point is missed	Write "X mg" Write "0.X mg"
MS MSO_4 and $MgSO_4$	Can mean morphine sulfate or magnesium sulfate Mistaken for each other	Write "morphine sulfate" Write "magnesium sulfate"

From The Joint Commission. *Facts about the official "do not use" list of abbreviations.* http://www.jointcommission.org/facts_about_do_not_use_list/. Accessed July 15, 2015.

need for distinct strategies to prevent the types of errors that occur with this concentrated form of insulin.

B.　Surgical Errors

The risk for errors associated with surgery is somewhat unique. The perceived sense of urgency in the operating room environment, use of interchangeable teams, and pressure to complete procedures on time bring together a variety of environmental and systems factors that can promote errors.[25] Successful procedures require a mixture of technical skills, good communication among teams, and adequate decision-making. **"Wrong surgery"** (meaning the procedure was performed on the wrong patient or on the wrong site, or the wrong surgery was undertaken) is surprisingly common, despite national efforts to eliminate this problem. Other problems include retained objects (e.g., surgical sponges or instruments) and failure to take appropriate precautions to prevent surgical site infections using established guidelines for care (e.g., giving antibiotics prior to surgical incision). While many factors contribute to surgical errors, a number of studies have identified risk factors. One such study found that the leading system factors were inexperience/lack of technical competence (41 percent), and communication breakdown (24 percent).[26] The same study reported that cases with technical errors (54 percent) were more likely than those without technical errors to involve safety challenges in multiple phases of care, multiple personnel, lack of technical competence/knowledge, and patient-related factors.[26]

C.　Diagnostic Errors

Despite advances in imaging and laboratory evaluation, diagnostic errors have remained common despite efforts to improve patient safety. **Diagnostic error** is defined as: "the failure to (a) establish an accurate and timely explanation of the patient's health problem(s) or (b) communicate that explanation to the patient."[27] It is estimated that 5 percent of patients receiving outpatient care in the United States will experience a diagnostic error, and postmortem examination research suggests that diagnostic errors contribute to 10 percent of patient deaths.[27] Diagnostic errors have been reported to account for 17 percent of preventable errors, and represent the most common reason for a paid malpractice claim in the ambulatory setting.[5,6,28]

According to the 2015 comprehensive IOM report, *Improving Diagnosis in Healthcare,* diagnostic errors will affect nearly every person at some point during his or her life and require increased attention as a major cause of significant morbidity and mortality.[27] Increasing emphasis has been placed on overdiagnosis, overtesting, and overtreatment as newer and more sensitive diagnostic modalities become available. Diagnosis and treatment of clinically insignificant diseases exposes patients to unnecessary morbidity and mortality. Many times, communication and teamwork errors are major contributors to surgical and diagnostic errors, and have increasingly been recognized as critical to the prevention of safety errors. The recent IOM report, *Improving Diagnosis in Healthcare,* outlined eight goals for reducing diagnostic errors.[27] These include the following:

1. Facilitate more effective teamwork in the diagnostic process among health care professionals, patients, and their families.
2. Enhance health care professional education and training in the diagnostic process.
3. Ensure that health information technologies (IT) support patients and health care professionals in the diagnostic process.
4. Develop and deploy approaches to identify, learn from, and reduce diagnostic errors and near misses in clinical practice.
5. Establish a work system and culture that supports the diagnostic process and improvements in diagnostic performance.
6. Develop a reporting environment and medical liability system that facilitates improved diagnosis through learning from diagnostic errors and near misses.
7. Design a payment and care delivery environment that supports the diagnostic process.
8. Provide dedicated funding for research on the diagnostic process and diagnostic errors.
9. Implementation of these core goals would not only reduce diagnostic errors, but also many other medical errors and go a long way toward improving patient safety.

D.　Transitions of Care Errors

Transitions of care, times when patients are moved from one setting of care or practitioner to another, are high-risk times for errors to occur (discussed in Chapter 3). Whether this involves a physical movement of a patient (e.g., from the intensive care unit to the floor) or a handover of responsibility from one team or practitioner to another, a transition point is a time when information about a patient can be lost, misinterpreted, or misconstrued. Many of the challenges around ensuring successful transitions of care are representative of the fact that traditionally our health systems have not been designed for high reliability. To ensure that information is not lost, experts recommend the use of a structured handoff tool or checklist. This can prevent failure to mention a pending study when signing out a patient or not passing along a key piece of information.

Adapted from I-PASS Handoff Curriculum Materials (http://www.ipasshandoffstudy.com), best practices to ensure a high-quality handoff include the following[29]:

1. Unambiguously transfer both information and responsibility.
2. Identify a protected time and space to initiate the handoff.
3. Use a standardized format or a shared mental model.
4. Ensure that patient information is up-to-date, accurate, and relevant.
5. Establish clear roles during the handoff.
6. Use closed-loop communication to ensure receipt and understanding of knowledge.

E. Teamwork/Communication Errors

As health care has become increasingly complex, effective teamwork and communication is becoming even more essential for the delivery of safe, high-quality health care. Communication errors have been identified as the root cause of almost 70 percent of all reported sentinel events, with 75 percent of these resulting in a patient death.[30] Medicine has traditionally functioned in a rigid hierarchical system, but increasing attention has been placed on improving teamwork that values the contributions and input from all team members. Multiple obstacles can contribute to ineffective team performance including changing team membership, time pressures, varying communication styles, fatigue, inadequate information sharing, lack of role clarity, and intensity and volume of workload.

It has been increasingly recognized that many of these challenges were shared by the aviation industry and subsequently overcome by crew resource management where emphasis was placed on decreasing the **authority gradient,** a term used to describe the psychological distance between a worker and a supervisor.[31] Effective communication is complete, clear, concise, and timely. **Situational awareness** of the changing clinical status or environment enables adaptation to the emerging situation and maintenance of a shared mental model, allowing team members to work toward the same goal. Programs such as TeamSTEPPS developed by the Department of Defense utilize standardized communication behaviors such as briefings, debriefings, checklists, and critical language to create a culture that encourages all members of the team to speak up in the interest of patient safety.[32] Manufacturers, such as Toyota, have employed a process in which all workers can stop the manufacturing line to immediately fix a problem and prevent an error.[33] In this process, each individual worker is empowered to pull the "Andon cord" to notify management of a quality concern through incorporation of signal lights to detect where the problem has

occurred. Health care settings have begun to employ this "stop the line" strategy to encourage all health care workers, from administrative staff such as housekeeping and food services to clinical staff such as nurses and doctors, to alert the team to the patient safety concern before any harm is incurred by the patient.

IV. FACTORS RELATED TO HEALTH PROFESSIONALS

While we can readily evaluate systems and processes for opportunities to improve safety, there remain human components to errors that are more difficult to evaluate and address. The study of this human component and how decisions are made is termed **cognitive science.** Classifying these errors into categories, including inadequate medical knowledge, incomplete data collection, and poor decision-making, can help identify areas for future improvement (Table 5.3).[34]

Every patient is unique, requiring decisions to consider that uniqueness. When patients present to the emergency department, they are assessed or triaged based on a constellation of questions, their initial appearance, and just a few key pieces of information. In addition to the caregiver needing a solid foundation of medical knowledge, the process by which they interpret this information and make a decision about urgency and severity is equally important. To make these judgments, people use a set of constructs known as **heuristics** and **biases.** A **heuristic** is a pattern, or "rule of thumb," that we use to approach a problem. A **bias** is a tendency to think one way or have a "gut feeling" about a situation, and it originates in your unconscious. Both can be helpful or harmful in certain circumstances.

Intuition is a key skill for predicting when a patient is critically ill or what complication may occur, especially when time is of the essence. We gain this intuition through pattern recognition. With increased exposures, we create memories of how certain diseases progress in most patients. When similar patients or problems are encountered in the future, we subconsciously begin to match the old experiences with the new and apply what we have seen to the present. On a positive note, these biases and heuristics allow us to quickly make decisions. While largely effective, they can also cause us to fail through the use of an incorrect decision tree. We may discount information about the patient that did not fit our expected pattern or persist in treating along a standardized pathway, even when the patient is not responding, because similar patients in the past did improve. Cognitive scientists have identified a number of biases that guide how we make decisions. Understanding and recognizing them in our daily decision-making allows us to overcome the potential for bias to result in patient harm. Common biases impacting health care providers include the following:

1. **Availability bias:** Overestimating the probability of something that is relatively easy to recall. Judging the likeliness of an event by how readily we recall it, not by careful assessment of all data.
2. **Confirmation bias:** Selective gathering and interpretation of evidence confirming a diagnosis while ignoring contrary information. Tendency to seek out information that affirms our choice and discount information that is contradictory.

Table 5.3 Examples of Cognitive Contributions to Errors

Category	Type	Definition	Example
Faulty knowledge	Knowledge base inadequate or defective	Insufficient knowledge of the relevant condition	Providers not aware of Fournier gangrene
	Diagnostic skills inadequate or defective	Insufficient diagnostic skill	Missed diagnosis due to misread electrocardiogram (ECG)
	Therapeutic skills inadequate or defective	Insufficient therapeutic skill	Patient suffers adverse event because not warned of potential side effects
Faulty data gathering	Ineffective, incomplete, or faulty workup, history, or physical examination	Problems in collecting, organizing, or coordinating patient's interview, examination, tests, and consultations	Delayed diagnosis of drug-related lupus; failure to consult the patient's old medical records
	Faulty test or procedure techniques	Standard test/procedure is conducted incorrectly	ECG leads reversal prompts wrong diagnosis of myocardial infarction
	Failure to screen	Failure to perform indicated screening	Missed colon cancer due to failure to obtain a colonoscopy
Faulty synthesis information processing or verification	Faulty context generation	Lack of awareness/consideration of aspects of patient's situation relevant to diagnosis	Missed perforated ulcer in a patient presenting with chest pain and laboratory evidence of myocardial infarction
	Failure to order or follow up on appropriate test	Lack of appropriate testing to confirm a diagnosis or action based on the result	No further imaging after a chest radiograph first reveals a small nodule
	Failed heuristics or "rules of thumb"	Appropriate rule of thumb not applied or overapplied under inappropriate circumstances	Diagnosis of bronchitis in a patient later found to have a pulmonary embolism
	Faulty interpretation of a test result	Test results are read correctly, but incorrect conclusions are drawn	Missed diagnosis of *Clostridium difficile* in a patient with a negative stool culture

3. **Omission bias:** Reluctance or avoidance of taking action out of fear of being held responsible for the outcome.
4. **Commission bias:** Tendency toward action rather than inaction.
5. **Hindsight bias:** Believing we accurately predicted the outcome of an event, when the correct outcome is known, reducing our ability to learn from the past.
6. **Regret bias:** Overestimating the probability of a diagnosis with severe possible consequences because of anticipated regret if the diagnosis were missed.
7. **Recency bias:** Accessing recent information more readily than older information, even if the older information is more relevant.
8. **Anchoring bias:** Making a decision based on initial start points or impressions and failing to change despite further information.
9. **Aggregate bias:** Believing this scenario is unusual or atypical, leading a physician or other health care professional to ignore guidelines.
10. **Search-satisfying error:** Discontinuing a search for an answer when coming across a finding.
11. **Sunk–cost-effect/bias:** So much has been invested in a decision that a physician or other health care professional persists with it.

Human errors can also occur because of physical errors. Undoubtedly, our patients expect that we arrive to work each day awake, alert, and focused on their needs. Yet the realities of human life mean we may be stressed, ill, fatigued, and less focused than we could be. When the need to provide 24-hour care and make rapid decisions in which another person's life is at stake is added in, the risk for patient errors becomes more likely. In response to such concerns, the Accreditation Council for Graduate Medical Education (ACGME) has restricted work hours for resident physicians and trainees.

However, practicing physicians are expected to self-assess levels of fatigue, weighing the risk of their own fatigue that could result in an error against the risk of transitioning care to different providers who may not know the patient. First instituted in 2003, resident duty hour restrictions have undergone a series of changes based on research and outcomes evaluations to strike a balance among the sometimes competing forces of continuity of patient care, education, and patient safety.[35]

While other high-stakes industries, such as the aviation industry, have legislated work and wellness policies, health care has not done so for a number of reasons. Individual skill sets and specialties can be scarce resources, meaning that there may not always be another physician to whom a fatigued physician can transition care of a particular patient. For example, a newborn infant is born with a severe congenital birth defect and rapidly becomes unstable, and evaluation suggests that they will only survive with emergency surgery to address the defect. The institution only has one pediatric surgeon trained to correct this defect, but they have just finished operating for nearly 30 hours without rest. The risks of transferring a patient to a different hospital or to a less specialized caregiver must be weighed against delaying care or provision of care by a fatigued physician at risk of making a human error.

Perhaps the greatest human error contributing to patient harm is failure to communicate with the patient, the family, and other professionals involved in the patient's care. The Joint Commission asks all member institutions to thoroughly evaluate unanticipated events resulting in death or serious injury to a patient and report their findings. A review of these sentinel events shows that communication errors are the most common error, playing a role in more than 60 percent of events.[30] Not only does poor communication contribute to adverse events, good communication results in lower patient

Surgical safety checklist

Before induction of anesthesia
(with at least nurse and anesthetist)

Has the patient confirmed his/her identity, site, procedure, and consent?
☐ Yes

Is the site marked?
☐ Yes
☐ Not applicable

Is the anesthesia machine and medication check complete?
☐ Yes

Is the pulse oximeter on the patient and functioning?
☐ Yes

Does the patient have a:
Known allergy?
☐ No
☐ Yes

Difficult airway or aspiration risk?
☐ No
☐ Yes

Risk of >550 mL blood loss (7 mL/kg in children)?
☐ No
☐ Yes, and two IVs/central access and fluids planned

→

Before skin incision
(with nurse, anesthetist, and surgeon)

☐ **Confirm all team members have introduced themselves by name and role.**

☐ **Confirm the patient's name, procedure, and where the incision will be made.**

Has antibiotic prophylaxis been given within the last 60 minutes?
☐ Yes
☐ Not applicable

Anticipated critical events

To surgeon:
☐ What are the critical or non-routine steps?
☐ How long will the case take?
☐ What is the anticipated blood loss?

To anesthetist:
☐ Are there any patient-specific concerns?

To nursing team:
☐ Has sterility (including indicator results) been confirmed?
☐ Are there equipment issues or any concerns?

Is essential imaging displayed?
☐ Yes
☐ Not applicable

→

Before patient leaves operating room
(with nurse, anesthetist, and surgeon)

Nurse verbally confirms:
☐ The name of the procedure
☐ Completion of instrument, sponge, and needle counts
☐ Specimen labeling (read specimen labels aloud, including patient name)
☐ Whether there are any equipment problems to be addressed

To surgeon, anesthetist, and nurse:
☐ What are the concerns for recovery and management of the patient?

This checklist is not intended to be comprehensive. Additions and modifications to fit local practice are encouraged.

Fig. 5.3 **WHO surgical safety checklist.**[39] (Reprinted with permission from the World Health Organization. http://apps.who.int/iris/bitstream/10665/44186/2/9789241598590_eng_Checklist.pdf.)

morbidity and mortality.[36] Communication failures in medicine are often linked to the hierarchical nature of the health care environment. The physician has traditionally been positioned at the pinnacle of the hierarchy, with the communication divide between them and the nurses and other staff being quite wide. While it remains necessary to have a leader of a team, the team will function more effectively if its members are not afraid to speak out and warn of a potential risk to the patient. The term **flattening the hierarchy** refers to creating an environment in which all members of the team feel safe in providing input, are valued for speaking up, and are not deprecated for doing so.[37] By permitting free flow of information up and down the leadership chain, many potential adverse events can be thwarted.

Communication can be enhanced by the use of structured conversations at critical junctures in care. Many medical centers use a tool called **SBAR** for communication during transitions of care and critical events.[38] SBAR stands for Situation, Background, Assessment, and Recommendation. The speaker first describes the current situation—*Mr. Saunders has developed sudden onset of shortness of breath.* Additional details are then provided. The second component is the background pertinent to the current situation—*He has a history of COPD and CHF. Yesterday he underwent emergency surgery for a blood clot in his leg.*

He had bleeding resulting in his anticoagulation medication being held. The key information needed to put the current situation into context is provided. This is followed by an assessment—*I am concerned he is having a pulmonary embolus. He may also be in congestive heart failure from all the fluid given during surgery.* The final component is the recommendation—*Please come assess the patient. I can call for a chest radiograph in the meantime.* This standard format allows for clear and concise information to be transmitted under what may be a stressful situation.

The surgical "time out" is another example of structured communication. In 2008, the WHO published a free checklist with just 19 items to be reviewed at the preoperative, intraoperative, and postoperative stages of a surgical procedure to reduce the number of surgical complications occurring around the world (Fig. 5.3).[39] With over 234 million operations occurring annually around the world and an estimated one half million deaths from these operations deemed to be preventable, the "Safe Surgery Saves Lives" multinational endeavor sought to improve both morbidity and mortality from preventable human errors.[40] In the first major study looking at patient safety before and after implementation of the checklist, major complications were decreased on average by 36 percent, deaths by 47 percent, and infections by about the same.[41] The unexpectedly impressive results led some critics to argue that the results were too good to be true. However, a meta-analysis of studies employing the WHO checklist has confirmed their findings, showing a marked decrease in surgical complications (risk ratio 0.59), particularly in studies in which compliance with the checklist was high.[42] It is not often that a free tool that takes less than 2 minutes to apply to a patient can save millions of lives. Yet there remains some reluctance among physicians and nurses regarding checklist implementation. In one study, despite the expectation of 100 percent utilization of the checklist, it was incompletely used in 60 percent of surgeries and not utilized at all in 10 percent.[43] This emphasizes the importance of changing both the individual and organizational culture to implement patient safety methodologies, even when the technology to do so is provided at no cost.

Structured forms of communication and pathways for patient care can be very effective for decreasing risk, but humans can occasionally be remarkably adept at adapting and then circumventing these processes. When providers repeatedly use a shortcut that deviates from a protocol, accept lower standards due to time or resource constraints, or conform to a different level of expectation, a new normal is created. This deviation from standards and policy on a recurrent basis without resistance is referred to as **normalization of deviance.** For example, a patient monitor sounds an alarm 10 times in 1 hour, and the nurse notes each time it is a false alert requiring the alarm to be silenced. The eleventh time, the alarm is silenced without looking at the screen. This is a normalization of deviance, which could put the patient at grave risk if the eleventh alarm was detecting an arrhythmia. The nurse has fallen prey to bias. A more appropriate response would be to review the screen for the eleventh time, followed by an investigation into how the monitor settings or patient leads might be adjusted to cease triggering the false alarm. The probability of an adverse event arising from normalization of deviance is inevitable unless the culture of the institution values addressing problems in real time.

Although it is clear that many system and human factors contribute to medical errors, there remains a need for both individuals and institutions to be held responsible for safety. A fine line exists between holding individuals accountable for errors and blaming the system for all adverse events. In his description of "Just Culture," James Reason distinguishes between inadvertent human error and egregious disregard of safety.[13] A **Just Culture** is one in which every employee advocates for an environment where safety concerns can be addressed in a nonpunitive manner with willingness to address underlying causes. Individuals who provide unacceptable or negligent care resulting in harm should be held responsible for their actions. However, institutions embracing a Just Culture will thoroughly evaluate the circumstances and mitigating factors surrounding the event with an eye toward improvement before blaming individuals.[44]

V. COMMUNICATING WITH PATIENTS AFTER ADVERSE EVENTS DUE TO MEDICAL ERRORS

Medical errors can be devastating for the affected patients, families, caregivers, and organizations, but each of these stakeholders has a very different perspective. While many patients experience physical trauma after a medical error, the emotional trauma for the patients and family members can be decreased by respectful, empathetic communication with the health care provider.[45] Patients and their families are fearful of further harm and need information about the injury incurred and future health care needs. Patients experiencing open communication and support from physicians and other health care professionals are more likely to continue the patient-provider relationship after experiencing a medical error.[46] Patients and families are more likely to pursue litigation if they feel the provider was not caring and compassionate.[46] Failure to disclose a medical error to a patient and his or her family results in frustration, anger, and suspicion that erodes the patient-physician relationship and hinders further medical care, leaving the patient not only injured from the adverse event, but potentially secondarily injured from avoidance and fear of further treatment. In addition, patients may be forced to pursue litigation to deal with the financial impact of an injury.

Due to embarrassment, fear of punitive action, and concerns of loss of professional respect, physicians and other health care professionals frequently withdraw after an error occurs.[47,48] Traditional medical culture that emphasizes "error-free practice" tends to create an environment that precludes open discussion of errors and organizational learning.[49] The lack of transparency between patients and physicians erodes the therapeutic relationship, leading to dissatisfaction for both patients and physicians.[50] Physicians and other health care professionals experience a significant amount of guilt in response to medical errors, but the majority have little experience with open disclosure of errors. Without the opportunity to disclose the error and re-establish an honest therapeutic relationship, health care providers may develop deleterious methods of coping or even choose to leave medicine after being involved in a medical error. Patients want to be assured that their providers are truly sorry for the error and want to understand how providers will ensure that other patients will not experience a similar outcome. In addition, experiences from the University of Michigan Health System and Veterans Affairs suggest that malpractice claims may be reduced through early disclosure.[50–52] Both patients and physicians require resources to deal with the emotional stress precipitated by medical errors.

When a patient has been harmed, health care professionals, in consultation with the health system's department of quality, should approach the situation with transparency and provide honest communication to patients and families. Full disclosure of a medical error includes: 1) providing an explanation of why the error occurred; 2) an apology; 3) an explanation of how the health impact will be minimized, including an explanation of how this will impact their future care; and 4) a discussion regarding actions that will be taken to minimize the chance for future recurrence to other patients.[53,54] The patient should receive a straightforward account of how the error occurred without placing blame or making accusations. The physician and other members of the care team should acknowledge and take responsibility for their roles in the error when appropriate. It is impossible to predict how all patients will respond to full disclosure and apology following an adverse event resulting in significant harm. Patients report feeling a mixture of emotions including sorrow, anxiety, depression, and frustration at the prospect that the error was preventable, but they are more likely to accept an apology when it is offered with expressions of remorse, sincerity, and a willingness to discuss the next steps in treatment.[53] While these expressions will be uncomfortable for those involved and perhaps difficult to hear, it is essential to remain attentive, listen actively, and demonstrate understanding, concern, and empathy for the patient's self-interests. These actions will help achieve the goal of rebuilding confidence in the health care providers and begin the healing process. Many patients will be grateful for the transparent and honest nature of full disclosure accompanied by a sincere apology. Many patients appreciate the opportunity to voice their concerns and feel empowered by offering solutions to prevent the error recurrence.

Open error disclosure is an essential component of improving patient safety through organizational learning while simultaneously supporting the healing process. Communication with the patient and his or her family should be open and occur regularly following error disclosure. The initial disclosure may be overwhelming for patients, but will inevitably lead to additional questions after they have time to process the information. Many institutions have patient-provider liaisons who provide a consistent relationship and communication schedule among the family, the providers, and the organization. Most importantly, health care providers should continue to provide treatment and avoid withdrawing from the patient due to embarrassment or guilt.

VI. SECOND VICTIMS

Health care providers are nearly universally impacted by involvement in an adverse event, even if they were not primarily responsible, making them the **second victims** of an adverse event or medical error. The emotional effect from adverse events affects the entire organization and requires skillful management with compassion and empathy. An organization that effectively supports second victims will facilitate honest discussion with health care providers as they describe their involvement in adverse events. Shame, humiliation, and fear of punishment often isolate providers after they are involved in a poor outcome, especially if they are viewed by their colleagues as being primarily responsible for the error. Organizational support of front-line providers through formal procedures to support second victims involved in the adverse event is essential.[55,56] Institutional openness and discussion of error and training in disclosure can help providers navigate difficult situations. Support services, including psychological counseling and peer support, are important in providing clinicians with effective coping strategies and cautions against maladaptive mechanisms.

VII. REPORTING SYSTEMS

Error reporting systems are an important part of improving health care practice. They can be either voluntary or mandatory, and each has a distinct set of advantages and disadvantages. **Voluntary reporting systems** often receive error reports from providers who are directly involved in the event, as opposed to **mandatory reporting systems,** which typically receive error reports from a designated person who often is not directly involved in the error. When a report is generated from a person who has only secondhand knowledge of an event, important details necessary for an event analysis may be omitted.[57] Voluntary reporting systems are ubiquitous across health care systems and commonly implemented using a Web-based secure data-collection process. Mandatory reporting systems include both federal and state

efforts. The United States Food and Drug Administration (FDA) medical device error reporting system requires hospitals and surgical facilities to submit reports to the FDA of suspected medical device–related deaths or serious injuries. Additionally, as of 2014, 26 states plus the District of Columbia have mandatory reporting systems for events that lead to a patient death or serious injury.

Reporting systems are most effective when they are perceived as neutral and designed to facilitate the improvement of patient safety. Voluntary systems are often perceived as more credible, and providers often place a higher level of trust on how information that is submitted will be used. This is in contrast to many mandatory reporting systems, in which there is often a sense among practitioners that blame is likely to be assigned when an event is submitted. Mandatory reporting is typically required for serious events (see Table 5.3) including death, retained foreign object after surgery, radiation overdose, or transfusion error.[58,59] Initially these events were coined **Never Events** that focused on shocking, largely preventable actions such as wrong site surgery or retained sponges that should never occur. Eventually, the National Quality Forum has expanded this Serious Reportable Events list to include serious and usually (but not always) preventable events divided into six categories: surgical, product or device, patient protection, care management, environmental, and criminal. According to Joint Commission standards, a **sentinel event** is a patient safety event that reaches a patient and results in death, permanent harm, or severe temporary harm (Table 5.4).[60] These events are deemed sentinel events because they signal the need for immediate investigation and system improvement to protect the patient and prevent further harm. While the Joint Commission does not require reporting of sentinel events, reporting is strongly encouraged to provide expertise during the event review and contribute to a transparent safety culture.

The success of reporting systems is almost entirely dependent on the ability of the system to facilitate process improvement and error identification. Additionally, since 2008 the federal government through the Centers for Medicare and Medicaid Services (CMS) has stopped paying for the extra costs associated with a growing list of serious preventable errors, and a growing list of payers have adopted similar payment policies. In coming years, both physician and hospital payments will be linked to quality and safety metrics established by the CMS and other payers. Many errors have been identified and corrected as a result of reporting systems, including errors that originate outside of the direct care environment such as medical device problems and drug manufacturing errors.

VIII. RISK ASSESSMENT AND MITIGATION

The prevention of medical errors and adverse events can be approached with a variety of strategies. One important concept is that of risk assessment and mitigation. Risk management can be thought of as occurring in a continuous cycle beginning with assessment of risk, system evaluation, management or mitigation of the identified risks, and then assessment of the impact of the interventions (Fig. 5.4). Assessment of risk begins with an objective evaluation that considers the probability that an event will occur, as well as the potential impact of a given event. The approach to prevention of a rare, but catastrophic event (e.g., a large earthquake or performing surgery on the wrong patient) is often different from the approach to managing a common, but less devastating error (e.g., not following up on routine laboratory tests or administering a medication orally instead of intravenously).

In assessing risk, it is important to consider the many factors that influence our health systems. These include the work environment, team and individual factors, and characteristics specific to a given patient. Using this type of framework, one can consider a systematic approach to risk assessment and ultimately the development of mitigation strategies that can include the adoption of policies or protocols, addition of training requirements, or putting into practice other safety initiatives such as the implementation of checklists or customized electronic reminder systems. To be effective, however, these strategies should be informed by a thorough understanding of the system to which they are being applied and the specific risk(s) they are designed to alter.[15]

IX. EVALUATION OF NEAR MISSES AND ERRORS

Evaluation of near misses and errors is an important part of improving the care delivery process and ensuring ongoing patient safety. The IOM report, *Patient Safety—Achieving a New Standard of Care* describes many of the aspects of event analysis, and many resources have been developed to facilitate the evaluation process.[61] Table 5.5 outlines the key steps of an event analysis.

The overall goal of an event analysis is to understand the underlying causes that led to a particular event. Once commonly referred to as a **root cause analysis,** most experts in the field now refer to these activities as an **event analysis,** rather than a root cause analysis because of the recognition that many events have more than one underlying cause.

Tools commonly used in an event analysis include process mapping, a cause-and-effect diagram (also called a *fishbone* or *Ishikawa diagram*), and key driver diagrams. Each facilitates an understanding of the various factors that contributed to a given event. A **process map** is a visual representation of a process showing how a sequence of events leads to a given outcome. Created on paper, electronically, or even using sticky notes, a process map can be used to identify the current state of a process—a key step in selecting changes or identifying areas for improvement. A cause-and-effect diagram shows the specific causes of an event, often categorized into groups such as people, processes, equipment, and environmental factors. A cause-and-effect diagram is powerful because it can reveal key relationships among a number of variables impacting a process. Finally, a key driver diagram shows the relationship among the aim of a process, the primary drivers that contribute to the aim, and the secondary drivers that impact the process but are necessary for the primary drivers.

A key point in the evaluation of near misses and errors that cannot be overstated is that the intent is to identify solutions to problems without assigning blame to particular individuals. Although human factors play an important

Table 5.4 The National Quality Forum's Health Care Serious Reportable Events (2011 Revision)

Surgical Events

Surgery or other invasive procedure performed on the wrong body part
Surgery or other invasive procedure performed on the wrong patient
Wrong surgical or other invasive procedure performed on a patient
Unintended retention of a foreign object in a patient after surgery or other procedure
Intraoperative or immediate postoperative/postprocedure death in an American Society of Anesthesiologists Class I patient

Product or Device Events

Patient death or serious injury associated with the use of contaminated drugs, devices, or biologics provided by the health care setting
Patient death or serious injury associated with the use or function of a device in patient care, in which the device is used for functions other than as intended
Patient death or serious injury associated with intravascular air embolism that occurs while being cared for in a health care setting

Patient Protection Events

Discharge or release of a patient/resident of any age, who is unable to make decisions, to other than an authorized person
Patient death or serious disability associated with patient elopement (disappearance)
Patient suicide, attempted suicide, or self-harm resulting in serious disability, while being cared for in a health care facility

Care Management Events

Patient death or serious injury associated with a medication error (e.g., errors involving the wrong drug, wrong dose, wrong patient, wrong time, wrong rate, wrong preparation, or wrong route of administration)
Patient death or serious injury associated with unsafe administration of blood products
Maternal death or serious injury associated with labor or delivery in a low-risk pregnancy while being cared for in a health care setting
Death or serious injury of a neonate associated with labor or delivery in a low-risk pregnancy
Artificial insemination with the wrong donor sperm or wrong egg
Patient death or serious injury associated with a fall while being cared for in a health care setting
Any stage 3, stage 4, or unstageable pressure ulcers acquired after admission/presentation to a health care facility
Patient death or serious disability resulting from the irretrievable loss of an irreplaceable biological specimen
Patient death or serious injury resulting from failure to follow up or communicate laboratory, pathology, or radiology test results

Environmental Events

Patient or staff death or serious disability associated with an electric shock in the course of a patient care process in a health care setting
Any incident in which a line designated for oxygen or other gas to be delivered to a patient contains no gas, the wrong gas, or is contaminated by toxic substances
Patient or staff death or serious injury associated with a burn incurred from any source in the course of a patient care process in a health care setting
Patient death or serious injury associated with the use of restraints or bedrails while being cared for in a health care setting
Radiological events
Death or serious injury of a patient or staff associated with introduction of a metallic object into the MRI area

Criminal Events

Any instance of care ordered by or provided by someone impersonating a physician, nurse, pharmacist, or other licensed health care provider
Abduction of a patient/resident of any age
Sexual abuse/assault on a patient within or on the grounds of a health care setting
Death or significant injury of a patient or staff member resulting from a physical assault (i.e., battery) that occurs within or on the grounds of a health care setting

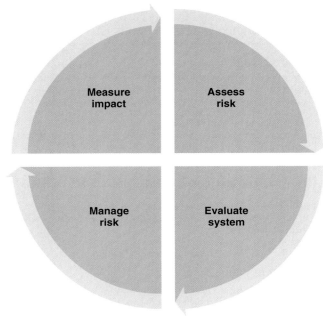

Fig. 5.4 **The cycle of risk management.**

Table 5.5 The Steps of an Event Analysis

Step 1: Awareness of the event	All health care workers must be empowered to recognize and report an event or a near miss. Additionally, systems should be implemented to enable routine analysis of significant events.
Step 2: Information gathering	Collect as much factual information as possible. Sources should include the medical record and interviews with staff involved in the incident.
Step 3: Facilitated team meeting	An effective team meeting will include a detailed discussion of the event, respecting the opinions of all present and avoiding the assignment of blame.
Step 4: Analyze the event	Answer these four fundamental questions: • What happened? • Why did it happen? • What have we learned from this event? • What should we change moving forward?
Step 5: Implement a change	Depending on the event analysis, it may be decided that no action is needed. However, often there are gaps in processes identified that are amenable to change. These changes should be implemented by a designated person and their implementation monitored.
Step 6: Report out	In order to ensure that others can benefit from the knowledge gained, a formal report should be generated and shared.

Adapted from NHS Education for Scotland and the National Patient Safety Agency. *Significant event analysis: guidance for primary care teams.* http://www.nrls.npsa.nhs.uk/resources/?entryid45=61500.[62]

role in adverse events, they are rarely the only factor. While it is important to ensure adequate accountability, there is an important distinction between ensuring that protocols and standards are adhered to and making negative statements about an individual involved in a given situation. Blame can quickly erode trust and teamwork.

X. MORBIDITY, MORTALITY, AND IMPROVEMENT CONFERENCES

For over 100 years, morbidity and mortality (M&M) conferences have been a longstanding venue in which to objectively discuss and learn from adverse events. Born from early efforts to examine surgical errors, these conferences are now an important place across all specialties where improvement opportunities can be discussed in a confidential manner protected by peer-review legal protections. Many institutions have renamed these meetings from M&M to MM&I (morbidity, mortality, and improvement) to emphasize the desire to focus on creating system-level improvements. Now an ACGME requirement, these conferences have evolved into standardized recurring meetings where clinicians involved in a given case can share their experiences with an eye toward creating system-level improvements.[63]

XI. PATIENT SAFETY IMPROVEMENT STRATEGIES

Only after the "how" and "why" of an adverse event are understood can systems and processes to prevent recurrence be created. The foundational concepts of quality improvement are introduced here, but Chapter 6 will provide significantly more detail on these principles. Two of the most common methodologies for prevention of errors include standardization and constraint. In standardization, the expectation of normal is clearly defined, and all team members are expected to meet the requirements without exception. In creating standards, care is taken to simplify processes, use technology or equipment to minimize human error, and reduce the probability of cognitive errors. Standards should be created by those closest to their use, flexible enough for wide applicability, and easily understood for training and implementation. Examples of successful application of standards to health care include the Joint Commission's "Do Not Use List" (see Table 5.1) and the WHO Surgical Safety Checklist (see Fig. 5.3).[22,39] At a local level, many institutions develop **clinical pathways** or protocols to standardize the care of disease processes, allowing all team members to care for a patient using guidelines resulting in similar care.

While requiring some loss of autonomous decision-making, the use of such protocols has been shown to improve outcomes, reduce complications, and even lower the cost of care. In the 1980s, Toyota's manufacturing process was so streamlined and standardized that people came from around the world to observe their techniques. Their system of simplification with repetition became known as **Lean,** and soon industries far and wide were applying Lean to their own processes.[64] The health care industry soon followed suit and began applying these same concepts to patient care in efforts to prevent harm, improve throughput, and enhance value.

Patient safety can also be improved through **constraint,** creation of limitations in a system. Known in other industries as "force functions," a constraint requires a person to slow down at a critical juncture and complete certain steps or goals to proceed with the intended action. For example, if a hospital decided to employ the WHO Surgical Safety Checklist prior to every invasive procedure, they might set up the constraint that the nurse cannot provide the equipment for beginning the procedure until the checklist is completed. Another common example is the requirement that two medical professionals confirm blood type, cross-match, and the patient's identification prior to transfusing blood. Policies utilizing constraints are intended to create situational awareness, a recognition that an event with increased potential for harm is about to occur, and all focus should be on prevention of such harm.

Constraint can also occur through external forces, including governmental and regulatory agencies. The FDA conducted an analysis of adverse events related to medical device failures from 1985 to 1989. The FDA determined that nearly half of all recalls related to these devices occurred due to poor product design, inclusive of software errors. As a result, Congress empowered the FDA through the Safe Medical Devices Act of 1990 to create and enforce manufacturing processes and standards for medical devices aimed at improving patient safety.[65]

XII. CHANGING THE FUTURE OF PATIENT SAFETY

Apart from culture change, perhaps the greatest opportunity for improving patient safety lies in advances in technology. The use of handheld computers (e.g., smartphones) has fundamentally changed the way humans interact with each other. These same technologies are already beginning to alter and enhance the way health care providers interact with patients. Interoperable electronic medical records can improve the accuracy and availability of information leading to improved diagnosis and treatment through broad access to records and results in diverse medical settings. Warnings and alerts embedded in electronic systems can minimize human error by calling attention to potential drug interactions. The same protocols created through standardization can guide the novice caregiver through the orders needed for a particular care pathway.[66] Though digital technology can also create new types of errors and risks, their promise for improvement overshadows their flaws.

Advancements in medical research also enhance patient care leading to improved safety. A range of devices from bar codes on patient identification bands to "smart" insulin pumps that evaluate blood glucose to determine appropriate dosing without human interaction all have the potential to protect patients from harm. In designing such devices, the interface of the instrument with the patient and health care provider is critical. Engineers play an important role in the design and redesign of medical devices from the perspective of safety. For example, many patients have been harmed by the accidental connection of enteral feeds to an intravenous line in error. It is not uncommon for a critically ill patient to have six or more intravenous lines with associated pumps adjacent to a feeding pump all clamped to the same pole. Envisioning this scenario makes it easy to understand how tubing can be connected to the incorrect delivery line. Simply due to tradition and norms, all of these medical devices use the same size and shape connections—a setup for error. In 2013, the International Organization of Standardization developed and engineered a new design and standard for enteral devices.[67] Once fully implemented, enteral and intravenous connections will no longer be compatible, virtually eliminating the potential for intravenous and enteral devices to be erroneously connected. It is through these and similar technologies that health care will become safer.

Perhaps the greatest impact on patient safety will come from changes in the education of physicians and other health care professionals and the culture of medical delivery. Traditional education of health care providers emphasizes the medical knowledge necessary for patient care with a paucity of training in how to ensure safe delivery of care. Recognition of the importance of incorporation of the concepts of systems-based care, interprofessionalism, leadership, and communication for the prevention of medical errors has led to incorporation of these topics into medical school and residency curriculums to varying degrees. This textbook is an effort to provide the reader with these core concepts in recognition of the value of melding core scientific knowledge with health care systems science for fundamentally changing the way professionals are trained.

In 2012, Eastern Virginia Medical School became the first to require completion of the Institute for Healthcare Improvement (IHI) Open School Basic Certificate program on quality, patient safety, and related delivery skills for graduation, and scores of medical schools have since followed suit.[68] The IHI Open School program is available without fee to medical students, residents, and faculty and lays the foundation for improved delivery of safe patient care. More extensive curricular change can be found in other medical schools where education in patient safety is fully integrated into the coursework alongside medical knowledge.[69,70] By teaching these skills at the onset of medical education as integral to patient care, the culture of safety and blame can be changed for the better. Through these efforts, it is hoped that all health care professionals enter practice understanding their essential role in creating a patient-centered and team-based approach to patient safety.

XIII. CHAPTER SUMMARY

Faced with overwhelming evidence that our health care system is causing harm, significant effort is underway to make it safer. These measures include recognition that most errors occur largely due to system errors, though human error is commonly the focus of blame. Efforts must be made at both the individual, local, and even international level to create and implement tools for evaluating and preventing episodes of patient harm. Research utilizing reporting systems and enhanced technology have the potential to mitigate errors on a larger scale in the future. Through the use of standardization in communication, error assessment, and awareness of human infallibility, a culture of vigilance for errors can supplement current prevention efforts and improve the safety of our health care systems. Providing the right care for every patient at the right time requires that all members of the health care team understand errors and error prevention while being committed to creating solutions to improve patient care.

QUESTIONS FOR FURTHER THOUGHT

1. What is the difference between an error and an adverse event?
2. What is the difference between a latent error and an active error, and how do they potentially interact in leading to an adverse event?

3. How does the operating room environment itself increase the risk for errors, and what interventions can be put in place to mitigate that risk?
4. How can medical education have an impact on reducing the cognitive errors that can ultimately lead to patient harm?

Annotated Bibliography

Brennan TA, Leape LL, Laird NM, et al. Incidence of adverse events and negligence in hospitalized patients. Results of the Harvard Medical Practice Study. *N Engl J Med.* 1991;324:370–376.

The Harvard Medical Practice Study was designed to study the incidence of injuries resulting from medical management, negligence, and malpractice. More than 30,000 charts were reviewed from a large, randomized sample of medial patients discharged from New York hospitals in 1984. The study revealed a high incidence of adverse events and negligence, with adverse events occurring in 3.7% of all hospitalizations and 27% of these adverse events due to negligence.

Kohn LT, Corrigan J, Donaldson M, eds. *To Err Is Human: Building a Safer Health System. Committee on Quality of Healthcare in America. Institute of Medicine.* Washington, DC: National Academies Press; 2000.

Issued in 1999 by the Institute of Medicine, this landmark report cited the high frequency and costs of medical errors and provided impetus for growth of the patient safety movement by bringing patient safety issues to the forefront of public concern. Based on multiple studies, it concluded that between 44,000 and 98,000 people die each year as the result of medical errors. The report described the epidemiology of errors and concluded that the majority of errors in medicine are attributable to faulty systems. The report called for a comprehensive approach to improved systems of care by health care providers, consumers, payers, governmental agencies, and accreditation bodies.

Lazare A. Apology in medical practice: an emerging clinical skill. *JAMA.* 2006;296(11):1401–1404.

The author describes that an effective apology is the logical next step after disclosure of a medical error. He suggests that apologizing for a medical error can promote healing and strengthen relationships between health care providers and patients. An apology should include an acknowledgment of the offense, an explanation, an expression of remorse, and reparation. The author offers 10 mechanisms through which apologies promote healing.

Reason J. Human error: models and management. *BMJ.* 2000;320:768–770.

The author describes the concepts of human error and explains that human error can be viewed in either a persons approach or a systems approach. He went on to describe the Swiss Cheese model of system failure that recognizes error is inevitable and every step in a process (such as health care delivery) has the potential for failure, with each layer of the system serving as a defensive layer to identify and catch the error before harm reaches the patient. High-reliability organizations focus on transitioning from a persons approach to a systems approach.

Wachter RM, Pronovost JP. Balancing "no blame" with accountability in patient safety. *N Engl J Med.* 2009;361:1401–1406.

The authors in this commentary explore the relationship between blame and accountability and why enforcement of standards for physicians tends to be weak. They propose a balance that can promote a safety culture and safe patient care. In this perspective, the authors, who are two patient safety leaders, describe noncompliance with hand washing as a pointed example of a physician behavior that can be dealt with by holding providers accountable for failure to adhere to a safety standard.

References

1. World Health Organization. *Patient Safety Curriculum Guide: Multiprofessional Edition.* http://apps.who.int/iris/bitstream/10665/44641/1/9789241501958_eng.pdf; 2011. Accessed December 14, 2015.
2. Emanuel L, Berwick D, Conway J, et al. What exactly is patient safety? In: Henriksen K, Battles JB, Keyes MA, et al., eds. *Advances in Patient Safety: New Directions and Alternative Approaches (Vol. 1: Assessment).* Rockville, MD: Agency for Healthcare Research and Quality; 2008. http://www.ncbi.nlm.nih.gov/books/NBK43629/.
3. Kohn LT, Corrigan J, Donaldson M, eds. *To Err Is Human: Building a Safer Health System.* Committee on Quality of Healthcare in America. Institute of Medicine. Washington, DC: National Academies Press; 2000.
4. Brennan TA, Leape LL, Laird NM, et al. Incidence of adverse events and negligence in hospitalized patients. Results of the Harvard Medical Practice Study. *N Engl J Med.* 1991;324:370–376.
5. Leape LL, Brennan TA, Laird N, et al. The nature of adverse events and negligence in hospitalized patients. Results of the Harvard Medical Practice Study II. *N Engl J Med.* 1991;324(6):377–384.
6. Leape LL. Error in medicine. *JAMA.* 1994;272:1851–1857.
7. Global Burden of Disease 2013 Mortality and Causes of Death Collaborators. Global, regional, and national age-sex specific all-cause and cause-specific mortality for 240 causes of death, 1990–2013: a systematic analysis for the Global Burden of Disease Study 2013. *Lancet.* 2015;385(9963):117–171.
8. James JT. A new, evidence-based estimate of patient harms associated with hospital care. *J Patient Saf.* 2013;9(3):122–128.
9. Van Den Bos J, Rustagi K, Gray T. The $17.1 billion problem: the annual cost of measurable medical errors. *Health Aff (Millwood).* 2011;30(4):596–603.
10. Von Laue NC, Schwappach DL, Koeck CM. The epidemiology of medical errors: a review of the literature. *Wien Klin Wochenschr.* 2003;115(10):318–325.
11. Reason J. *Human Error.* New York: Cambridge University Press; 1990.
12. Leape LL, Bates DW, Cullen DJ, et al. Systems analysis of adverse drug events. *JAMA.* 1995;274(1):35–43.
13. Reason J. Human error: models and management. *BMJ.* 2000;320:768–770.
14. Chassin MR, Loeb JM. High-reliability health care: getting there from here. *Milbank Q.* 2013;91(3):459–490.
15. Collins SJ, Newhouse R, Porter J, et al. Effectiveness of the surgical safety checklist in correcting errors: a literature review applying Reason's Swiss Cheese model. *AORN J.* 2014;100(1):65–79.
16. Vincent C, Taylor-Adams S, Stanhope N. Framework for analysing risk and safety in clinical medicine. *BMJ.* 1998;316(7138):1154–1157.
17. Vincent C. Understanding and responding to adverse events. *N Engl J Med.* 2003;348(11):1051–1056.
18. Lesar TS, Briceland L, Stein DS. Factors related to errors in medication prescribing. *JAMA.* 1997;277(4):312–317.
19. *Preventing Medication Errors: A $21 Billion Opportunity.* Washington, DC: National Priorities Partnership and National Quality Forum. https://psnet.ahrq.gov/resources/resource/20529; December 2010. Accessed November 15, 2015.
20. Aspden P. Institute of Medicine (US) Committee on Identifying and Preventing Medication Errors. *Preventing Medication Errors: Quality Chasm Series.* Washington, DC: National Academies Press; 2007.
21. Bates DW, Cullen DJ, Laird N, et al. Incidence of adverse drug events and potential adverse drug events. Implications for prevention. ADE Prevention Study Group. *JAMA.* 1995;274:29–34.
22. The Joint Commission. Facts about the official "do not use" list of abbreviations. http://www.jointcommission.org/facts_about_do_not_use_list/; June 30, 2015. Accessed November 15, 2015.
23. Institute for Safe Medication Practices. ISMP list of high-alert medications in acute care settings. https://www.ismp.org/tools/highalertmedications.pdf; 2014. Accessed November 30, 2015.
24. Santell JP, Hicks RW. Medication errors involving geriatric patients. *Jt Comm J Qual Patient Saf.* 2005;31(4):233–238.
25. Sarker SK, Vincent C. Errors in surgery. *Int J Surg.* 2005;3(1):75–81.
26. Rogers SO, Gawande AA, Kwaan M, et al. Analysis of surgical errors in closed malpractice claims at 4 liability insurers. *Surgery.* 2006;140(1):25–33.
27. National Academies of Sciences, Engineering, and Medicine. *Improving Diagnosis in Health Care.* Washington, DC: National Academies Press; 2015.

28. Bishop TF, Ryan AK, Casalino LP. Paid malpractice claims for adverse events in inpatient and outpatient settings. *JAMA*. 2011;305:2427–2431.

29. Starmer A, Spector N, Srivastava R, et al. I-PASS, a mnemonic to standardize verbal handoffs. *Pediatrics*. 2012;129(2):201–204.

30. Joint Commission on Accreditation of Healthcare Organizations. Sentinel event statistics. http://www.jointcommission.org/sentinel_event_statistics/; June 29, 2004. Accessed January 15, 2016.

31. Salas E, Wilson K, Burke CS, et al. Does crew resource management training work? An update, an extension, and some critical needs. *Hum Factors*. 2006;48(2):392–412.

32. Agency for Healthcare Research and Quality. TeamSTEPPS: strategies and tools to enhance performance and patient safety. http://www.ahrq.gov/professionals/education/curriculum-tools/teamstepps/index.html. Accessed January 20, 2016.

33. Teich ST, Faddoul FF. Lean management—the journey from Toyota to healthcare. *Rambam Maimonides Med J*. 2013;4(2):e0007.

34. Graber ML, Franklin N, Gordon R. Diagnostic error in internal medicine. *Arch Intern Med*. 2005;165(13):1493–1499.

35. Accreditation Council on Graduate Medical Education Task Force on Quality Care and Professionalism. The ACGME 2011 duty hour standards: enhancing quality of care, supervision, and resident professional development. http://www.acgme.org/acgmeweb/Portals/0/PDFs/jgme-monograph[1].pdf; 2011. Accessed January 25, 2016.

36. Young GJ, Charns MP, Desai KR, et al. Patterns of coordination and clinical outcomes: a study of surgical services. *Health Serv Res*. 1998;33(5):1211–1236.

37. Hughes A, Salas E. Hierarchical medical teams and the science of teamwork. *Virtual Mentor*. 2013;15(6):529–533.

38. Haig KM, Sutton S, Whittington J. SBAR: a shared mental model for improving communication between clinicians. *Jt Comm J Qual Patient Saf*. 2006;32(3):167–175.

39. World Health Organization. WHO Surgical Safety Checklist. http://apps.who.int/iris/bitstream/10665/44186/2/9789241598590_eng_Checklist.pdf; 2009. Accessed January 10, 2016.

40. World Alliance for Patient Safety. The second global patient safety challenge: safe surgery saves lives. The World Health Organization. http://www.who.int/patientsafety/safesurgery/knowledge_base/SSSL_Brochure_finalJun08.pdf; 2008. Accessed January 21, 2016.

41. Haynes AB, Weiser TG, Berry WR, et al. A surgical safety checklist to reduce morbidity and mortality in a global population. *N Engl J Med*. 2009;360(5):491–499.

42. Bergs J, Hellings J, Cleemput I, et al. Systematic review and meta-analysis of the effect of the World Health Organization surgical safety checklist on postoperative complications. *Br J Surg*. 2014;101(3):150–158.

43. Fourcade A, Blache JL, Grenier C, et al. Barriers to staff adoption of a surgical safety checklist. *BMJ Qual Saf*. 2012;21(3):191–197.

44. Wachter RM, Pronovost JP. Balancing "no blame" with accountability in patient safety. *N Engl J Med*. 2009;361:1401–1406.

45. Dulclos C, Eichler M, Taylor L, et al. Patient perspectives of patient-provider communication after adverse events. *Int J Qual Health Care*. 2005;17(6):479–486.

46. Levinson W, Roter D, Mullooly J, et al. Physician-patient communication: the relationship with malpractice claims among primary care physicians and surgeons. *JAMA*. 1997;277(7):553–559.

47. Wu A. Medical error: the second victim. *BMJ*. 2000;320:726–727.

48. Gallagher TH, Waterman AD, Ebers AG, et al. Patients' and physicians' attitudes regarding the disclosure of medical errors. *JAMA*. 2003;289(8):1001–1007.

49. Wilf Miron R, Lewenoff I, Benyamini Z, et al. From aviation to medicine: applying concepts of aviation safety to risk management in ambulatory care. *Qual Saf Health Care*. 2003;12:35–39.

50. Kachalia A, Kaufman SR, Boothman R, et al. Liability claims and costs before and after implementation of a medical error disclosure program. *Ann Intern Med*. 2010;153:213–221.

51. Kraman SS, Cranfill L, Hamm G, et al. John M. Eisenberg Patient Safety Awards. Advocacy: the Lexington Veterans Affairs Medical Center. *Jt Comm J Qual Improv*. 2002;28(12):646–650.

52. Kraman SS, Hamm G. Risk management: extreme honesty may be the best policy. *Ann Intern Med*. 1999;131:963–967.

53. Lazare A. Apology in medical practice: an emerging clinical skill. *JAMA*. 2006;296(11):1401–1404.

54. Massachusetts Coalition for the Prevention of Medical Errors. When things go wrong: responding to adverse events. http://www.macoalition.org/documents/respondingToAdverseEvents.pdf; 2006. Accessed January 22, 2016.

55. Seys D, Wu AW, Van Gerven E, et al. Health care professionals as second victims after adverse events: a systematic review. *Eval Health Prof*. 2013;36:135–162.

56. Stewart K, Lawton R, Harrison R. Supporting "second victims" is a system-wide responsibility. *BMJ*. 2015;350: h2341.

57. Mahajan RP. Critical incident reporting and learning. *Br J Anaesth*. 2010;105(1):69–75.

58. Liang BA. Risks of reporting sentinel events. *Health Aff (Millwood)*. 2000;19(5):112–120.

59. National Quality Forum. Serious reportable events in healthcare—2011 update: a consensus report. Washington, DC: National Quality Forum; 2011.

60. The Joint Commission. Patient safety systems. http://www.jointcommission.org/assets/1/18/PSC_for_Web.pdf; 2016.

61. IOM report. Patient safety—achieving a new standard for care. *Acad Emerg Med*. 2005;12(10):1011–1012.

62. NHS Education for Scotland and the National Patient Safety Agency. Significant event analysis: guidance for primary care teams. http://www.nrls.npsa.nhs.uk/resources/?entryid45=61500. Accessed November 1, 2016.

63. Deis JN, Smith KM, Warren MD, et al. Transforming the morbidity and mortality conference into an instrument for systemwide improvement. In: Henriksen K, Battles JB, Keyes MA, Grady ML, eds. *Advances in Patient Safety: New Directions and Alternative Approaches (Volume 2: Culture and Redesign)*. Rockville, MD: Agency for Healthcare Research and Quality (US); 2008.

64. Institute for Healthcare Improvement. Going Lean in health care. IHI Innovation Series white paper. http://www.ihi.org/resources/pages/ihiwhitepapers/goingleaninhealthcare.aspx. Accessed February 6, 2016.

65. United States Food and Drug Administration. Human factors implications of the new GMP rule overall requirements of the new Quality System Regulation. http://www.fda.gov/MedicalDevices/DeviceRegulationandGuidance/HumanFactors/ucm119215.htm. Accessed January 25, 2016.

66. Koutkias VG, Mcnair P, Kilintzis V, et al. From adverse drug event detection to prevention. *Methods Inf Med*. 2014;53(6):482–492.

67. Stay Connected. New global design standards for enteral device feeding connections. http://stayconnected.org. Accessed February 4, 2016.

68. Institute for Healthcare Improvement Open School. More medical and nursing schools to require IHI Open School Basic Certificate. http://www.ihi.org/education/ihiopenschool/resources/Pages/MoreMedicalAndNursingSchoolsRequireBasicCertificate.aspx. Accessed January 15, 2016.

69. Institute of Healthcare Improvement Open School. Systems change: with innovation grant and the Open School, Brody School of Medicine changes education. http://www.ihi.org/education/ihiopenschool/resources/Pages/SystemsChangeBrodySchoolOfMedicine.aspx. Accessed February 6, 2016.

70. American Medical Association. *Med Schools Focus on Quality Improvement, Patient Safety*. http://www.ama-assn.org/ama/ama-wire/post/med-schools-focus-quality-improvement-patient-safety; 2016. Accessed November 1, 2016.

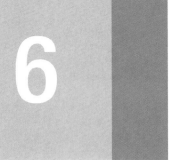

6

Quality Improvement

Jordan M. Kautz, MD, Niti S. Armistead, MD, and
Stephanie R. Starr, MD

This chapter defines quality improvement (QI) in health care and the relationship of quality to the value equation (see Chapter 4) and to patient safety (see Chapter 5). It summarizes the importance of measuring quality beyond QI alone. It defines types of quality measures and data sources as well as their limitations. It describes the most commonly used QI methods in health care (Model for Improvement, Plan-Do-Study-Act, Lean, and Six Sigma). The most common issues in health care quality (clinical decision support, standardization, equipment redesign and forcing functions, front-line engagement of clinical microsystem teams, leadership, and change management) are described, along with successful interventions to address each one. Lastly, the relationship between QI and scholarship is highlighted.

I. QUALITY IMPROVEMENT IN HEALTH CARE

A. Definition

Quality improvement (QI) in health care has been defined as the combined and unceasing efforts of everyone (health care professionals, patients, their families, researchers, payers, planners, and educators) to make changes that will lead to better patient outcomes (health), better system performance (care), and better professional development (learning). Taken this way, QI encompasses all of the changes made to improve health and health care delivery. As such, QI should be interwoven into the daily activities of all health professionals, as each professional really has two jobs when he or she comes to work every day: to do his or her work and to improve his or her work.[1] Colloquially, QI is often considered to be one of those methodologies appropriated from other industries (e.g., *Lean* from Toyota, *Six Sigma* from Motorola, among others) and applied to health care. For some, the most useful definition in practice is from the Agency for Healthcare Research and Quality (AHRQ): systematic and continuous actions that lead to measurable improvement in health care services and the health status of targeted patient groups. It must be remembered, though, that while all improvement involves change, not all change produces measurable improvement.

B. Relationship to Value and Patient Safety

It would be difficult to find a patient who does not expect or want quality health care and also assume that this presumes safe care. Quality and safety are not synonymous, however. In addition, any discussion of quality care generally necessitates a discussion of cost and value. Chapter 4 provides a detailed discussion of value in health care, including the links between quality and safety, and defines health care value as the quality of care divided by the total cost of care. Quality can be further defined as the combination of patient outcomes, safety, and service. Chapter 4 also highlights the six dimensions of quality of the Institute of Medicine: care that is safe, timely, effective, efficient, equal, and patient-centered (or STEEEP).[2] It discusses the well-documented dissonance between US health care spending and many measures of quality. Given this, health professionals must recognize early in their training that QI efforts should not focus solely on considerations of cost, but also of distributive justice and resource utilization.

Chapter 4 suggested five actions that health professionals can and should take to provide high-value (and therefore high-quality) care.

1. Understand the benefits, harms, and relative costs of interventions.
2. Decrease or eliminate the use of interventions that provide no benefit and/or may be harmful.
3. Choose interventions and care settings that maximize benefits, minimize harms, and reduce costs.
4. Customize care plans with patients that incorporate patients' values and address their concerns.
5. Identify system-level opportunities to improve outcomes, minimize harms, and reduce health care waste.

If a service is overused (such as daily complete blood count testing in stable inpatients or advanced imaging in acute low back pain), a QI approach would provide a useful and necessary framework to reduce waste. By contrast, if a service is deemed to be of value (such as use of a series of specific steps shown to decrease the risk for central-line–associated blood stream infections), the focus of the QI effort is likely to be change management, implementation, and support, not reducing cost. This chapter then will touch on constructs of value, waste, and patient safety, but will aim to discuss QI more broadly without specific emphases. Given the topic breadth, Chapter 5 is dedicated to a discussion of patient safety. The scope of this chapter is the use of QI interventions in health care improvement up to the health care organization level; the dynamics and changing complexities of the US health care system at large are addressed in Chapter 3. There are other methodologies and tools for improving quality (such as systems engineering and human factors analysis) that are beyond the scope of this chapter.

II. QUALITY MEASUREMENT

A. Measuring Quality

Earlier chapters have highlighted many gaps in health care, including the Institute of Medicine's dimensions of quality discussed earlier. Gaps in health care can be recognized or measured at multiple levels: a front-line care delivery team (clinical microsystems), a hospital or clinic (mesosystem), or a health care system (macrosystem), regionally or nationally. Existing gaps in health care quality may be unrecognized, recognized or "seen" but not measured, measured and used internally for local health care improvement efforts, measured and published as health care improvement or health services research, or measured and publically reported.

Not everything in health care can be measured, so it is important to prioritize which gaps must be closed in order to decide what should be measured. Meaningful data are needed to stimulate change, and measurement is needed to know if improvement has occurred. Measurement moves health care from opinion-driven to data-driven decision making. It is the key to dispelling deeply ingrained assumptions and generalizations as well. Any discussion of QI must therefore include an explanation of quality measures. In general, quality is measured for the following reasons:

- *Measuring quality enables teams to identify what works and what does not work in health care (through health care improvement efforts and/or research).* Measuring health care quality is essential to not only evaluating the performance of the health system and the care experience, but also to driving necessary improvement where the delivery of care falls short of expectation or desired outcomes. There are reasons other than QI to measure quality.
- *Measuring quality helps consumers (patients and their families) make informed choices about their care.* Health care decisions are complex, and patients face a variety of choices. Measuring and reporting the quality of health care can help patients get the information they need in order to make decisions about where and when to seek health care.
- *Measuring quality influences payment by holding health plans and providers accountable for providing high-quality health care.* Tying accreditation, certification, public reporting, and financial incentives (or penalties) to the quality of health care can encourage health plans and providers to deliver the best care possible.
- *Measuring quality promotes a culture of safety by preventing overuse, underuse, and misuse of health care.* Overuse and misuse of health care services (procedures, tests, and medications) can lead to preventable complications and death. Measuring health care quality helps to ensure that patients receive the right care at the right time, the first time, every time.
- *Measuring disparities in health care delivery and outcomes maintains focus on all dimensions of quality.* Racial and ethnic minorities routinely face more barriers to care and receive poorer quality care. Measuring health care quality can help us understand the effectiveness of care that diverse populations receive, which can help policymakers target improvements and hold providers accountable.[3]

B. Types of Quality Measures

Within the last 2 decades especially, measurement in health care has come to embody an emerging principle of "while some is good, more is not necessarily better and may be harmful." Clearly measurement is important. How else will the United States know where it is, how it is performing in relationship to others, and where the country wants to go? But measurement and reporting can expend tremendous time and resources. There are nuances to interpreting quality measures, making interpretation difficult for health care professionals as well as lay individuals. For example, a brief review of hospital mortality rates by practice leaders in a specific hospital may not consider to include variables such as risk adjustment (i.e., how sick the patients were to begin with) and expected mortality (preventable death). For some measures, it may not be clear whether it is good to be high, low, or somewhere in-between (e.g., C-section rates). And the proliferation of measures has created a signal-to-noise problem. What does the United States need to focus on to have the greatest impact on patient care and well-being?

This is by no means a new issue. Widely regarded the father of quality measurement in health care, Avedis Donabedian took up this topic nearly one half century ago and provided a framework for understanding how we might measure and understand quality in health care: structure, process, and outcome.[4]

- *Structural* measures are often accessible and "concrete" measures. Examples include nurse-to-patient ratios in the intensive care unit, numbers of advanced practice providers attaining certain credentials, and the number of monitored beds in a facility. Structural measures are used when it is known that care settings meeting certain standards are more likely to provide higher-quality care; they are easier to capture and most revealing when deficiencies are found.[5] The major limitation is that the relationship between structure and outcomes is not often well established. Also, just because a specific infrastructure exists does not mean that the system actually uses the capability. Thus, it may not be clear if a structure measure truly results in better patient health such as for electronic health records (EHRs).

- *Process* measures generally refer to assessments of activities carried out by health care professionals to deliver services. Examples include the percentage of patients with symptomatic or asymptomatic left ventricular (LV) dysfunction (LV ejection fraction <40 percent) who are placed on angiotensin-converting enzyme (ACE) inhibitors, the percentage of patients receiving prompt antibiotics after recognition of sepsis, or the percentage of 2-year-olds in a primary care population receiving vaccinations in line with national practice guidelines. Good process measures should always be backed by evidence that can reliably link the process measured with improved outcomes. Process measures also have limitations, in part because evidence-based process measures are not available for many areas of care. Process measures tend to focus on preventive care and management of acute or chronic disease, but are difficult to identify for areas such as teamwork and organizational culture. They may not capture the true quality of care delivered by an individual provider, as different health professionals may contribute to varying degrees to the care that is being measured.[5]

- *Outcome* measures are generally defined as the health state of a patient resulting from health care. It is helpful to consider two types of clinical outcome measures: intermediate outcome measures and long-term outcome measures. Intermediate outcome measures reflect changes in physiology that lead to longer-term health outcomes. Examples of intermediate outcomes include blood pressure, body mass index, and laboratory tests such as hemoglobin A1c or low-density lipoprotein (LDL) cholesterol. Long-term outcome examples include quality of life, occurrence of a myocardial infarction or stroke (types of unwanted events that can cause morbidity), and mortality. Long-term outcome measures are those measures that patients are most willing to pay for (i.e., perceive as most valuable, or relevant). They are the measures that health care professionals and teams most want to improve. While Donabedian supports outcomes measures as the ultimate validation of the effectiveness and quality of medical care, they may not be practical in cases in which the outcome is rare, failures are evident only years after a procedure or other health care intervention, and when outcomes are subject to sample size considerations. Outcome measures are also subject to a variety of influences, not always easily captured and not always obviously related to the systems or processes of care, such as 30-day readmission rate.[5] This is why process measures (that are linked by evidence to good clinical outcomes) are often used instead as "proxies" for health outcomes.

Table 6.1 provides an example of structure, process, and outcome measures that hospitals might use in an effort to limit one unwanted health care event: hospital-acquired blood infections after intravenous lines are placed in large (or central) veins (central-line–associated blood stream infections, or CLABSIs).

More recently, *patient experience* measures have been developed and used to give feedback to health professionals and systems on patients' experiences of their care, including the interpersonal aspects of care. These measures may assess many other aspects of care, ranging from the clarity and accessibility of information from providers, whether teams provide patients' test results, and how quickly patients are able to get appointments for urgently needed care. Patients with better care experiences are often more engaged in their care, more committed to treatment plans, and more receptive to medical advice.[5]

C. Sources of Data

At the core of any QI initiative is data, which is needed to define the extent of the problem and to assess the impact of improvement. Just as there are a variety of QI methodologies, there are many types and sources of data that can be utilized in a QI effort. Data may range from large databases with national and international scope to back-of-the-envelope counts. The

Table 6.1 Examples of Structure, Process, and Outcomes Measures to Help Decrease Unwanted Health Care Events (Central-Line–Associated Blood Stream Infections) in an Intensive Care Unit

Measure Type	Focus of Assessment	Criterion	Standard
Structure	Expertise in central-line placement	Percent of ICU providers participating in simulation-based training and annual competency assessment	100 percent of ICU providers participate
Process	Use of central-line "bundle" (series of steps performed for each central line placed)	Percent compliance with all elements of the bundle for all ICU patients with a central line	At least 95 percent compliance with all bundle elements
Outcome	Incidence of CLABSI	Number of CLABSIs per 1000 catheter days in ICU patients	Zero CLABSIs

CLABSI, Central-line–associated blood stream infection; *ICU*, intensive care unit.

big categories of data sources include administrative data, abstracted data, and surveillance data as well as data from direct observation, surveys, the EHR, and registries.

Perhaps the most well-known example of *administrative* data is the Medicare Provider Analysis and Review file (Med-PAR), which contains data from claims for services provided to beneficiaries admitted to Medicare certified inpatient hospitals and skilled nursing facilities. It contains details on demographics as well as diagnoses, procedures, and discharge disposition, including death and re-admissions. These data are analyzed and repackaged in numerous public websites comparing and grading facilities, in formulas for value-based purchasing and other federal programs linking performance to reimbursement, and also provide a rich source of data for research purposes. While the MedPAR data are often 3 or more years old, hospitals typically have internal access to these data within weeks after patients are discharged from the hospital. The data are not real-time, but can guide efforts aimed at improving hospital-based clinical outcomes by querying specific diagnoses (e.g., sepsis, stroke, pneumonia) to determine outcomes such as mortality, length of stay, resource utilization, discharge status (e.g., home, facility, hospice), or by extracting codes classified as "complications" (e.g., iatrogenic pneumothorax or accidental puncture or laceration) to conduct further evaluations.

Data that are *abstracted* from patient records can provide more clinical detail than administrative data based on claims. While coding and claims data allow for analysis related to outcomes (such as mortality, re-admissions, and cost) and even regional and/or national trends with regard to variations, they do not provide detail on clinical practice such as compliance with evidence-based standards of care. For example, the use of beta blockers during both acute and long-term management of myocardial infarction reduces mortality, yet reports have indicated that they are prescribed appropriately only in a minority of cases. Chart abstraction is needed to determine if eligible patients received the recommended treatment or if it was withheld for an acceptable reason (presuming that this is documented in the chart). Determining compliance with recommended practice in this manner is time and labor intensive and is, therefore, reserved for more prevalent conditions associated with morbidity and mortality (e.g., myocardial infarction, heart failure, stroke, pneumonia, and sepsis) for which endorsed best practices are available.

Many organizations and professional societies have developed *registries* focused on specific populations (such as trauma, cancer, and stroke) or procedures (cardiac surgery, all surgical care, and cardiopulmonary resuscitation). Data is abstracted into a standard tool, submitted to a central clearinghouse, and subsequently analyzed. The advantage of registry data over claims data is the clinical details that are often available in registries, including functional status after an event such as stroke or joint replacement surgery. As with data abstraction and direct observation, the disadvantage of registry data is the labor-intensive process to build and maintain the registry. In addition, many registries come with significant fees. In the future, the use of registries may be facilitated and made more efficient as EHRs and other clinical databases are able to transmit data to registries electronically.

Surveillance data is data that are collected and analyzed in order to understand the health of a population and do not focus on individual patients or clinical encounters. The most common surveillance efforts in hospitals are related to surveillance for hospital-acquired infections. The collection of these data is independent of the clinical care and the decision making of the provider of the record. Instead, system reports of patient populations (such as those patients with central lines or urinary catheters hospitalized within a specific time period) and test results (such as positive blood or urine cultures) are collected and analyzed based on criteria developed by an oversight body such as the Centers for Disease Control and Prevention.

The most common *survey* data in health care is data on patient satisfaction, now more commonly referred to as *patient experience*. While there are many ways to survey patients, the standardized tool mandated for hospitalized patients is the Hospital Consumer Assessment of Healthcare Providers and Systems (HCAHPS) survey. Surveys can also be used for other purposes as varied as measuring employee engagement or safety culture. A major challenge with all survey data is ensuring adequate response rate.

EHRs have great potential to provide quality data at the level of individual patients, all patients for a given provider, and all patients in a system across the continuum of care. The challenges using EHRs for meaningful quality reporting include difficulty with extracting information in free text form, invalid reports resulting from incomplete input of needed data, and lack of compatibility between EHRs and with other data systems used in gathering and analyzing quality data.

While most quality data is gathered from patient records, administrative codes, and tests/results, some behaviors are best collected via *direct observation*. Hand hygiene compliance is one such measure. Washing hands is generally accepted as a low-cost, low-risk intervention that can help reduce transmission of infections to patients. While proxy measures like soap usage may suggest the level of hand hygiene, the most legitimate way of measuring hand hygiene compliance among health care workers is to directly observe whether or not employees wash their hands. Similar to abstracted data, direct observation is labor intensive, and the challenge is ensuring that there are adequate observations to make data meaningful.

III. QUALITY REPORTING

A. Perspectives of Different Stakeholders

As discussed earlier, there are a number of reasons why quality is measured: helping patients and their families make informed choices about their care, influencing payment by holding health plans and professionals accountable for providing high-value care, ensuring patient safety, measuring disparities in care delivery and clinical outcomes, and identifying what works in health care and improvement. It is therefore not surprising (and is important to pause and consider) how and why different stakeholders in the health care system might rank the importance of various quality measures. Measurement is critical, but the interpretation, the context, and the impact of measures requires a broader understanding of the complexities of the health care system. In general, patients and families care most about clinical outcomes such as mortality (life and death), morbidity (functional status, pain or other limitations), and overall quality of life. Employers would agree but are focused more on the costs of care for employees than the employees themselves.[6] These rankings are not necessarily static over time. With an increased focus on costs of care and the impact of costs on society broadly, as well as increased out-of-pocket costs by patients,[7] stakeholders may share more similar rankings over time.

B. Examples of Publically Reported Measures

There are thousands of endorsed health care quality measures in the United States. These can be searched using the AHRQ National Quality Measures Clearinghouse[8] via a number of search filters or categories, including measure type (structure, process, outcome, and patient experience), patient demographics (age and gender), care setting, organization that has endorsed the measures, health care professional role (nurses, clergy, pharmacists, and physicians), data source (EHRs, public health data, and billing data), and Institute of Medicine's dimensions of quality. It is helpful to learn about several of the most commonly used publically reported measures.

Many quality measures are developed and disseminated at a national level by the federal government and its partners. The Centers for Medicare & Medicaid Services (CMS) core measures[9] are developed by a collaborative that includes health insurers, CMS leaders, and the National Quality Forum (NQF), a not-for-profit, nonpartisan health care improvement organization. Core measures seek to aid in promotion of evidence-based measurement for QI, consumer decision making, and value-based payment. CMS partnered with AHRQ to develop the HCAHPS,[10] the tool used most commonly to survey hospitalized patients on their care experience. Patients and health care organizations can benchmark quality at the state[11] or hospital level.[12] Commonly used patient safety measures include the National Patient Safety Goals from the Joint Commission[13] and AHRQ's Patient Safety Indicators.[14]

Although many quality measures focused initially on hospital care, the number of measures for the outpatient setting (such as MN Community Measurement[15]), transitions of care across settings, and a wider range of health conditions are increasing. For example, in recent years there has been an increased focus on outpatient safety, health care disparities, and measures for geriatric and pediatric patients. In addition to other sources of publically reported measures, there are private benchmarking organizations that provide quality measures to the public, including the University HealthSystem Consortium, The Leapfrog Group, and Healthgrades.

C. The Future of Quality Measurement and Reporting

Many challenges remain in the quest to appropriately, feasibly, and reliably measure the quality of health care. The Affordable Care Act requires (as outlined in the National Quality Strategy) performance in six priority domains of quality: patient experience and engagement, population and community health, safety, care coordination, cost, and efficiency.[16] Efforts to improve quality measurement must include a transition to using more broad-based, meaningful, and patient-centered care over an episode of care rather than dependence on the use of setting-specific, narrow "biopsies" or snapshots of process measures such as use of aspirin at the time of hospital discharge for heart attack patients. Efforts

must also include identification of important measures, retirement of measures that have been consistently achieved, combining measures in a portfolio that addresses multiple stakeholder needs, and adoption of these measures across public and private payment systems.[17]

Experts have suggested that a number of steps are needed to raise the bar to improve health outcomes. These steps would ideally include using clinical measures with information focused on care (in lieu of limited information based on billing data) that are harmonized (same measures with the same definitions used elsewhere in the system), measuring outcomes broadly for all patients (rather than for small segments of patients receiving selected care) all of the time (i.e., efficient data collection via the EHR versus labor-intensive data abstraction).[18]

CASE STUDY 1

The Keystone Study looked at 103 intensive care units (ICUs) in Michigan and aimed to reduce the median and mean rate of catheter-related blood stream infections utilizing a central-line bundle with the following components: hand washing; using full-barrier precautions during central-line insertion; cleaning the site with chlorhexidine; avoiding the femoral site if possible; and removing unnecessary catheters. This project was successful, but what are the questions that need to be asked and answered to identify why it was successful and how the success may be replicated in other settings?

While one could conclude that use of this checklist in any ICU could lead to the same results, reading the methodology of the study more closely reveals a bundle of interventions beyond the ones stated in this case study. The department also used a daily goal sheet to improve clinician-to-clinician communication, implemented interventions to reduce the incidence of ventilator-associated pneumonia, and attempted to improve unit-level safety culture. Those involved in this study also engaged local champions, encouraged partnering with local hospital-based infection-control practitioners, delivered extensive education, revamped central-line kits, proposed "emergency stops," engaged in daily rounds discussion, and involved C-suite–level leadership. The authors themselves note that they "did not evaluate the relative effectiveness of the separate components of the intervention." Can you identify the key challenges of this study and devise ways to make it more likely that useful conclusions will emerge?

IV. QUALITY IMPROVEMENT METHODS

There are a variety of QI methodologies currently utilized in health care, and they have more similarities than differences. Some have advantages in their simplicity (e.g., Plan-Do-Study-Act or PDSA), while others tap into experience from other industries (e.g., Toyota Lean model). Some health care organizations choose to declare allegiance to a single methodology (e.g., Six Sigma), while many others will have a more blended or context-specific approach. Some health care delivery problems require more precision (i.e., preventing wrong site surgery and ensuring that newborn babies go home with the right parent), necessitating choice of one method (such as Six Sigma) over another. While it is fairly typical to have a core group of experts, some level of training and familiarity with these principles in front-line leadership is critical for successful utilization of these methods. Many use the term *method* to refer to the higher-level view of the entire QI philosophy or approach and use the term *tool* to refer to specific (smaller-scale) approaches to one small part of a larger QI initiative or project. Of course, at the heart of any QI effort are data. In order to close gaps and improve care delivery with any methodology, the improvement team must clearly define the gap they seek to close and the data needed to determine if they have succeeded.

A. Model for Improvement

The Model for Improvement is the most commonly used QI approach in health care and was popularized by the Institute for Healthcare Improvement (IHI) as a framework to guide improvement efforts.[19] This framework is meant to work in concert with any QI methodology that an organization may be using and involves two parts. Part one requires that the team start by answering the following three critical questions before the team tests change ideas using QI methods during part two. The three questions that can be answered in any order are as follows:[20]

1. What are we trying to accomplish?
2. How will we know that the change is an improvement?
3. What changes can we make that will result in an improvement?

As a Chinese proverb states, "The beginning of wisdom is to call things by their proper name." Question 1 is about defining the problem and the *aim* of the improvement exercise. The aim should be measurable, time-specific, and clear in scope and population impacted. A commonly used acronym for goal setting is to use the SMART (Specific, Measurable, Attainable, Relevant, and Time-bound) framework. It is critical to clearly define the scope of the project to ensure that the target goal truly is attainable with the available time and resources. Question 2 is about defining the appropriate measures to track success. As previously stated, all improvement involves change, but not all change will lead to improvement. Defining measures (with baseline and target) and tracking progress in time is critical to determine if change results in improvement. Finally, question 3 involves identifying key changes that will be tested. These ideas can come from various sources including front-line workers, experiences of others, publications, or innovations.

From defining the problem to testing change ideas, a critical element of any successful QI effort is getting the right people on the improvement team. Teams vary in size and composition but generally need a diversity of roles and disciplines to be represented. For example, if a team is pulled together to decrease wait time in a clinic, in addition to physicians, representation from nurses, receptionists, schedulers, information technology, facilities, and perhaps even ancillary services such as laboratory or radiology, depending on structure and function of that clinic, is important. Team composition does not need to be unnecessarily complicated, and it is crucial that, once appointed, all team members find their participation to be valuable to the aim.

In summary, selecting the right team, clearly defining the problem/aim, establishing quantifiable measures, and selecting ideas for change are all crucial prerequisites before any change can be implemented. Once the team is ready to implement a change idea, then one of the QI methodologies is used to test it in a methodical manner. The most commonly used testing tool in the Model for Improvement is PDSA.

B. Plan-Do-Study-Act

After planning is completed, the QI project is ready to start performing tests of change.[21] PDSA cycles provide the simplest structure for iterative development of change, either as a standalone method or as a part of wider QI approaches like Model for Improvement.[22] The Plan phase of PDSA defines the specifics of the change intervention (who, what, where, and when) and also plans the data collection. Most of this will likely already have been covered during the planning steps described earlier in the Model for Improvement. If PDSA is utilized as a standalone tool, the elements related to defining aim, assembling the right team, defining measures of success, and outlining change interventions all occur in the Plan phase. The test of change begins during the Do phase. The fundamental principle of the PDSA cycle is to rapidly test small-scale pilot(s). It is critical to document obstacles so they can be addressed in subsequent cycles.

During the Study phase, the team analyzes the results using predetermined process, outcomes, and balancing metrics. In the Act phase, the QI team adapts intervention(s) based on results of the Study phase and incorporates the findings into planning cycle to test the next or revised change based on what was previously learned (Fig. 6.1).

The number of PDSA cycles needed varies on the complexity of the initiative. Run charts provide an easy way of tracking progress over time and impact of each cycle. Through this data-driven iterative process, decisions can be made about which of the originally proposed changes actually result in improvement, will get implemented on a larger scale, and ultimately become the new way of doing work.

C. Lean

Principles of Toyota Production System (TPS) have been applied to other industries, including health care, in the form of Lean methodology. Taiichi Ohno, a Toyota Motor Corporation engineer, is credited with creation of TPS, which is based on maximizing efficiency by eliminating waste ("muda" in Japanese). Waste, or non–value-added activities, from a business perspective do not add to the financial margin or customer experience and therefore need to be eliminated. The following seven types of health care waste have been identified[23]:

1. Waste of overproduction (largest waste)
2. Waste of inventory or stock at hand
3. Waste of rework (e.g., assembly mistakes)
4. Waste of movement (e.g., poor work area ergonomics)
5. Waste associated with waiting (e.g., patients waiting to be seen for appointments)
6. Waste of processing (e.g., outdated policies and procedures)
7. Waste of transport or handling

Lean tools aim to eliminate every form of waste and simplify and maximize value by putting the right processes in place. The first step in improvement is to identify all the steps in the current state, which is best accomplished by bringing a cross-section of workers from service chief to front-line staff together and develop a common understanding of what the current state or the current process actually looks like. This process of drawing out all the steps involved in completing a task is called *process mapping*. Since most professionals are focused on their task, it is often eye-opening to review the full picture together. This highlights the importance of ensuring that each step in the

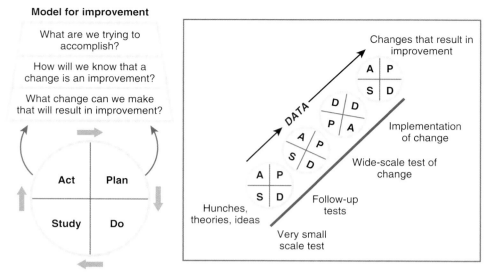

Fig. 6.1 **Model for improvement and PDSA.** (From Associates in Process Improvement. www.apiweb.org. Accessed March 17, 2016.)

process is represented by someone on the team who routinely does the work. The team then seeks to improve performance by removing all steps that do not create value.

Fig. 6.2 is an example of two process maps and shows how wasted steps can be reduced in an existing process to improve efficiency and timeliness in processing laboratory specimens.

Value stream mapping (VSM) is a more complex Lean tool. This detailed process map includes estimates of time taken for each step and the quality of the work done at each step. Value is always determined from the perspective of the customer (typically the patients in health care). Lean tools such as VSM are often used to decrease turnaround time for services (e.g., laboratory or radiology) or improving throughput through a busy area (e.g., emergency department).

When clinical teams seek to improve their productivity (e.g., increase the number of completed surgical procedures in a given day), they often initially plan to build more structure such as operating rooms to increase their output. Lean teaches that work is either value added (i.e., something that patients will pay for, such as having an ultrasound performed), incidental work (such as billing and coding by physicians), and waste. If there is significant existing waste in the process to start, building more structure will magnify the waste. Lean tools might have provided more capacity by eliminating waste, such as is shown in Fig. 6.3.

By redesigning workflow, Park Nicollet Medical Center (Minneapolis, Minnesota) eliminated the need for patient wait rooms in their new ambulatory clinic. Instead of scheduling patients in "batches" (e.g., five patients assigned to five rooms at one time), patients were checked in using the concept of continuous flow.[23]

Another key concept in Lean methodology relates to standardization and eliminating inappropriate variation in practice. As discussed in Chapter 3, there is a needed balance between eliminating variation and individualizing care for patients. Health care can never be 100 percent standardized, but by eliminating variation that does not add value (e.g., for 80 percent of situations), the system creates capacity for tailoring the situation for the remaining work (20 percent). At that same institution discussed earlier, orthopedic surgeons

were shown case carts with all the instruments and supplies they had ordered for total hip and total knee replacement surgery each with a price tag attached. The surgeons were unaware of the variability in use of instruments and supplies for the same procedures and the cost impact. Through discussion, there was a 60 percent reduction in the number of instruments. The exercise was expanded to general surgery, and the net effect reported was that 40,000 fewer items per month that needed to be sterilized.

D. Six Sigma

Like Lean, Six Sigma originated in the manufacturing industry in the mid-1980s in the Motorola corporation.[23] While both methodologies focus on eliminating waste, Lean emphasizes removal of all unnecessary and wasteful steps. Six Sigma focuses on eliminating variation by minimizing defects in a process. *Defect* is defined as any instance in which a product or outcome is not within acceptable standards. Examples can include harmful events like wrong site surgery or wasteful events like wrongly labeled laboratory specimens. "Sigma" is a statistical unit that compares how many standard deviations a process is performing when compared to perfection. Level of sigma performance (scale 1 to 6) correlates with the defect per million opportunities (DPMO), which, in turn, allows calculation of the defect or error-free rate (Table 6.2). DPMO is essentially observed defect rate extrapolated to every 1 million opportunities. When a process is functioning at Six Sigma level, there are 3.4 defects per 1 million opportunities (DPMO), yielding an error-free rate of 99.9996 percent (i.e., virtually error-free). While an error-free rate of 99 percent may seem excellent, that is where airline performance for lost luggage is typically rated and is considered inadequate simply given the high number of opportunities. It may not be feasible to achieve Six Sigma in every process, but the methodology challenges preconceived notions regarding improvement.

Six Sigma performance is achieved through systematic steps to help identify and address root causes. The five steps are Define, Measure, Analyze, Improve, and Control

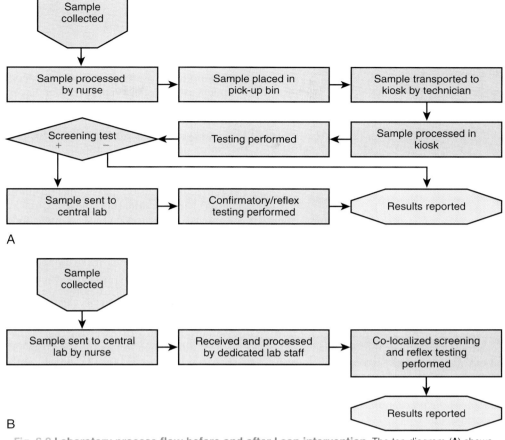

Fig. 6.2 Laboratory process flow before and after Lean intervention. The top diagram (**A**) shows the step in processing laboratory specimens before Lean was used to streamline the process; the bottom diagram (**B**) shows the final process after the improvements were made. (From White BA, Baron JM, Dighe JS, Camargo CA Jr., Brown DF. Applying Lean methodologies reduces ED laboratory turnaround times. *Am J Emerg Med.* 2015;33:1572–1576.)

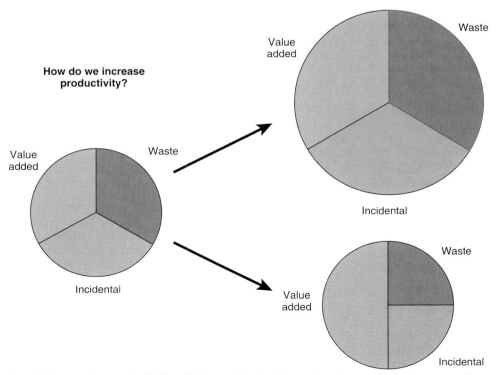

Fig. 6.3 Increasing productivity with Lean. Note that if waste is not removed from the process, then the waste is magnified if more resources are given to expand the process.

Table 6.2 Sigma Levels

Sigma Level	Defects per Million	Yield
1	690,000	31%
2	308,000	69.20%
3	66,800	93.320%
4	6,210	99.3790%
5	230	99.9770%
6	3.4	99.99966%

(DMAIC). During the Define phase, the improvement team creates a project charter, which describes the scope, purpose, goals, and stakeholders for the project. It is important that all members of the QI team agree on these details of the project before moving forward. The Measure phase is the second step, when the team develops a plan for data collection, including details related to the target defects, and collects baseline data on how the process is performing.

Health care professionals have a tendency to jump to solutions before ensuring that all on the team have accurate information about what is actually occurring before any improvements are designed or implemented. In addition to drawing out a process flow as described earlier, there are other QI tools available to help accomplish this step. Some examples include the following:

1. Drawing out a cause-and-effect or fishbone diagram that can narrow down root causes by collecting contributing factors in some broad categories (e.g., people, equipment, environment, supplies).
2. Conducting time and motion studies that typically direct observation of a task and the time it takes (e.g., time spent by a nurse during a shift for completing required documentation).
3. Completing a SWOT (Strengths-Weakness-Opportunity-Threat) analysis.

In the Analyze stage, the baseline is analyzed using statistical and other QI tools to ascertain the reasons for the defects. The use of specific QI tools (such as the Five Whys[24]) helps ensure that the team adequately understands what is contributing to the defects (quality gap). Many health care professionals on a QI team are quick to suggest solutions to the quality gap before the gap has been adequately defined, the baseline (pre-intervention) performance has been measured, and the team has sufficiently considered the key factors or reasons for the gap. Those new to QI might find it helpful to consider a response to the question, "If you have 1 hour to save the world, how would you spend that hour?" Some have attributed this answer to Albert Einstein: "I would spend 55 minutes defining the problem and then 5 minutes solving it."[25]

After the baseline data (or performance) is analyzed, the team develops creative solutions or interventions that are implemented in the Improve phase. During this fourth step, post-intervention data is collected (often at multiple points) to identify which interventions are most effective.

In the fifth and final stage, the Control phase, processes are developed to ensure that successful interventions are adopted as new standards and that reverting to old processes is impossible. Mechanisms to monitor compliance with new processes are also developed during this stage.

E. Lean Six Sigma

The Lean and Six Sigma strategies have been combined into a methodology known as Lean Six Sigma, so that a joint implementation may overcome weaknesses of either system when implemented alone. Lean offers standard solutions to common problems by focusing on the value stream and the customer, but is seen as weak on organizational infrastructure and analytical tools. Six Sigma includes a strong emphasis on defining defects using QI tools, but is often perceived as too complex.[26] Combining both approaches provides a framework for evaluating workflows to ensure efficiency and value (Lean) and a focus on measuring and eliminating errors (Six Sigma).[27] In combination, these approaches foster an environment that focuses on measurement and rapid continuous improvement.

There is belief that Lean, Six Sigma, Lean Six Sigma, and PDSA are vehicles to sustained levels of high-quality health care, but whether widespread adoption of these methodologies in health care will be effective is an open question. Systematic reviews of PDSA,[22] Lean, Six Sigma,[28] and Lean Six Sigma all report a lack of rigorous evaluation in health care. Furthermore, there is a clear lack of adherence to the principles of QI methodologies, such as PDSA applications reported without any iterative cycles of change and Six Sigma studies reported without error rate calculations sigma levels. It is therefore difficult to ascertain whether a particular method is effective in health care.

In summary, no one QI method has proven superior to others in the health care setting, and no one method is ideal for all situations. Using a QI methodology ensures a standardized and rigorous approach to closing gaps without missing a crucial step. The underlying principles of analysis, measurement, and review are consistent across all methodologies, and the disciplined application of all steps is far more important than the choice of the specific method (Table 6.3).

V. COMMON QUALITY ISSUES AND SUCCESSFUL INTERVENTIONS

Thus far we have learned that successful QI interventions clearly define the problem (quality gap), measure baseline and post-intervention performance, establish the existing and desired processes, use QI methods and tools in a disciplined manner, and use iterative testing of small-scale change. The subset of change ideas that lead to desired outcomes are often combined into a finalized protocol or proven set of recommendations and ready for widespread dissemination.[21] All too often, widespread expansion of a quality initiative does not yield the desired outcomes, leading to disappointment, cynicism, and continued suboptimal care because success often hinges on adoption and behavior change by front-line providers who, in turn, often view it as "one more thing to do" or the "flavor of the month." Just providing the methods and telling people to do something does not ensure that it will be done. In order to maximize the chance of successful implementation of any initiative, it is important to leverage the system that supports humans in doing their best work. Several such strategies are highlighted in the sections that follow.

Table 6.3 Summary of Specific Quality Improvement Approaches

Methodology	Plan, Do, Study, Act (PDSA)	Lean	Six-Sigma
Focus	Structured planning and testing of solutions	Eliminate waste across service lines to improve quality, workflow, and value	Statistical-based problem solving and improvement
Primary target	Piloting improvements	Workflow	Large problems and variation
Approach	Plan Do Study Act	Value Value stream Flow Pull Perfection	Define Measure Analyze Improve Control
Primary result	Improvement through small tests of change	Reduced flow times	Uniform process output

A. Clinical Decision Support

A clinical decision support (CDS) system links patient data with stored knowledge in a database and provides suggestions to providers to improve the care they deliver.[29] Given the volume and complexity of clinical information, CDS systems leverage the power of the EHR to link that knowledge to an individual patient problem and inform physicians and other health care professionals in real time regarding how to translate that knowledge into patient care. CDS can take the form of a medication order support (e.g., prompting adjustment for diminished renal function), order sets that incorporate recommended practices (e.g., pneumonia or sepsis care, reminders to discontinue catheters or monitors, or critical laboratory notifications). On occasion, CDS systems can result in alert fatigue and even cause harm by delaying treatment. One potential cause for delay would be the use of hard-stop to avoid harmful consequences (e.g., drug-drug interaction in medication prescribing software). A seemingly well-intended alert can be interruptive, and efforts to bypass for legitimate and unanticipated circumstances can cause direct patient harm. Similarly, the issue of alert fatigue arises from a high number of clinically insignificant alerts that consume time and cause mental distraction. Increasing specificity of alerts by employing mechanisms to prevent unnecessary notifications (such as ensuring that a patient is on enteral nutrition before suggesting an intravenous-to-oral medication change) can help decrease clinically insignificant alerts.

B. Standardization: Protocols and Order Sets

Traditional approaches to diagnosing and treating patients have relied upon physicians making decisions based on their education and training and the application of that clinical knowledge. One consequence of this individualized approach has been wide variation in care, some of which may be acceptable based on patient-specific or system factors, but sometimes is clearly unacceptable. One way to address unacceptable variations in care is through the use of protocols and order sets. For certain conditions, best practices can be built into algorithms or protocols that drive the front-line providers to deliver those processes as long as clinical criteria are met. Embedding these best practices into the EHR so the standard choices are ordered by the provider via order entry is done by use of order sets. Protocols can be very specific (e.g., a hypoglycemia protocol that directs the nurse to administer the precise dosage of dextrose for blood sugar <50 mg/dL) or more comprehensive as has been done in recent efforts related to care redesign.[30]

C. Equipment Redesign and Forcing Functions

Overreliance on memory and dependence on education (and re-education) of staff is not an effective QI strategy. All too often, especially when things get busy, staff juggling multiple priorities will miss critical steps, make errors, and risk causing harm to patients. One example of this has been staff accidently connecting enteral tube feeds to intravenous catheters. Instructing staff to "be more careful" would be less effective than getting catheters for which the connector is incompatible with the incorrect receiver. This is an example of equipment redesign that makes it impossible for a human to erroneously make an incorrect connection. An example of "forcing function" would be to make it impossible for a provider to complete entering orders on a patient unless they have addressed critical elements like code status and prophylaxis for deep venous thrombosis. As discussed earlier, forcing functions in the EHR can have unintended consequences and need to be utilized with caution.

D. Front-Line Engagement and Team-Based Care

Any QI effort requiring behavior change by front-line providers requires an understanding of factors associated with successful behavior change. Too many great ideas fail to take hold because the individuals most impacted don't see the value or, worse, believe the change to be detrimental to safety, quality, or efficiency. Input from front-line staff in every aspect of care redesign is vital to fostering ownership. Additionally, ensuring that staff receive adequate feedback once an initiative is underway helps ensure follow-through and hardwiring of the new practice. Audit and feedback is one strategy used in the belief that health care professionals are prompted to modify their practice when their performance is inconsistent with the desired target.[31] While it can indeed be effective, the effectiveness seems to depend on baseline performance and how the feedback is provided. For example, feedback is more likely to be effective if the feedback is delivered by a supervisor or trusted colleague, provided multiple times, delivered in both verbal and written form, and includes an explicit target and action plan. The challenge in every QI project is not simply developing a good intervention but ensuring its successful execution. That is where front-line engagement and teamwork become vital.

E. Leadership and Board Accountability

Quality and safety as organizational priorities must start from the top, and for most hospitals the top is a board of trustees. Ensuring that leadership is working tirelessly to improve outcomes and remove barriers for front-line staff to do their best work is a key responsibility of the board. This notion was popularized when included as a key element of the Institute of Healthcare Improvement's (IHI's) 5 Million Lives Campaign. This campaign was aimed at reducing incidents of harm in hospitals, and the one nonclinical intervention included was to fully engage the governance leadership in quality and safety. This intervention was more commonly known as "Getting Boards on Board."[32] In a previous era, hospital boards were primarily responsible for the organization's financial status and reputation. From a more modern view, boards, in partnership with executive leadership, set system-level expectations and accountability for safety and quality. The interventions that translate this core responsibility into action include setting specific aims to reduce harm and improve quality; reviewing data and hearing stories that put a human face to data; fostering an environment of transparency, continuous learning, and support of patients, families, and staff; and, finally, establishing executive accountability, including holding the executive team accountable for achieving clear QI goals.

F. Change Management

Virtually all QI efforts involve making a change at some scale. People have varying responses to change: from innovators and early adopters to laggards (the last to adopt an innovation). In addition to front-line engagement, a key element of successful QI efforts includes the early identification of champions. The champions are typically from the early adopters group. Much of the change needed involves changing behavior, which, in turn, gets to the importance of connecting to motivation, making the right thing easy to do, offering reward and recognition in a meaningful way (which is not always financial), and fostering an environment of engagement for all.

VI. QUALITY IMPROVEMENT AND SCHOLARSHIP

There are distinct differences between how QI and other health care improvement projects are executed and how scholarly activities are typically conducted. An unfortunate and unhappy tension between QI activity (improving processes of care) and scientific knowledge (improving clinical evidence) was highlighted in an editorial by Don Berwick in 2008 in which he discussed the limitations of the oft-glorified randomized controlled trial (RCT) to address all needed learning.[33] He explained why the traditional RCT model cannot be directly applied to many health care improvement attempts. Most system improvements (such as rapid response teams for deteriorating hospitalized patients) are complex and have many components, requiring social change. The effectiveness of systems (and therefore of system improvements) relies in part on leadership, changing environments, organizational history, and many other factors. Understanding (and clearly reporting) the context, therefore, in which health care improvements are studied and reported is critical. The setting (or context) in which improvement takes place is important to understanding its effectiveness (or the lack thereof). At the same time, there must be necessary rigor when assessing the success or failure of QI initiatives in order to decide whether the interventions should be disseminated and adapted to other settings.

The most widely known and accepted standards for publishing health care improvement initiatives are the Standards for Quality Improvement Reporting Excellence (SQUIRE) 2.0 Guidelines.[34] Indeed, many health care improvement teams now use these guidelines to help plan as well as execute and report their projects. An in-depth discussion of the opportunities to improve the rigor of health care improvement scholarship is beyond the scope of this chapter, but several common themes are included in the following paragraphs.

There are frequent inconsistencies in the description of and adherence to QI methodologies in the literature (when compared to how they are actually used in practice). For example, a systematic review of the application of the PDSA method found that many studies utilizing and reporting PDSA use fail to include key features of the methodology (such as iterative cycles, prediction-based test of change, small-scale testing, use of data over time, and documentation).[22] This is not a problem with the tool, per se, but with its use.

QI and other health care improvement teams are not effective at telling their stories. The SQUIRE 2.0 guidelines highlight several important ways in which QI can and should be different from traditional research, including context. In addition, the intervention may and likely will change throughout the study in response to feedback, continuous data analysis, and interaction with the context. The SQUIRE 2.0 guidelines emphasize the importance of facilitating this change so we can advance the science and know what works, rather than remaining focused on a fixed intervention that does or does not work.

Health professionals are not good at understanding the stories QI teams have to tell. There are many issues in interpreting evidence from a QI study, including whether the intended interventions actually occurred, data quality was assessed, follow-up was sufficiently long to allow for a drift in clinical behavior, and all patient-important outcomes are considered.

VII. CHAPTER SUMMARY

Quality improvement (QI) in health care includes any effort (small or large scale) to improve health care delivery, outcomes, or both. QI is part of the health care value equation defined in Chapter 4 (quality of care divided by cost over time) and includes patient safety, (addressed separately in Chapter 5). Quality is measured in order to improve care, help consumers make choices, and influence payment of health care professionals and organizations in order to improve care.

There are several types of quality measures, including structural, process, outcome, and patient experience measures. Each has its strengths and weaknesses, and a combination is required to help ensure quality care. Measures are taken from many data sources, each with its strengths and weaknesses, including administrative data, abstracted data from patient records, data from registries, surveillance data on populations of patients, survey data, EHR data, and directly observed and recorded data.

Each stakeholder group in health care varies how it ranks the importance of quality measure types. Many measures are publically reported and can be obtained at the national, state, or local (i.e., by hospital) level. Many necessary changes are anticipated in how quality measures are developed, adopted, and used in the future.

The Model for Healthcare Improvement and PDSA are two commonly used QI methods in health care. Other commonly used QI methods (Lean and Six Sigma) originated in the manufacturing industry and have been applied to health care problems. Use of one method over another varies frequently by institution, by the quality gap each QI team is seeking to close, or both.

Successful QI interventions for common health care problems have included clinical decision support systems, protocols and order sets, equipment redesign and forcing functions, front-line engagement and team-based care, leadership and board accountability, and change management.

There are distinct differences between traditional scientific research and QI scholarship. Use of the SQUIRE 2.0 guidelines, the current benchmark for publishing QI interventions, both to plan and disseminate projects can help teams improve the rigor of QI scholarship.

QUESTIONS FOR FURTHER THOUGHT

1. What are five things individual physicians can do in their practice to help provide high-value care to their patients?
2. Why is it important to measure health care quality, and how might the measurement results be useful to different stakeholders (patients, payers, institutional leaders, and public health officials)?
3. What are the four types of quality measures and their strengths and limitations?
4. What quality improvement method—a PDSA cycle, Lean, or Six Sigma—would be most appropriately applied to improving patient experience during the activities that comprise a doctor's appointment (related to time spent waiting to see the physician, having laboratory tests drawn, and filling a prescription)? What method might be better to identify and reduce errors within the same processes?
5. What are some things that can be done in terms of enabling technology, system processes, or leadership qualities to enable quality and safety improvement efforts to succeed?

Annotated Bibliography

Batalden P, Davidoff F. What is "quality improvement" and how can it transform healthcare? *Qual Saf Health Care*. 2007;16(1):2–3.
The authors highlight the domains of interest in quality improvement, selected tools and methods used to close specific quality gaps, and the knowledge systems involved in health care improvement.

Donabedian A. The quality of care: how should it be assessed? *JAMA*. 1988;260(12):1743–1748.
This sentinel article summarizes the initial national discussion on measuring health care quality.

Glasgow JM, Scott-Caziewell J, Kaboli P. Guiding inpatient quality improvement: a systematic review of Lean and Six Sigma. *Jt Comm J Qual Patient Saf*. 2010;36(12):533–540.
This systematic review summarizes what is known about the effectiveness of Lean and Six Sigma in health care, as well as the limitations of the existing literature.

Institute of Medicine. *Crossing the Quality Chasm: A New Health System for the 21st Century*. https://www.iom.edu/Reports/2001/Crossing-the-Quality-Chasm-A-New-Health-System-for-the-21st-Century.aspx. Published March 1, 2001. Accessed January 22, 2016.
This white paper classifies the types of quality gaps (dimensions of quality) that health systems must target in their health improvement efforts, and lays out the road map for how to improve US health care quality.

Taylor M, McNicholas C, Nicolay C, Darzi A, Bell D, Reed J. Systematic review of the application of the plan-do-study-act method to improve quality in healthcare. *BMJ Qual Saf*. 2014;23:290–298.
This systematic review summarizes what is known about the effectiveness of Plan-Do-Study-Act cycles in health care, as well as the limitations of the existing literature.

References

1. Batalden P, Davidoff F. What is "quality improvement" and how can it transform healthcare? *Qual Saf Health Care*. 2007;16(1):2–3.
2. Institute of Medicine. *Crossing the quality chasm: a new health system for the 21st century*. http://www.nap.edu/catalog/10027/crossing-the-quality-chasm-a-new-health-system-for-the. Published March 1, 2001. Accessed January 22, 2016.
3. Families USA. *Five ways measuring the quality of health care is good for consumers*. http://familiesusa.org/blog/2014/01/five-ways-measuring-quality-health-care-good-consumers. Published December 15, 2015. Accessed March 17, 2016.
4. Donabedian A. The quality of care: how should it be assessed? *JAMA*. 1988;260(12):1743–1748.
5. Families USA. *Measuring health care quality: an overview of quality measures*. http://familiesusa.org/sites/default/files/product_documents/HSI%20Quality%20Measurement_Brief_final_web.pdf. Published May 2014. Accessed March 17, 2016.
6. Ransom SB, Joshi M, Nash DB. *The Healthcare Quality Book: Vision, Strategy And Tools*. Chicago, IL: Health Administration Press; 2004.
7. Schoen C, Radley D, Collins SR. *Commonwealth Fund. State trends in the cost of employer health insurance coverage, 2003–2013*. http://www.commonwealthfund.org/~/media/files/publications/issue-brief/2015/jan/1798_schoen_state_trends_2003_2013.pdf. Published January 2015. Accessed March 17, 2016.
8. Agency for Healthcare Research and Quality National Quality Measures Clearinghouse. http://www.qualitymeasures.ahrq.gov/search/advanced-search.aspx. Accessed March 15, 2016.
9. *Centers for Medicare and Medicaid Services (CMS) core measures*. https://www.cms.gov/Medicare/Quality-Initiatives-Patient-Assessment-Instruments/QualityMeasures/Core-Measures.html. Accessed March 15, 2016.
10. *CAHPS hospital survey*. http://www.hcahpsonline.org/home.aspx. Accessed March 15, 2016.
11. Agency for Healthcare Research and Quality. *National healthcare quality and disparities reports, state view*. http://nhqrnet.ahrq.gov/inhqrdr/state/select. Accessed March 15, 2016.
12. Hospital Safety Score. http://www.hospitalsafetyscore.org/. Accessed March 15, 2016.
13. The Joint Commission. *National patient safety goals*. http://www.jointcommission.org/standards_information/npsgs.aspx. Accessed March 15, 2016.
14. Agency for Healthcare Research and Quality. *Patient safety indicators*. http://www.qualityindicators.ahrq.gov/modules/psi_overview.aspx. Accessed March 15, 2016.
15. Minnesota Community Measurement. http://mncm.org/. Accessed March 15, 2016.
16. US Department of Health and Human Services. *2012 Annual progress report to Congress: national strategy for quality improvement in health care*, 2012. http://www.ahrq.gov/workingforquality/nqs/nqs2012annlrpt.pdf. Accessed March 15, 2016.

17. Conway PH, Mostashari F, Clancy C. The future of quality measurement for improvement and accountability. *JAMA*. 2013;309(21):2215–2216.

18. Panzer RJ, Gitomer RS, Greene WH, Webster PR, Landry KR, Riccobono CA. Increasing demands for quality measurement. *JAMA*. 2013;310(18):1971–1980.

19. Agency for Healthcare Research and Quality Practice Facilitation Handbook Module 4: Approaches to Quality Improvement. http://www.ahrq.gov/professionals/prevention-chronic-care/improve/system/pfhandbook/mod4.html. Accessed March 17, 2016.

20. Institute for Healthcare Improvement. http://www.ihi.org/resources/Pages/HowtoImprove/default.aspx. Accessed March 17, 2016.

21. Schriefer J, Leonard M. Patient safety and quality improvement: an overview of QI. *Pediatr Rev*. 2012;33(8):353–359.

22. Lau CY. Quality improvement tools and processes. *Neurosurg Clin N Am*. 2015;26:177–187. http://dx.doi.org/10.1016/j.nec.2014.11.016.

23. Associates in Process Improvement. www.apiweb.org. Accessed March 17, 2016.

24. White BA, Baron JM, Dighe JS, Camargo Jr CA, Brown DF. Applying Lean methodologies reduces ED laboratory turnaround times. *Am J Emerg Med*. 2015;33:1572–1576.

25. iSixSigma. *Determine the root cause: the 5 whys*. http://www.isixsigma.com/tools-templates/cause-effect/determine-root-cause-5-whys/. Accessed March 15, 2016.

26. Quote Investigator. http://quoteinvestigator.com/2014/05/22/solve/. Accessed March 21, 2016.

27. Koning H, Verver J, Heuvel J, Bisgaard S, Does R. Lean Six Sigma in healthcare. *J Healthc Qual*. 2006;28(2):4–11.

28. Glasgow JM, Scott-Caziewell J, Kaboli P. Guiding inpatient quality improvement: a systematic review of Lean and Six Sigma. *Jt Comm J Qual Patient Saf*. 2010;36(12):533–540.

29. DelliFraine J, Wang Z, McCaughey D, Langabeer J, Erwin C. The use of Six Sigma in health care management: are we using it to its full potential? *Health Manage Q*. 2013;22(3):210–223.

30. Beeler PE, Bates DW, Hug BL. Clinical decision support systems. *Swiss Med Wkly*. 2014;144:w14073. http://dx.doi.org/10.4414/smw.2014.14073.

31. Ivers N, Jamtvedt G, Young J, et al. Audit and feedback: effects on professional practice and healthcare outcomes. *Cochrane Database Syst Rev*. 2012;Jun:6.

32. Conway J. Getting boards on board: engaging governing boards in quality and safety. *Jt Comm J Qual Pt Safety*. 2008;34(4):214–220.

33. Berwick DM. The science of improvement. *JAMA*. 2008;299(10):1182–1184.

34. Ogrinc G, Davies L, Goodman D, Batalden P, Davidoff F, Stevens D. SQUIRE 2.0 (Standards for Quality Improvement Reporting Excellence): revised publication guidelines from a detailed consensus process. *BMJ Quality and Safety*. 2015. http://dx.doi.org/10.1136/bmjqs-2015-004411. [Epub ahead of print.]

7

Principles of Teamwork and Team Science

Jason Higginson, MD, MA, and Donna M. Lake, PhD, RN, MEd

LEARNING OBJECTIVES

1. Understand the importance of teams to health systems science.
2. Define what composes a team and the hallmarks of effective teams.
3. Understand the relationship between teams and interprofessional practice.
4. Understand the theoretical considerations important to team education.

Health care is undergoing a revolution, moving from a lone provider model to one that embraces the recognition that the system of care is the essential element to the health of patients. The goals of the Triple Aim, improving quality, outcomes, and costs of health care delivery for patients and populations, requires teamwork and an understanding of team science. Teams working toward a common goal can improve health outcomes for individuals and communities. An understanding of teams, their structures, and critical elements will enable health professions students to fully engage in this critical component of the future of health care. This chapter outlines for health professions students the basic framework by which teams are formed, educated, and trained. This understanding of teams will be reinforced by a discussion of how interprofessional collaboration is the cornerstone of future health professions education. Focusing on both the theory and practice of team science will equip students with the necessary knowledge to be effective members and leaders of teams.

CHAPTER OUTLINE

I. INTRODUCTION—TEAMS, A CRITICAL ASPECT OF HEALTH SYSTEMS SCIENCE

In any human endeavor where complexity and multiple variables coexist with significant consequences for failure, risk is mitigated when teamwork and team performance are a focus of attention. The focus of this chapter is on teams, teamwork, **team science**, and interprofessional collaborative practice and their relationship to health care and **health systems science** (HSS). Effective teams and team membership are crucial elements to success in any undertaking that involves more than one individual. **High-reliability organizations (HROs)** operate in complex, hazardous environments making few mistakes over long periods of time. HROs are increasingly becoming a focus in HSS because of the recognition that they represent a model approach to HSS. A key aspect of HROs is their focus on teams.[1]

As noted in Chapter 2, the goals of HSS are improving understanding and application of the principles, methods, and practice of improving quality, outcomes, and costs of health care delivery for patients and populations within systems of medical care. Teams are an integral component of HSS. Applying lessons on teams from high-reliability organizations can inform those interested in HSS in the incorporation of teams and teamwork into health care environments. Notable HROs often studied for their incredible record of safety and attention to teamwork are aviation, naval nuclear propulsion, and civilian nuclear power generation. Cases studied in these environments demonstrate that failures are rarely the result of the actions of a single individual but are often the result of collective systems failures.[2] The root of these failures is often the result of elements of poor team performance such as communication failure, poor interpersonal interaction, and lack of role clarity.

The landmark Institute of Medicine report *To Err Is Human* found that potentially 98,000 preventable deaths occurred in the United States annually due to medical error.[3] One of the key recommendations from this report was the need to "establish interdisciplinary team training programs, such as simulation, that incorporate proven methods of team management." Understanding the attributes and theory behind team science will better prepare health care professions students to incorporate a team-centered focus into their career and will lead to significant improvement in achieving the goals of the Triple Aim—health for all individuals (population health), an ideal experience for all patients as they interface with the system (including quality and satisfaction), and achieving both at the lowest possible cost (reducing the per capita cost of health care).

II. THE PROMISE OF INTERPROFESSIONAL PRACTICE

The individual expert model prevalent today in health care must be transformed to a model that crosses disciplines, generations, professions, and groups—to a more team-based collaborative partnership, which will produce efficient, timely, high-quality, compassionate, and patient-centered care.

Teams are now recognized as a crucial element in HSS. Health care delivery systems involve numerous interfaces and patient handoffs among many health care professionals for any given patient regardless of the context of care. For example, in a 3-day hospital stay, a patient may interact with as many as 30 different professionals, including physicians, nurses, x-ray and laboratory technicians, nutritional staff, and transport team members. Team collaboration is essential to ensure that the diverse group of professionals interacting with patients on a daily basis integrates their activities with the patient's best interest at the center of their actions. Collaborative teamwork in health care is commonly referred to as **interprofessional practice.** The promise of interprofessional practice is "when multiple health workers from different professional backgrounds work together with patients, families, caregivers, and communities to deliver the highest quality of care."[4]

The growing complexity of health care mandates the need for team science education at all levels from health professions students to seasoned health professionals as it provides the basis for overhauling the health care system and improving health outcomes for individual patients and populations of patients. A growing plethora of publications over the last 3 decades has called for significant changes in health care systems due to the recognition that the United States is not achieving the best health outcomes for individuals or whole populations, yet the United States spends an exorbitant amount for poor-quality health care.

Interprofessional collaboration is universally noted to be a critical component to improve outcomes in health care. This recognition resulted in the Institute for Healthcare Improvement's (IHI) formulation of the Triple Aim: improving the patient experience of care, improving the health status of communities, and reducing the per capita

cost of health care.[5] The US health care system is the most costly in the world, accounting for 17 percent of the gross domestic product, with estimates that this percentage will grow to nearly 20 percent by 2020, yet with comparatively poorer outcomes.[6] The IHI developed the Triple Aim initiative as a statement of purpose, and it became the organizing framework for the United States' National Quality Strategy to improve health systems as it relates to high cost and poor clinical outcomes. The Center for Creative Leadership Model White Paper, *Collaborative Healthcare Leadership: Six part model for adapting and thriving during a time of transformative change* outlined "there is a need for rapid innovation and adaption to change, which will require collaborative, interdependent culture and solutions that cut across functions, regions, and professions."[7]

A. Defining Teams

What defines a team? Over the last half century, much work in the social sciences has been focused on defining what makes a team and what elements contribute to effective team performance. The National Academy of Sciences in 2015 released *Enhancing the Effectiveness of Team Science,* which aimed to summarize the state of this varied literature.[8] They identified the widely accepted definition of a team as *two or more individuals brought together by an organization who are working or interacting (face-to-face or virtually) on one or more institutionally important common goals or tasks and are assigned different roles and responsibilities while embedded in an encompassing organizational system with linkages to the broader system or task environment.*

Why are teams defined in this way? The prevailing heuristic that leads to this conclusion on the definition of a team is the input-process-output model developed by McGrath.[9] By studying groups of individuals working together, it becomes clear that input factors such as individual personalities and identities, individual skill, team task definition, and team structure and size alter the functioning of the team. Processes such as how teams are assembled and composed and the rules that govern interaction modulate many of the inputs and result in the team's ultimate output effectiveness (Fig. 7.1).

B. High-Performing Teams

Team effectiveness is defined by evaluating whether a team achieves its goals. References about effective teams in the medical literature frequently derive conclusions and parallels from studies of teams that function in fields other than

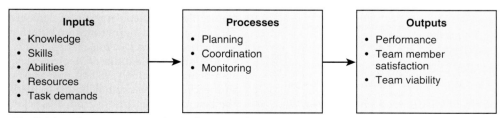

Fig. 7.1 Inputs-processes-outputs framework. (From King H, Battles J, Baker D, Alonso A. TeamSTEPPS™: Team Strategies and Tools to Enhance Performance and Patient Safety. In: Henriksen K, Battles JB, Keyes MA, Grady ML. *Advances in Patient Safety: New Directions and Alternative Approaches [Vol. 4: Technology and Medication Safety].* Washington, DC: Agency for Healthcare Research and Quality; 2008. http://www.ncbi.nlm.nih.gov/books/NBK43770/. Accessed December 29, 2015.)

health care. Given the unique nature of health care, it is important to note that these parallels should be reviewed with caution. The study of teams in health care is an area open to continued investigation as health care contains nuances that may alter the prevailing operational theories of team performance. Nonetheless, many common elements have been identified as characteristics of high-performing teams.[8]

First, teams with a shared understanding of their goal have been demonstrated to be significantly more effective than those without a universal understanding of their goal. If all members understand the output they are trying to achieve, it is more likely that efforts will be directed toward that goal. Second, clear definitions as to members' roles (i.e., role clarity) are another essential element in team effectiveness. By focusing on role clarity, teams are able to efficiently deploy the various skills that exist and reduce duplication of efforts to achieve defined goals. Third, team cohesion and low levels of conflict are critical to effective team performance. Teams must be cohesive and limit friction among members to ensure that effort by all will be utilized for goal achievement. When friction and disunity take hold, effort is often wasted or team members limit their participation. Building team cohesion results in trust among team members, facilitates task engagement, and facilitates team citizenship, all of which result in improved effectiveness. The elements of team effectiveness related to patient safety and quality improvement are displayed in Table 7.1.

Table 7.1 Teamwork Overview Quality and Patient Safety

Aspects of Teamwork	Examples of Safety-Relevant Characteristics
Quality of collaboration	Mutual respect Trust
Shared mental models	Strength of shared goals Shared perception of a situation Shared understanding of team structure, team task, team roles, etc.
Coordination	Adaptive coordination (e.g., dynamic task allocation when new members join the team; shift between explicit and implicit forms of coordination; increased information exchange and planning in critical situations)
Communication	Openness of communication Quality of communication (e.g., shared frames of reference) Specific communication practices (e.g., team briefing)
Leadership	Leadership style (e.g., value contributions from staff, encourage participation in decision-making) Adaptive leadership behavior (e.g., increased explicit leadership behavior in critical situations)

From King H, Battles J, Baker D, Alonso A. TeamSTEPPS™: Team Strategies and Tools to Enhance Performance and Patient Safety. In: Henriksen K, Battles JB, Keyes MA, Grady ML. *Advances in Patient Safety: New Directions and Alternative Approaches (Vol. 4: Technology and Medication Safety)*. Washington, DC: Agency for Healthcare Research and Quality; 2008. http://www.ncbi.nlm.nih.gov/books/NBK43770/. Accessed December 29, 2015.

C. Leading Teams

The effectiveness of a team is a function of both its assembly and subsequent leadership.[10] Leadership is not the focus of this chapter and will be discussed in more depth in Chapter 8, but this chapter will examine the basic elements as they pertain to teams now. Reflection on observed styles of leadership by health professions students can help draw the link between observed team performance and leadership performance. Leadership can be loosely defined as the behavior of an individual or group that directs the activities of a group or organization toward a desired goal. Leading requires a diverse array of talents: vision, strategy, resource allocation, operational tactics, professionalism, inspiration, integrity, emotional intelligence, and mission-mindedness, to name but a few of the necessary qualities. Over the last century, many theories regarding effective leadership have been explored and developed, often in fields other than health care. However, understanding the various leadership models that have emerged can inform the growing health care leader as to potential approaches to leadership.[11]

First, there is the transformational leader who encourages goal achievement through mobilizing the team to selfless service in the pursuit of the team goal. This leadership type often relies on charisma to encourage and inspire team members to join the mission. This model of leadership relies heavily on the leader's vision and powers of persuasion. While this may be an effective leadership style, it may not suit every leader's abilities, and some question its utility in health care as the health system seeks mission-mindedness and agendas that center on patient's desires as opposed to goals being set by those in health care leadership.

Second, there is the transactional leader, which is based largely on reward and penalties. In this form of leadership, the leader sets goals, and team members are either rewarded or suffer consequences if goals are not met. This model of leading is very prevalent in health care and the easiest to establish because the motivation for the team is extrinsic. Goals, penalties, and rewards are provided and set by the leader. Some argue that the extrinsic nature of the transactional model is its greatest weakness. In health care, it is commonly recognized that most people are internally motivated to care for people, and the transactional method has the potential to undermine that motivation.

The third leadership style to consider is that of the adaptive leader. An adaptive leader is one who confronts hard realities with truth. This leadership style is one in which core beliefs and values are emphasized and focused on to influence change. An adaptive leader focuses on organizational justice (i.e., "telling it like it is"). This can be an effective leadership style because it allows team members to gain a clear understanding as to where they stand and how they are doing. Some argue that this approach is a key element of trust building. Further, it is argued that the candidness of this approach encourages teams to have full engagement in problem solving as all members are aware of where problems lie and are more likely to come to collaborative solutions. It takes a great deal of emotional intelligence to lead by this method, and some argue that the hard conversations involved with leading this way may not always result in a motivated team due to individual sensitivities among team members.

Finally, there is the servant leader, who is focused on the needs of others, particularly those on the team. This leadership style is characterized by a leader who listens to team members, empathizes with them, and encourages and enables them to reach their full potential. This leadership style is thought by some to serve health care well, although some question if a lack of an imperative for results inhibits the servant leader in the current metric-driven health care environment.

The reality of considering various leadership models is that in most contexts some elements from each will be necessary. Each leader and team will be unique and require different techniques to achieve team goals. Leadership of a team can be approached in a myriad of ways, and no one approach or person will be suited to every situation. However, what is generally accepted is that effective leaders foster an environment in which mutual respect and support develop, a common vision and goal for the team is established, communication is appropriate, and conflict is managed within the team.

The science defining what constitutes effective leadership is difficult to evaluate, as leadership is difficult to define and measure. Regardless of the strategies employed, leading a team requires a balance of coaching and directive approaches. Knowing team dynamics, understanding the change process, and bringing the best out of individuals contribute to effective team functioning. Making the study of leadership an aim in health professions education will allow students to think more deeply about leadership, hone and practice leadership skills, and reflect on their strengths and weaknesses.

D. Constructing Teams

As much as the leader influences the effectiveness of a team, the team members are equally important. Selecting team personnel is an important process, and individual members must possess the knowledge, skills, and attitudes to accomplish the defined goal. However, team membership is not always a completely volitional process. Often team members are drawn from the already assembled workforce. Outlining the essential attributes required of the team prior to team assembly is a critical step in developing a successful team. Thought should be employed in explicitly defining what the goal will be and what tasks will need to be accomplished and by whom. Clear expectations as to the requisite knowledge, skills, and attitudes should be applied to team selection. Identifying who will be empowered to perform the various tasks needed to achieve the goal will inform decisions as to membership needs. In most circumstances in which teams are drawn from already established work pools, it is incumbent that leaders take into account the various knowledge, skills, and attitudes of those assigned to the team and ascribe roles that are commensurate with the talents available.

Choosing the appropriate team size is equally important to membership as it relates to effectiveness. Team size influences communication patterns as well as the ability to meet, assign tasks, and redirect activity toward goal achievement. After the team is assembled, some thought should be employed to define the operational rules of the team: when and how communication and meetings will occur, method for reaching decisions, and who possesses decision-making rights. Understanding team growth and dynamics will allow a leader to anticipate and respond to the challenges faced while leading a team.

Case Study 1

The discharge of orthopedic surgical patients on Unit 5B is frequently delayed due to late and/or incomplete discharge orders from the medical team. This delay in the timeliness of the discharge process results in patient confusion regarding departure from the medical faculty and causes increased patient frustration with a prolonged discharge process. In addition, the delay in discharge creates bottlenecks and delays in the pharmacy, delaying discharge medication retrieval and preventing or truncating nurse discharge teaching. Finally, as an added problem, the backup results in a lack of bed availability for new surgical patients on this unit.

Who are the members of the interprofessional health care team involved in this process?

What are the possible consequences of the poorly functioning team on Unit 5B beyond those stated in this case study?

Where could this process be improved and by whom?

How could this health care team improve its effectiveness and provide a positive patient experience?

The interprofessional team in this situation is everyone involved in the care of the patient (doctors, nurses, and pharmacists) and the patients themselves. Breakdown in this discharge process can have significant ramifications for the patient. Medical errors can occur due to the patient not being fully informed as to discharge instructions and medication use. Patients could suffer significantly and become frustrated with the increasing risks of delayed and rushed discharges. Staff discord could mount as the ability to complete assigned tasks becomes more challenging due to wasted time waiting for orders to initiate tasks. The process of discharge requires multiple levels of communication and will require the formation of a team among all involved. First, the medical team can define and communicate the patient goals/factors that will result in discharge following admission or surgery. Predefining the goals and communicating them to other staff on the team can allow for anticipation of possible discharges. Once anticipated, staff can be proactive in requesting discharge orders once a patient meets predefined parameters, instead of waiting for the medical team to re-evaluate the patient. Secondly, communication between the pharmacy and the physician/nursing team can establish a mechanism to review the patient's medications and anticipate potential discharge orders prior to actual discharge. This process can allow early ordering and teaching of medication information, reducing the rush on the day of discharge and likely improving communication. Decreasing wait time, patient knowledge, and setting and meeting expectations through these processes have been demonstrated to reduce errors and increase patient satisfaction.

E. Stages of Team Development

Health professionals and more specifically health professions students are frequently joining new teams as part of their everyday experience. Teams constantly change and progress through well-recognized stages. Reflection on the stages of team development can provide insight for health professions students as they examine the teams they join. Students may note that their experiences on highly effective teams are a reflection of a team that is mature in team development, and this may contrast with dysfunctional teams that are low performing and have yet to build trust and team cohesion.

There are four well-established stages of team development:

- **Stage 1—Forming:** exploration and building trust
- **Stage 2—Storming:** attitude changes, competitiveness and tension, disunity
- **Stage 3—Norming:** satisfaction, respect development, decision-making
- **Stage 4—Performing:** high level of interaction, performance increased and optimized, and confidence within the team[1]

In stage 1, team members are identified, group goals are set, and the members begin to understand the capabilities of the various team members. Once the team is formed, stage 2 begins and roles and responsibilities are delineated, and patterns of communication are established. This can be one of the more difficult phases to progress through, as there are numerous points where tension and disunity can develop. It is important to note that leadership is essential in this phase to ensure open communication despite conflict, or tension becomes the norm. This will help to maintain those valuable to the team as team members and prevent transitions of the disgruntled to the sidelines. It must be noted that this does not mean that harmony and consensus must reign but that collegiality in the face of disagreement must become the norm.

Stage 3 begins when team trust is established. This allows for effort toward achieving the team's goals to begin. During this stage, team members come to understand that they can rely on one another's abilities and can disagree openly with maintenance of mutual respect. Finally, the last stage is that of a mature team where a shared common goal has been established, trust is a norm, and productive work is performed with efficiency.

Not all teams mature through these stages. However, growth through these stages will result in teams that exhibit backup behavior in which team members compensate for each other, manage conflict within the team, regularly provide feedback, and self-correct.[1] The definition of an effective team is *a goal-driven group of individuals with a common shared mental model for success that exhibit mutual aid and trust and who are able to achieve its desired end state.*

III. TEAMS AND COLLABORATION

Zwarenstein and colleagues reviewed the existing literature relevant to interprofessional collaboration and noted measurable changes in patient outcomes when structured processes for interaction and collaboration were initiated.[12] Their findings highlight a key concept in evaluating teamwork: Is organized collaboration teamwork? Often in the literature, the concepts of teams, teamwork, and collaboration are used synonymously.[13]

For the most part, this is a reasonable approach, but it is important to note that the commitment to a common goal may not be as strong or made as explicit in a collaborative setting as it is with a clearly defined team. Recall that the definition of a team makes explicit that the group objective is a common goal, whereas in collaboration some goals may overlap, but individuals may not share the same priority. In HSS, there is an overarching goal for collaborative efforts: health for all individuals, an ideal experience, and achieving both at the lowest possible cost. Given this context, studies citing outcomes for interprofessional collaboration in health care are relevant to evaluating team performance. Zwarenstein and colleagues note in their review of the collaborative practice literature that there is a relatively low sample size of studies, and many interventions have yet to be replicated, but the evidence that exists suggests collaboration does improve outcomes.

IV. EVALUATING TEAMS AND TEAMWORK

Specifically demonstrating the connection between teamwork and actual patient outcomes or successful goal achievement, as noted, remains challenging.[14] The reason for this difficulty is that evaluation of teamwork requires quantification of complex behaviors that do not in and of themselves directly correlate to the desired outcome,[15] but the utilization of a validated and reliable scoring tool can provide valuable feedback to a team and redirect the efforts of teams. There are numerous tools available. The key considerations in tool selection are determining if the selected tool is applicable to the team environment it will be used to evaluate.[16]

The main domains generally evaluated by the available tools examine one or more of four aspects of teamwork and/or team training: attitude, comprehension, behavior, and process. As discussed earlier, a high-functioning team has a shared vision for success, and this can readily be measured by assessing the attitudes and understanding of team members in relation to team goals. There is growing literature demonstrating that awareness of goals does alter patient outcomes. A good example comes from infection-control research demonstrating that knowledge of hygiene goals such as hand washing will increase rates of hand washing and decrease nosocomial infections. The behavioral assessment tools available usually measure communication and coordination between team members. While these are clearly important elements of teamwork, the available literature is not as robust regarding the measured effect on health outcomes. The literature that does exist in this area is often from the procedural specialties and does demonstrate improved performance with better communication from team members. However, it is likely safe to assume, and there is growing evidence to support the notion, that higher levels of communication and coordination are desirable in all areas and will improve outcomes and increase value in health care. Finally, process assessments measure rates at which teams complete or utilize a prescribed process. Again, these have been demonstrated in procedural specialties such as surgery, anesthesia, and intensive care to improve coordination of efforts, increase role clarity, and enhance care delivery.

Regardless of the noted difficulty in measuring team performance, it is generally acknowledged that evaluating the function of teams is an important aspect of improved patient safety and quality of care. Tools available to health system leaders increase every day and are available and applicable in numerous environments in which teams operate in health care.

CASE STUDY 2

Dr. Johnson is a solo family physician who works in a rural area. He prides himself on his dedication and commitment to maintaining his practice at the cutting edge of evidence-based medicine. He no longer admits his patients to his local hospital because it has moved to a hospitalist model; he still follows their progress while admitted and sees them in his office once discharged. Recently, he has noted wide variation in management of his patients with regard to medication use and length of stay. He feels that he could make some suggestions to the hospitalist team since he is current on the literature and is in the unique position of seeing the variation that exists.

Is there a need for a team in this situation?

What should be the goal of the team?

How might a team help?

How should Dr. Johnson approach forming a team with the hospitalists?

Who should lead this team, what factors might decide this choice?

There is a need to form a team in this situation. The goals of HSS are to improve individual patient and population outcomes, better patient experiences, and increase value of care. Dr. Johnson's recognition of the wide variation of practice among the hospitalists suggests that there is likely an opportunity to improve both individual and population outcomes. A team approach to this problem could help align everyone's efforts, build consensus as to best practices, and alert people to alternative opinions within the group. This level of alignment can improve inpatient care by ensuring that practice is based on evidence and decreasing staff confusion through a common approach. Outpatient care will likewise benefit as the bond and communication to the inpatient area will likely improve through team interaction. Dr. Johnson's approach to forming a team with the hospitalists will be critical to achieving success. How Dr. Johnson frames the issue will determine interest levels and commitment. It is critical to not alienate the hospitalists through accusations, but to solicit help in solving a problem. In health care, forming teams often involves getting people to rally behind a shared common aspiration. Dr. Johnson should frame this as intending to improve patient outcomes. In this situation, choosing a leader is critical. Often leaders are assigned by organizations; here there is no mandate to form a team thus no clear leader. Leadership will reside in whoever is passionate about the task at hand. Dr. Johnson, having identified the problem and having concern for the outcome, is an obvious choice. However, Dr. Johnson's role as leader may change as the work progresses if others are interested or the work to be done is more on the inpatient side.

V. UNDERSTANDING HEALTH SYSTEMS, SYSTEMS THINKING, AND TEAMS

Systems thinking is a crucial element of any HSS endeavor, as described in Chapter 2. Systems thinking allows recognition, understanding, and synthesis of the complex interdependencies and relationships within a functional system like health care. The components of a system are the constantly changing workings of a multilayered organization. The ability to recognize patterns and repetitions of daily interactions and how they work together in accomplishing a specific purpose is essential to maximizing the outcome of those interactions.[17] Systems thinking allows the formation of linkages among disparate areas of activity in health care to advance the overarching goal of HSS: improving outcomes, patient experience, and value in health care. Competency in HSS requires that health professions students understand how patient care relates to the health system as a whole and how to use the system to improve the quality, experience, and value of patient care. Health professions students are therefore expected to demonstrate an awareness of and responsiveness to the larger context and system of health care, as well as the ability to call effectively on other resources in the system to provide optimal health care.[18]

The ability to proficiently perform within the context of a health system as part of a team and the ability to utilize the full health care team is essential to HSS. Overall, the systems thinking HSS competencies for health professions students include the following:

- Work effectively and understand the microsystem they inhabit.
- Understand how their microsystem interacts with other microsystems in the formation of a mesosystem and macrosystem.
- Understand where and how patients encounter the health care system.
- Understand community-based components of the system.
- Understand population health.
- Understand health care finance, reform, and value-based care.

All of these competencies require teamwork.

A. Teamwork and the National Landscape

Teamwork and teams are now widely regarded by national organizations as a critical element of the national approach to quality and patient safety. Various agencies are defining how teamwork relates to their diverse activities including: regulation and policy, education, clinical practice standards, professional networks, and community outreach.

The Health Resources and Services Administration (HRSA), an agency of the US Department of Health and Human Services, is the primary federal agency charged with improving health and achieving health equity through access to quality services and a skilled health workforce. The HRSA directs its efforts by coordinating the efforts of 90-plus programs and more than 3000 grantees. One way HRSA has demonstrated the contribution of teams and systems thinking in patient safety and health outcomes is with its Patient Safety and Clinical Pharmacy Services Collaborative (PSPC).

The PSPC reported in May 2013 the results of a team-based initiative that included 344 teams of community health providers, representing more than 885 organizations of community-based health care providers across 48 States, the District of Columbia, Puerto Rico, and the Virgin Islands.[19] Team members represented community health centers, hospitals, and schools of pharmacy, nursing, and medicine. This PSPC teamwork initiative decreased adverse drug events that caused harm to patients, with an average improvement of 40 percent for a high-risk patient population between 2009 and 2010. Numerous different approaches to similar problems were observed reflecting different local needs. Success was achieved by allowing organizations participating in the initiative the ability to identify their own needs, their own delivery system, and key processes that needed attention. Another key finding was the importance of widening the definition of the team and including patients in the solutions. Patient needs and expectations were drivers of many of the team-based innovations.

B. Interprofessional Collaborative Practice and Competencies: Improving Health Care Through Relationships

A critical turning point in health over the last decade was the release of *Health Professions Education: A Bridge to Quality* by the Institute of Medicine,[20] which identified the core competencies needed for health care professionals of the future (Fig. 7.2). The report emphasized that health professionals should be educated to deliver patient-centered care as members of a team, emphasizing evidence-based practice, quality improvement approaches, and informatics.

The World Health Organization prepared a framework and definition for interprofessional education and collaborative practice that is widely accepted:

Interprofessional education occurs when students from two or more professions learn about, from, and with each other to enable effective collaboration and improve health outcomes. Once students understand how to work interprofessionally, they are ready to enter the workplace as a member of the collaborative practice team. This is a key step in moving health systems from fragmentation to a position of strength.[4]

This recognition that interprofessional education represented a critical aspect of the future of health care lead to the formation in 2009 of the Interprofessional Education Collaborative (IPEC) by six US education associations of health professions to promote and encourage constituent efforts that would advance substantive interprofessional learning experiences to help prepare future health professionals for enhanced team-based care and improved population health outcomes. The IPEC organizations represent allopathic and osteopathic medicine, dentistry, nursing, pharmacy, and public health. The IPEC created core competencies for interprofessional collaborative practice to guide curricula development across health professions schools. Examination of the IPEC core competencies can enhance understanding of the essential elements that will help an interprofessional team be successful.

IPEC core competencies for interprofessional collaborative practice include four domains. The first domain centers on changing the manner in which formation of professional identity is approached. The underlying philosophical principle guiding this is recognition that health care is an ethical pursuit. Situating the learner's ethical obligations around his or her role as a member of a health care team would advance interconnectedness among health care professions. Previously, professional identity formed in ways that fostered silos and separation of the various health professions, each with a separate perception of their ethical obligations. The IPEC advances the notion that emphasizing the common ethical imperative of collaborative practice and patient-centeredness will be critical in development of an interprofessional ethos in health care education, practice, and teams.

The second domain focuses on ensuring that health professions students understand and can articulate their roles and responsibilities and how these relate to the roles and responsibilities of others on the health care team. Diversity of capabilities is identified as the underpinning of functional teams. Further, the ability to evaluate and understand the capabilities of team members fosters an environment of trust and support. Inaccurate understanding of role scope and capabilities can lead to friction and poor team performance due to mismatched expectations and abilities.

The third domain focuses on communication among health professionals. It has long been known that

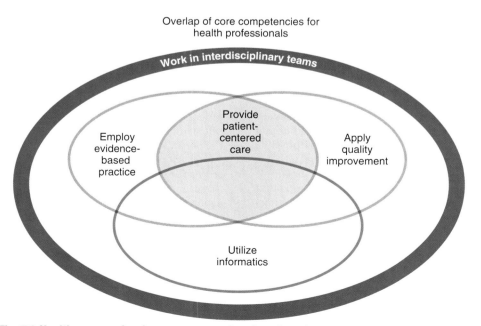

Overlap of core competencies for health professionals

Work in interdisciplinary teams

Employ evidence-based practice

Provide patient-centered care

Apply quality improvement

Utilize informatics

Fig. 7.2 **Health care professions core competencies.** (From Greiner A, Knebel E. *Health Professions Education: A Bridge to Quality.* Washington, DC: National Academies Press; 2003.)

communication is an essential element of teamwork. It is now becoming clear that communication among interprofessional teams is an essential element needed in health professions education. Communication patterns and abilities set the mode and manner of team interactions. Poor patterns that are heavy in non-shared jargon disrupt teamwork. Clear communication with a shared lexicon and mutually agreed pattern and method improves team functioning.

The fourth and last IPEC domain is teams and teamwork. Forming and functioning as a team is a complex task. Education for health professionals needs to focus on the elements of team performance shown to improve effectiveness. There is an imperative that health care move to a paradigm with shared accountability for the outcomes of the patients being cared for by the health care system. Shared accountability can be seen as setting a common team goal by which all members understand they have a role to play in the eventual outcome. For this notion to take root, shared problem solving, shared decision making, relinquishing of professional sovereignty with acceptance of group dynamics, and acceptance of shared expertise will be vital.

For the competencies contained in these four domains to become an integral part of health care teams, they must become part of the everyday environment in health care. This will begin to be the case when students of all the health care disciplines learn together routinely, practice as teams, and gain clinical skills in a team-focused environment. Institutions will need to make this a priority and develop faculty capable of leading the transition to team-based care. Students will need to be evaluated and mentored not only in the knowledge, skills, and attitudes necessary for their chosen career specialty, but also in their performance as a member of a team.

CASE STUDY 3

A neonatal intensive care unit's quality council is reviewing yearly quality data and discovers that the unit is performing very poorly in central-line–associated blood stream infections. Everyone is dismayed and turns to the medical director for guidance. The medical director immediately recognizes this as a major concern. She states up front that she is not sure how to solve the problem, but that addressing it is her top priority for the unit going forward. She immediately begins to alert everyone who works in the unit of the quality council's discovery and begins to solicit people who are interested in helping solve the problem and elicit their opinions for possible solutions. After forming the team, she discovers that a number of newly hired nurses do not know the unit policy for maintaining central lines. She also is informed that the pharmacy has recently changed vendors for total parenteral nutrition (TPN) and that the new vendor's TPN bags require a workaround by the nurses to connect to the unit's IV tubing. During a team meeting, her charge nurse informs her that she has a friend who works in a nearby unit that had the same issue and now has not had an infection in over 500 days. That unit has a bundle of interventions they are confident led to their success. What has the NICU director done well in this process? What stage is this team currently in in team formation? What is this team's way forward?

The NICU director has done a number of things well in leading this process. First, she was very responsive to the unit council's concerns regarding the infection problem, immediately raising the issue and soliciting help and solutions. Communication is a critical element of any successful team. The NICU director's communication resulted in numerous findings from the staff that may have a direct bearing on fixing the problem. Further, her communication with the team resulted in her charge nurse discovering another team with the same problem and a potential solution. That team is currently formed, has well-established communication and trust with many potential solutions in place, and is, therefore, entering the final stage of team development. The way forward for this team is to evaluate the information they have received, adapt that information to the local situation, communicate the plan to the unit, and enact the plan. The team has to manage the change process and ensure that points of tension and friction are promptly managed. Continual messaging of the overall goal is needed as well as keeping everyone well informed of intended changes. Establishing feedback mechanisms on the impact of the changes is also critical.

VI. TEAM TRAINING

A. Educating Teams—Theory

While teams are part of everyday experience, forming and maintaining effective teams is not routinely taught. Understanding the methods and theories by which people learn is an essential aspect of developing teams and teamwork. It is only part of the job to understand the competencies that are necessary for effective teams to operate. It is equally important to understand how those competencies are transmitted to health professions students and practitioners. Further, as discussed earlier, health care is only now realizing the need for health professions students to learn together before they can work together as a team.

Theories about learning are plentiful and have rich published explorations, which are beyond the scope of this chapter. However, it is important to note the basics of these theories, which inform how education on teams may be enhanced. There are broad categories of learning theory that need to be considered when thinking about interprofessional education (IPE); behaviorist theory focuses on the outcomes of learning or behaviors, cognitivist theory emphasizes the role of internal thought, and constructivist theory focuses on the person who is learning.[21,22]

Behaviorists posit that learning occurs through trial and error and experientially. Further, all learning results in outcomes that can be measured. Thus, IPE models that take a behaviorist approach often focus on what can be measured at the end of the education process and find methods to ensure that desired behaviors are learned. The learning may be reinforced by rewarding the desired behaviors. Using a behaviorist model can result in learners who exhibit significant behavioral change due to the inherent capacity of students to focus on what they know will be rewarded. However, some argue that this ignores an important element of education such as thoughtfulness about why actions are being taken. Behaviorist models can at times fail to reinforce reflection by students as to why they are doing what they are doing and the consequences of such learned behavior.

Cognitivist and constructivist theories, which address the process of learning and the learner, aim to establish higher-order skills that build patterns of problem solving and insight. These theories form the foundation for commonly used experiential learning models such as problem-based learning or inquiry-based learning. The tenets of these educational theories are reflected in the key assumptions of adult learning theory. These tenets state that adults are self-directed and independent, tap into previous experience to inform current learning, value learning that has a direct impact on their daily experience and problems, and respond to internal motivation above external motivation. Proponents of cognitivist/constructivist theory feel that students in these models will change their behavior because they have an awareness of the reasons behind the need for a given pattern of action.

It is likely that some coupling of all the various educational models will be necessary to develop best practices for education on teams to impact patient safety and quality in health care (Fig. 7.3). It will be equally important to be able to ensure that behaviors change through reward and feedback while simultaneously ensuring that students are equipped with the higher-order problem-solving abilities necessary to meet challenges that are not easily identified.

B. Educating Teams—Practice (Models for Medical Team Training)

As discussed earlier, recognition that teams are the base unit that will improve health care and achieve national patient safety objectives derives from work teaching teamwork in other industries. The easiest example to cite and the archetype most often followed for medical team training is that of commercial aviation. The flight industry has a fatal mishap rate of 0.2 lives lost per every 1 million miles of travel. This represents a 6-fold decrease in fatalities since the 1970s and is a remarkable achievement given that air travel has seen increasing volume over that same time period.[23] Aviation

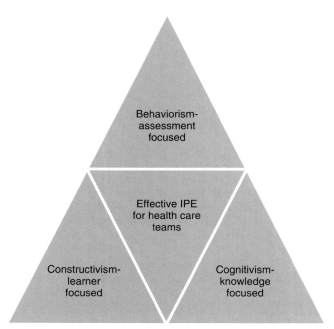

Fig. 7.3 Learning theory and effective interprofessional education.

adopted the team training model known as Crew Resource Management (CRM). CRM was a response by the aviation industry to an alarming number of fatal accidents that occurred in the late 1970s and early 1980s. The aim of CRM was to change the aviation industry culture from an individualistic pilot-centric culture to one that embraced the team concept of safety. No longer did all direction and corrective monitoring sit with one individual, the pilot, but the entire team was responsible for the safe operation of the aircraft. This was not an easy transition, and formation of team ethos did not occur by decree. An active process was necessary to change the industry standard; CRM became that standard. A similar shift is ongoing in health care.

Prior to the CRM movement, a pilot was solely evaluated on the technical skills of flying; performance as a team member was not evaluated. CRM utilized full team simulation to evaluate team performance, in particular, situational awareness, metacognition of team members (i.e., "do team members have insight into their thought patterns?"), shared mental models, and efficiency of resource management. These are all the hallmarks of functional teams. Another aspect of CRM is that it progresses through three phases. Phase one is indoctrination and awareness, characterized by development of a shared vision for safe operations of an aircraft, shared vocabulary, and shared expectations for interpersonal interaction and decision making. CRM also reframes outdated leadership expectations and focuses on standard operating procedures. Phase one is accomplished through didactic lectures, group discussion, and analysis of cases, and role-playing training/simulation exercises. Often CRM is modulated in response to surveys from crews as to areas of perceived need or poor performance.

Phase two is characterized by recurrent training. No matter how well executed the indoctrination is, ongoing reinforcement and practice is a key to successful CRM training. Further, team needs may change over time, and assessment and redirection is often needed to maintain team skills and focus.

Phase three is continuous reinforcement that is characterized by focusing on CRM concepts outside of the training environment. This is often accomplished by making the CRM concepts part of mishap reporting and standard performance evaluations. Applying the concepts this way sends the message that CRM is an important aspect of everyday operations.

The success of CRM in aviation has seen its adaptation to health care in the form of medical team training (MTT). The most common team-training method discussed in health care is Team Strategies and Tools to Enhance Performance and Patient Safety (TeamSTEPPS). TeamSTEPPS is derived from collaboration between the Department of Defense Patient Safety Program, TRICARE Management Activity, and Agency for Healthcare Research and Quality and was rolled out in 2006.[24] TeamSTEPPS focuses on many of the areas discussed in this chapter that lead to teams becoming high functioning. It has the broadest application of the various programs that exist because it is not based on any one health care discipline but is targeted at team concepts in general. The four main areas of focus are leadership, situation monitoring, mutual support, and communication (Fig. 7.4).

TeamSTEPPS is taught via a mixture of didactic lectures, discussions, and simulation events. Much like CRM, it is multistep process from initial training to sustainment (Fig. 7.5).

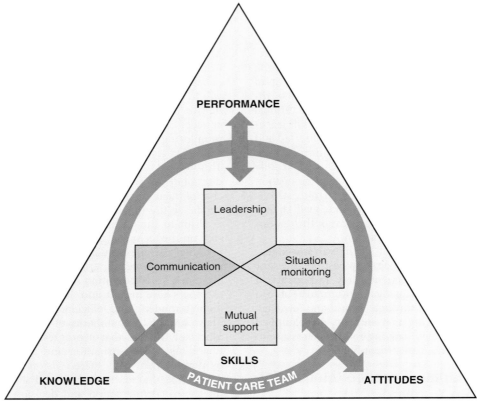

Fig. 7.4 **TeamSTEPPS instructional framework.** (From King H, Battles J, Baker D, Alonso A. Team-STEPPS™: Team Strategies and Tools to Enhance Performance and Patient Safety. In: Henriksen K, Battles JB, Keyes MA, Grady ML. *Advances in Patient Safety: New Directions and Alternative Approaches [Vol. 4: Technology and Medication Safety]*. Washington, DC: Agency for Healthcare Research and Quality; 2008. ht tp://www.ncbi.nlm.nih.gov/books/NBK43770/. Accessed December 29, 2015.)

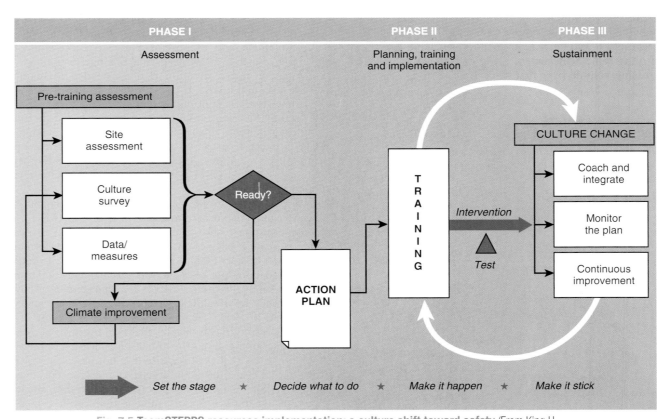

Fig. 7.5 **TeamSTEPPS resources implementation: a culture shift toward safety** (From King H, Battles J, Baker D, Alonso A. TeamSTEPPS™: Team Strategies and Tools to Enhance Performance and Patient Safety. In: Henriksen K, Battles JB, Keyes MA, Grady ML. *Advances in Patient Safety: New Directions and Alternative Approaches [Vol. 4: Technology and Medication Safety]*. Washington, DC: Agency for Healthcare Research and Quality; 2008. http://www.ncbi.nlm.nih.gov/books/NBK43770/. Accessed December 29, 2015.)

There are numerous other programs available for team training. Some of these are specifically focused and include Anesthesia Crisis Resource Management, which brings CRM concepts to anesthesia, and Team-Oriented Medical Simulation, which focuses on the entire operating room.

VII. CHAPTER SUMMARY

The study of HSS essentials, the third science, is increasingly recognized as equally important as learning the clinical and basic sciences. All three areas of expertise have equal applicability to health care's ultimate goal of delivering high-quality care as safely as possible. Outlined in this chapter are the critical pieces to forming and maintaining high-performing teams and the role teams play in interprofessional collaborative practice. Health care is evolving with the goal of improving patient care, experience, and value. These goals form the framework for HSS, and teamwork and team science are the critical connection between plans and execution in any health care setting. Attention to the aspects of teams, team functions, leadership, education, and training will be essential to achieving mastery of HSS and advancing the goals of high-quality and high-value patient care.

QUESTIONS FOR FURTHER THOUGHT

1. What is the definition of a team?
2. What are the qualities present on an effective team?
3. What are the four defined stages of team formation?
4. Why are teams critical to health systems science?

Annotated Bibliography

Cooke NJ, Hilton ML, eds. *Enhancing the Effectiveness of Team Science.* Washington, DC: National Academies Press; 2015.
This National Academy of Sciences report determines what is currently known about the processes and products of team science and the circumstances under which investments in team-based research are most likely to yield intellectually novel discoveries and demonstrable improvements in contemporary social, environmental, and public health problems.

Gordon S, Mendenhall P, O'Connor B. *Beyond the Checklist: What Else Health Care Can Learn from Aviation Teamwork and Safety.* Ithaca, NY: ILR Press; 2012.
An overview of teamwork and crew resource management strategies learned in aviation and applied to the medical setting.

Hopkins D. *Framework for Action on Interprofessional Education and Collaborative Practice.* Geneva: World Health Organization; 2010.
The Framework for Action on Interprofessional Education and Collaborative Practice highlights the current status of interprofessional collaboration around the world and identifies the mechanisms that shape successful collaborative teamwork.

Lekka C. *High Reliability Organisations: A Review of the Literature.* Derbyshire, United Kingdom: Health and Safety Executive Books; 2011.
Peer-reviewed papers that discuss the processes and practices in place in high-reliability organizations.

Zwarenstein M, Goldman J, Reeves S. Interprofessional collaboration: effects of practice-based interventions on professional practice and healthcare outcomes. *Cochrane Database Syst Rev.* 2009;Jul 8(3).
This review suggests that practice-based IPC interventions can improve health care processes and outcomes.

References

1. Baker D, Day R, Salas E. Teamwork as an essential component of high-reliability organizations. *Health Serv Res.* 2006;41(4 Pt 2):1576–1598.
2. Lekka C. *High Reliability Organisations: A Review of the Literature.* Derbyshire, United Kingdom: Health and Safety Executive Books; 2011.
3. Kohn LT, Corrigan JM, Donaldson MS. *To Err Is Human.* Washington, DC: National Academies Press; 1999.
4. Hopkins D. *Framework for Action on Interprofessional Education and Collaborative Practice.* Geneva: World Health Organization; 2010.
5. Stiefel M, Nolan K. *A Guide to Measuring the Triple Aim: Population Health, Experience of Care, and Per Capita Cost.* IHI Innovation Series white paper. Cambridge: Institute for Healthcare Improvement; 2012.
6. Centers for Medicare & Medicaid Services. NHE fact sheet. https://www.cms.gov/Research-Statistics-Data-and-Systems/Statistics-Trends-and-Reports/NationalHealthExpendData/NHE_Fact_Sheet.html. Updated March 26, 2012. Accessed December 29, 2015.
7. Browning H, Torain D, Patterson T. Collaborative healthcare leadership: a six-part model for adapting and thriving during a time of transformative change. Center for Creative Leadership. http://www.executivenursefellows.org/cms_docs/CollaborativeHealthcareLeadership.pdf. Issued September 2011. Accessed December 29, 2015.
8. Cooke NJ, Hilton ML, eds. *Enhancing the Effectiveness of Team Science.* Washington, DC: National Academies Press; 2015.
9. McGrath JE. *Social Psychology: A Brief Introduction.* New York: Holt, Rhinehart and Winston; 1964.
10. Fiore SM. Interdisciplinarity as teamwork: how the science of teams can inform team science. *Small Group Research.* 2008;39(3):251–277.
11. Trastek V, Hamilton N, Niles E. Leadership models in health care—a case for servant leadership. *Mayo Clin Proc.* 2014;89(3):374–381.
12. Zwarenstein M, Goldman J, Reeves S. Interprofessional collaboration: effects of practice-based interventions on professional practice and healthcare outcomes. *Cochrane Database Syst Rev.* 2009;Jul 8(3).
13. Yan X, Parker S, Manser T. Teamwork and collaboration. *Rev Hum Factors Ergon.* 2013:55–102.
14. Manser T. Teamwork and patient safety in dynamic domains of healthcare: a review of the literature. *Acta Anaesthesiol Scand.* 2009;53(2):143–151.
15. Whittaker G, Abboudi H, Khan S, Dasgupta P, Ahmed K. Teamwork assessment tools in modern surgical practice: a systematic review. *Surg Res Prac.* 2015;2015:494827.
16. Rosen M, Weaver S, Lazzara E. Tools for evaluating team performance in simulation-based training. *J Emerg Trauma Shock.* 2010;3(4):353–359.
17. Nelson E, Batalden P, Lazar J. *Practice-Based Learning and Improvement: A Clinical Improvement Action Guide Joint Commission Resource.* Oakbrook Terrace, IL: Joint Commission Resources; 2012.
18. Swing SR. The ACGME outcome project: retrospective and prospective. *Med Teach.* 2007;29(7):648–654.
19. Health Resources and Services Administration. *The National Quality Strategy.* http://www.ahrq.gov/workingforquality/pias/pspcpia.htm. Published 2015. Accessed December 29, 2015.
20. Greiner A, Knebel E. *Health Professions Education: A Bridge to Quality.* Washington, DC: National Academies Press; 2003.
21. Ertmer P, Newby T. Behaviorism, cognitivism, constructivism: comparing critical features from an instructional design perspective. *Performance Improvement Quarterly.* 2013;26(2):43–71.
22. Hean S, Craddock D, O'Halloran C. Learning theories and interprofessional education: a user's guide. *Learning in Health and Social Care.* 2009;8(4):250–262.
23. Gordon S, Mendenhall P, O'Connor B. *Beyond the Checklist: What Else Health Care Can Learn from Aviation Teamwork and Safety.* Ithaca, NY: ILR Press; 2012.
24. King H, Battles J, Baker D, Alonso A. TeamSTEPPS™: Team Strategies and Tools to Enhance Performance and Patient Safety. In: Henriksen K, Battles JB, Keyes MA, Grady ML, eds. *Advances in Patient Safety: New Directions and Alternative Approaches (Vol. 4: Technology and Medication Safety).* Washington, DC: Agency for Healthcare Research and Quality; 2008. http://www.ncbi.nlm.nih.gov/books/NBK43770/. Accessed December 29, 2015.

8

Leadership in Health Care

Sara Jo Grethlein, MD, Brian Clyne, MD, and
Erin McKean, MD, MBA

LEARNING OBJECTIVES

1. Understand the factors driving the leadership imperative in health care.
2. Describe the key competencies related to health care leadership.
3. Describe the pathways to formal leadership roles across multiple domains in health care.
4. Understand the concept of professional identity formation as it relates to leadership.

In considering how to best develop effective health care leaders, some fundamental questions arise: How is leadership best taught and learned? What leadership models or theories are most applicable to health care? How does health care *leadership* differ from *management,* and how do leadership and management intersect? Is health care leadership distinct from leadership in other industries? Are there distinguishing leadership competencies in a health care environment? What are the opportunities and pathways to health care leadership? This chapter will address these and other questions as the multifaceted topic of leadership in health care is explored.

CHAPTER OUTLINE

I. INTRODUCTION

The US health care system is undergoing disruptive change characterized by major shifts in the traditional models of care delivery, payment, and government regulation. Spiraling costs, inadequate access, inconsistent quality, increased competition, and the need for improved **population health** are just a few of the challenges facing modern health care. In response to these challenges and an increasingly complex system, the demand for effective leadership has never been higher. From the primary care physician leading a team in an office practice to the CEO tasked with managing a hospital system, many experts believe the future success of the health care industry will rest on how well it develops its leaders.

Many of these future leaders will be physicians and other health care professionals. According to a recent survey, 60 percent of hospitals plan to hire more physician leaders in the next 5 years.[1] Traditionally, physicians ascended to such leadership roles based on clinical skill, scholarly productivity, or research excellence. However, it is becoming clear that successful health care leadership requires more than clinical credibility or content knowledge. It demands creative thinking, an ability to work across disciplines, operational skills, and an understanding of organizational culture—topics notably absent from most health professional school curricula and residency training programs.

Despite a growing emphasis on preparing clinician leaders, some experts have speculated that deeply ingrained physician characteristics and the culture of medical training run counter to the leadership development that is now required. Consider the formative members of the pipeline—health care professional school applicants—whose early lives are filled with achievement and leadership potential. If leadership is valued highly by the profession, essential for the future of health care and vital for acceptance to our professional schools, how then does the health system end up with practicing health care providers who require intensive retraining as leaders? Some have speculated that typical personal characteristics such as competitiveness and independent-mindedness may neutralize leadership skills. For example, physicians typically value autonomy and are taught to act in the best interest of individual patients, and health care systems are hierarchical, rewarding personal achievements. This may not be the optimal foundation for leading change that requires collaboration, relational skills, emotional intelligence, and systems thinking. This might explain the recent proliferation of academies, courses, and degree programs designed to train (or intensively retrain) health care leaders.

II. THE HEALTH CARE LEADERSHIP IMPERATIVE

To confront the many challenges facing the US health care system, experts and organizations have pointed out the critical need for effective leadership. Physicians and other professionals are being called upon to develop and demonstrate the capabilities to lead health care transformation.[2–4] The Institute of Medicine (IOM) has described the need to "develop leaders at all levels who can manage the organizational and systems changes necessary to improve health."[5] The Association of American Medical Colleges (AAMC) has called for "new roles for physician leaders" and a "focus on organizational leadership in a new era of health care."[6] The American Association of Colleges of Nursing (AACN), along with other health care organization collaborators, introduced the Clinical Nurse Leader (CNL) nursing role in 2003.

At the same time, accreditation bodies are incorporating leadership competencies into their training and practice standards. For example, leadership has become an essential competency for medical students as described in the AAMC Core Entrustable Professional Activities for Entering Residency. Among the expected behaviors of medical school graduates is the ability to "provide leadership skills that enhance team functioning, the learning environment, and/or the health care delivery system."[7] In graduate medical education, the requirement to develop physician leaders is explicit. The Accreditation Council for Graduate Medical Education (ACGME) requires residents to demonstrate the ability to "work effectively as a member or leader of a health care team or other professional group."[8] In 2013, the AACN described entry-level competencies for all CNLs, including maintaining an outcomes-focus, interprofessional communication skills, and the ability to apply improvement science and systems theory.[9] The Royal College of Physicians and Surgeons of Canada's CanMEDS Physician Competency Framework was modified in 2015 to include "Leader" as one of the essential roles of physicians (Fig. 8.1).[10] This change from "Manager" to "Leader" in the CanMEDS framework reflects the emphasis on clinicians working collaboratively and "[engaging] with others to contribute to a vision of a high-quality health care system and take responsibility for the delivery of excellent patient care through their activities as clinicians, administrators, scholars, or teachers."

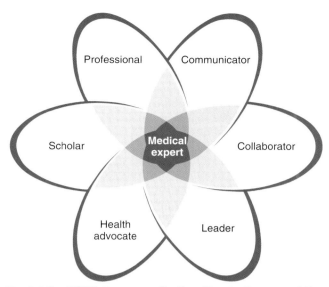

Fig. 8.1 CanMEDS diagram reflecting "Leader" as one of the essential roles of physicians. (Copyright © 2015 The Royal College of Physicians and Surgeons of Canada. http://rcpsc.medical.org/canmeds. Reproduced with permission.)

Distinction is often made between managers and leaders, with the commonly held belief that "Managers do things right. Leaders do the right things."[11] In this dichotomy, managers are portrayed as orderly, predictable figures who focus on structure, planning, and execution. Leaders, by contrast, are the visionary catalysts focused on defining purpose and executing change. In health care, managers are needed to identify efficiencies and improve operational structures, especially in the clinical setting. Leaders must be skilled at seeing connections and future opportunities in a rapidly changing and competitive landscape. While the core functions of managers and leaders may be different, significant overlap exists in their skill sets. Both are crucial to organizational success. Further, management skills and behaviors make leaders more effective.

III. WHO ARE HEALTH CARE LEADERS?

Traditional thinking in health care left "leadership" to administrators, relegating physicians and nurses to patient management or departmental/unit service roles. Fast forward to the current environment, where clinician leadership has been shown to improve patient outcomes, decrease clinical operational and capital expenditures, improve efficiency, and improve staff satisfaction and retention.[4,12] Barriers to such leadership have included the lack of leadership training, the lack of a common language in quality and leadership, the assumption that physicians will resist change, the undervaluing of the cumulative effect of incremental changes, and a lack of institutional culture that empowers front-line clinicians and staff. Changes to a deeply ingrained culture often require moments of crisis. The value crisis in health care has provided an opportunity to change how the health system thinks about and design leadership training in health care. Professional development to succeed in both formal, authority-based roles and informal, transformational leadership roles is necessary.

In the realm of formal administrative leadership, several collaboratives have emerged to represent groups of leaders. The Institute for Healthcare Improvement (IHI) Leadership Alliance[13] is a collaborative of health care leaders committed to the science of improvement and the **Triple Aim:** improving the experience of care, improving the health of populations, and reducing per capita costs of health care. Berwick and colleagues argue that "Leaders involved in health care must be actively and directly involved in catalyzing change needed to achieve the Triple Aim" because of contextual challenges in redesigning systems of care, rapid evolution of delivery innovations that outpace the development of national or state policies, the need for trusting relationships with the public, and bipartisan political gridlock that squelches authentic dialogue and progress.[14]

The IHI has proposed four mental models for health care leaders, nourished in the context of high-impact leadership behaviors.[15] The models were developed through expert interviews and a meeting of expert organizational leaders. The mental models include 1) individuals and their families as partners in care, 2) a focus on value (defined as quality per cost), 3) service alignment with payment systems, and 4) empowerment of all participants as improvers. Aligned with these new mental models for thinking about health care delivery, the high impact leadership behaviors that promote change are person-centeredness, front-line engagement, relentless focus, transparency (about results, progress, aims, and defects), and boundarilessness.

Person-centeredness requires considering the needs and values of patients, families, and communities, not single-mindedly focusing on disease statistics and dollars. Front-line engagement demands that leaders be present and transparent, sharing information and asking open questions while adapting to the needs of the team or organization. Relentless focus requires articulating a clear vision and aligning activities with priorities to achieve stated aims. Boundarilessness (without boundaries) is highly related to front-line engagement and transparency, sharing lessons learned and collaborating throughout a system or organization. These models and behaviors are thought to characterize true leaders in both formal and informal positions within health care.

The National Center for Healthcare Leadership (NCHL),[16] a US-based think tank of providers, system administrators, suppliers, and academics, is a nonprofit organization focused on the development of health care leaders in the formal administrative setting in order to improve health care delivery and population health. The NCHL offers structured coaching, executive fellowships, and consulting services aimed at improving the leadership capabilities of executives and their teams, regardless of background or path to leadership. The NCHL has specific initiatives on women's leadership and diversity leadership, attempting to understand the gaps in formal leadership expectations and prepare for these groups, as well as aiming to positively impact executive leadership diversity.

There is less literature and discussion about informal leadership in health care, though this does not reflect its relative importance. Non-administrative leaders often are experts in their respective fields with great potential to influence processes and behaviors. By definition, leaders must have followers. Followers need not be direct reports to a leader, and expert leaders of engaged followers very often are found outside of the executive suite. When these leaders are identified, empowered, and trained, they have the capacity to influence culture change and process improvement. Each day, there are countless examples of effective front-line leadership in health care. The system depends on individuals without formal titles stepping up to identify problems, take action, and initiate meaningful change. Students have shown leadership in speaking up to prevent wrong-sided surgery or wrong procedures from being performed. Dr. Mona Hanna-Atisha, a pediatrician in Flint, Michigan, stepped up to state government officials who initially dismissed her research showing a spike in lead levels in children after the switching of the Flint water supply.[17] Her persistence, coupled with courage and an intense patient-centered mindset, led to statewide changes and a national focus on health care disparities and environmental health. She embodied professionalism, outcomes-focus, team management, effective communication, and navigation of the politics in microsystems and macrosystems.

In an ideal health care environment, any member of the team is empowered to demonstrate situational leadership. As an example, a nursing student studying hospital-acquired infections became concerned that the computer keyboards on mobile workstations were the source of a recent *Clostridium difficile* outbreak on the medical wards. Assuming responsibility for improving the system, she gathered data and reframed the problem as both a patient safety issue and a financial concern for the hospital. She engaged key stakeholders in infection control and identified areas of best practice. She communicated her findings to the hospital leadership, appealing to them using persuasive firsthand patient stories. Ultimately, she gained support for implementing a solution—a modification to the hand hygiene policy that includes cleaning of all computer keyboards.[18] Students and staff who are in entry-level positions often question why they are being given leadership training or being exposed to a leadership curriculum. It is easy to underestimate the power of leading from within or influencing organizational behavior without holding a formal administrative role. This informal leadership influence can also be exerted by organizations. One excellent example comes from the American Medical Student Association (AMSA). Distressed by both observed examples of conflict of interest between the pharmaceutical industry and medical school faculty and staff and the lack of education around this issue, the AMSA began a PharmFree campaign in 2002 by gathering information about the relationships between institutions and the pharmaceutical industry. The organization hoped that by publicizing the identified potential conflicts of interest, they would encourage schools to limit gifts, advertising, and contact with sales representatives in order to minimize undue influence of commercial entities in medical decision making about therapeutic choices.[19]

Through this program, in 2006, the students invited each school to submit its policies and curriculum for evaluation and then published an 11-point PharmFree Score Card. High-profile schools scored poorly, and the publicity spurred change. The AMSA's efforts aligned with other initiatives. In 2008 the AAMC and in 2009 the IOM formally called for inclusion of conflict of interest education in the curriculum of medical schools. The AMSA has continued its leadership in this domain, publishing model curricula and updating the annual scorecard. The impact of this effort has expanded at many institutions where student input is now incorporated into both curriculum and policy formulation.[20]

After graduating from a prestigious residency program where she had been chief resident, Dr. Hogan completed a competitive fellowship in infectious diseases. She quickly earned a reputation for clinical excellence, strong research skills, and dedication to bedside teaching. She became the youngest division director and fellowship director in the institution before her recent promotion to chief academic officer. Almost immediately, Dr. Hogan was overwhelmed with the complexity of the job and began questioning her decision to join the executive ranks of the hospital's administration. She had inherited a staff with low morale due to conflicts between two key members of the group. There were also major budget constraints, programs facing loss of accreditation, and physicians in need of professionalism remediation. From her day-to-day schedule to long-term strategic planning, Dr. Hogan decided to take on every issue personally. She was frustrated to learn that her talents as a clinician and teacher were less relevant as she dealt with finances, human resource policies, conflict, and change initiatives. Things reached a critical point when the board voted to acquire a network of local hospitals to enhance clinical revenue and reduce outside competition. Dr. Hogan was charged with leading the integration of all educational programs in the system, a monumental undertaking. She knew that in order to be successful and advance in her career, she would need a new set of skills. Dr. Hogan enrolled in a leadership training course at the local business school and, over time, she learned to be as effective in the boardroom as she had been at the bedside.

Are health care professionals like Dr. Hogan prepared for leadership roles? What factors contribute to the demand for leadership skills among health care professionals? Can leadership skills be learned? If so, how do health care professionals go about acquiring foundational leadership skills? What are some common pathways to health care leadership?

IV. THE IMPORTANCE OF CLINICIAN LEADERSHIP

The American Association for Physician Leadership (AAPL) was founded in the 1970s in order to develop physician managers. The AAPL reported in a white paper that in 2014 only 5 percent of hospital leaders were physicians.[21] However, hospitals with physician executives take the top positions in national hospital rankings and disproportionally outperform other hospitals in cancer care, the management of digestive disorders, cardiology, and cardiac surgery. Physician-led hospitals on average score higher in performance management and Lean management. It is thought that this improved performance may come from great knowledge of the "core business." In almost all industries, executive leadership of companies or systems comes from the core business function domain. For example, executives in the competitive soft drink industry tend to have strong marketing and strategy backgrounds, while automobile industry executives tend to have a strong background in operations, engineering, or product development. Again, this intimate knowledge of the industry may provide a greater ability to create a vision, address core values, focus both on process and outcomes, strategize, assess data in context, communicate and empathize with stakeholders, and engage front-line leaders to execute a plan.

A 2013 McKinsey white paper also noted the critical importance of direct involvement of front-line clinicians and physician engagement. The authors estimate from their consulting experience in over 150 hospitals that if clinical operations were unchanged, nonclinical variable costs would need to be reduced 30 percent for an overall 5 to 10 percent reduction in operational costs. This would be nearly impossible. In other words, improvement in health care value cannot be fully achieved without changes to the actual delivery of clinical care. To achieve changes in clinical care, the actual participants in this care must be engaged, informed, and empowered.

V. GUIDING PRINCIPLES OF HEALTH CARE LEADERSHIP

The response to the "leadership imperative" in health care has been an explosion of training programs, targeting all levels of experience across the full range of disciplines. Many academic medical centers, major universities, and professional and specialty societies now sponsor leadership training programs.[22,23] Some are comprehensive and ambitious, like the United Kingdom's National Health Service (NHS), which established a health care leadership model and a developmental program for all health care providers.[24]

Although there is growing emphasis on leadership development, there is no clear consensus on what defines effective health care leadership, nor is there much evidence about best practices to guide training. As a result, programs emphasize a wide range of skills and vary in their methods.[25] Some heath care leadership programs stress quality improvement, while others emphasize technical competencies such as finance or strategic planning. Still others focus on clinical or academic development. The clinician leadership movement has evolved to the point where one can pursue very specific leadership training to enhance business acumen, communication skills, political sophistication, emotional intelligence, and many other targeted, core leadership skills.

Most contemporary leadership programs are organized by broad domains (e.g., direction-setting, working with others) further classified into the specific knowledge or skills desired of leaders. Several published studies have sought to identify the most important competencies for health care leaders. One study examined physician beliefs regarding leadership competencies and determined that interpersonal and communication skills, professional ethics and responsibility, and continuous learning and improvement were the most important.[26] Another study of physician leaders found that emotional intelligence and vision were among the fundamental competencies to being a successful physician leader.[27] Another study found that communication, ethics, and conflict resolution were the most highly rated competencies for health care leadership.[28] Stoller contends that having a service orientation, being collaborative and adaptable, being a change agent, having vision and initiative, and developing other competencies are especially important for effective health care leadership.[29] The Stoller model overlaps with the Feagin Medical Leadership Model from the Duke Institute for Health Innovation, which describes patient-centeredness as the core of health care leadership, followed closely by teamwork, selfless service, integrity, emotional intelligence, and critical thinking.[30]

Interprofessional leadership programs and those designed specifically for nurses, pharmacists, and health care administrators emphasize the same content areas as those targeted toward physicians.[31,32] One example is the Woodruff Leadership Academy at Emory University, which is designed for health care professionals from many disciplines. The content includes seminars on strategic thinking, personal awareness, negotiation, and conflict management, all within a health care context.[33] Nursing-specific leadership programs incorporate leadership theory and change management, with particular emphasis on teamwork and professional ethics.[34,35]

The NCHL has created a copyrighted model of "competencies required for outstanding health care leadership for the future." The Healthcare Leadership Alliance Model is an interprofessional model that emphasizes core leadership and management competencies developed through psychometric analysis and a modified Delphi technique using experts from different areas of health care administration. In this model, competencies are organized into domains of *transformation* (achievement orientation, analytical thinking, community orientation, financial skills, information seeking, innovative thinking, and strategic orientation), *people* (human resources, interpersonal understanding, professionalism, relationship building, self-confidence, self-development, talent development, and team leadership), and *execution* (accountability, change leadership, collaboration, communication skills, impact and influence, information technology management, initiative, organizational awareness, performance measurement, process management/organizational design, and project management).[36] The United Kingdom's Healthcare Leadership model includes nine dimensions (or domains), with detailed descriptions of leadership competencies within each dimension.[37] The Medical Leadership Competency Framework (MLCF), also developed by the United Kingdom's NHS, is centered on "delivering the service" and describes domains of shared leadership including setting direction, demonstrating personal qualities, working with others, managing services, and improving services.[38] There are four elements within each domain, and there are four competencies within each element. The tool is progressive, noting three distinct phases of leadership growth with relevant and timely learning opportunities: undergraduate, postgraduate, and continuing practice.

In 2011, Al-Touby proposed the Functional Results-Oriented Health Care Leadership model.[39] This model is directed toward "attaining excellent patient outcomes" and postulates that leadership must serve the predefined task, the team, and the individuals within the team, having a constant focus on exceptional results. In many ways, this model is similar to the Toyota Production System (TPS) model, emphasizing a central "purpose" of excellent patient outcomes. The TPS model is a model for manufacturing that has been applied to service industries, utilizing Lean production. More importantly than the use of Lean alone, the TPS model employs "A3 management," which emphasizes purpose (including the patient as the center of health care delivery), processes (continual pursuit of perfection and team-based problem solving), and people ("horizontal" and interprofessional thinking, individual empowerment and ownership of problem solving, and coaching without usurping the process).[40]

Based on the vast array of leadership models that exist in business and other industries, there is no universal skill set or proven formula for effective leadership. The same is true in the health care sector, though research and expert opinion suggest that certain qualities and skills are more advantageous in this realm. Demonstrating patient-centeredness, a service orientation, integrity, and strong relational skills are among the threshold competencies for effective health care leaders.

VI. INFLUENTIAL LEADERSHIP THEORIES

Cultures throughout history have celebrated leaders as heroic figures who possess special qualities. Emperors, generals, and business tycoons are depicted as having exceptional strength, courage, or brilliance resulting in positions of high status. As leadership became a topic of academic study in the early 20th century, the initial research focused on identifying the personality traits that distinguish these leaders from nonleaders. The "great man" theory and other trait theories of leadership suggested that charisma, self-confidence, intelligence, and extraversion made leaders different from everyone else. Subsequent research on behavioral theories sought to isolate the behavior patterns that distinguish leaders. Behaviorists focused on how leaders act and identified different leadership styles including people-oriented versus task-oriented. While trait theory implied that leadership is innate and predisposed, behavioral theory suggested that people could learn to be leaders by understanding how to behave and interact with others.

The notion that leaders are made rather than born sparked decades of further research attempting to describe and quantify leadership on many dimensions, but it remains an elusive subject from the point of academic study. Ultimately, effective leadership likely requires the right combination of personality traits, modifiable behaviors, and context. Several modern leadership theories—transformational, situational, and servant—align with commonly held beliefs about health care professionals and have dominated the physician leadership development movement. Other leadership theories and types exist, such as transactional leadership in which the leader alone sets goals along with rewards and penalties. Such hierarchical leadership roles are commonly seen in health care but generally lack alignment with behaviors known to empower patients and professionals and improve outcomes. For example, the Veterans Health Administration wait time scandal in the United States shed light on transactional leadership styles where impossible standards conflicted with professional obligations and available resources, leading to fear, falsification of records, and cover-ups.[41]

A. Transformational Theory

Transformational leadership theory is focused on how leaders stimulate others to transcend their own self-interests to reach higher-order goals or visions. Transformational leaders motivate others through raising awareness of idealized goals and through role modeling. The four *I*'s of transformational leadership as described by Bass include: idealized influence, inspirational motivation, intellectual stimulation, and individualized consideration.[42] Quinn describes transformational leadership functionally as being results-centered, internally directed (acting on values and with integrity), other-focused (committing to the collective good, even at personal cost), and externally open (adapting to feedback and the environment, taking appropriate risk).[43]

In health care, this might be demonstrated by guiding departmental leaders to work toward institutional success rather than solely their parochial goals. This could manifest as more prosperous units supporting less-profitable ones, sharing resources, or approving priorities that place other groups' needs before their own for the betterment of the entire organization.

B. Situational Theory

In situational leadership theory, effective leadership depends on selecting the right leadership style contingent on the followers or group context. Situational leaders shift among four behaviors depending on how willing and able followers are to complete a task: directing, coaching, supporting, or delegating.[44] In this model, the effectiveness of a leader is determined more by environmental factors, the characteristics of the followers, and the nature of the work at hand. Situational leadership requires attention to the needs of subordinates and the complexity of the task at hand. In the clinical context, leading a team to resuscitate a critical patient might require a combination of delegating, directing, and coaching, all in a matter of minutes. For hospital executives, leading a merger between two institutions may require a different style than responding to a public relations crisis such as a highly publicized patient safety issue.

C. Servant Theory

Servant leadership theory contends that a leader's influence derives from serving the needs of others. Characteristic behaviors of servant leaders include listening, empathizing, accepting stewardship, and actively developing others' potential.[45] Countless examples of servant leadership exist in health care, where professionals put aside self-interests in order to bring out the best in others. Front-line clinicians and primary care providers are often the archetype for servant leadership in health care—the image of a devoted clinician who delivers care directly to his or her patients and to the community. Others work to promote health equity and use their positions to advocate on behalf of those who cannot. Examples include public health leaders advocating for gun safety in order to prevent childhood injuries, or clinicians working to curb the epidemic of deaths from opiate abuse through prevention (i.e., improved provider education) and treatment programs.

VII. HEALTH CARE LEADERSHIP COMPETENCIES

Health care leadership competencies are the combination of observable and measurable knowledge, skills, abilities, and personal attributes that effective leaders demonstrate. Although this list is not exhaustive, competence in the following domains are frequently noted in the previously mentioned leadership models and appear to be required for managing change. The competencies may be arranged in the categories of foundational, self-management, team management, influence and communication, systems-based practice/management, and change management (or executing toward a vision) (Fig. 8.2).

A. Foundational Competencies Specific to Health Care

1. Maintaining Patient-Centeredness

Health care leaders often answer to multiple constituencies such as patients, staff, communities, and those with financial interests in the institutions they lead. Competing priorities are a routine challenge, and it is the responsibility of a leader to ensure that the best interest of patients remains central. The CEO of a hospital may be faced with making a decision about closing a financially unprofitable primary care clinic, or the dean of a medical school may have to select which educational or research priorities to nurture with limited resources.

2. Professionalism

Leaders serve as role models for their institutions and constituents. Demonstrating excellence in their professional field, commitment to ongoing professional development, and adherence to ethical and legal standards of practice allows a leader to serve as an example. Without the respect of those he or she serves, a leader cannot succeed. Consistent adherence to ethical standards, truth telling, and fairness are the fundamental attributes of leadership. Balancing competing interests can be a challenge to professionalism for leaders. Take the example of a health care worker with a substance abuse problem. If a leader accepts the disease model of addiction, how does he or she simultaneously respect the rights of the recovering professional and the safety of patients? Should a patient come to harm due to care provided by an impaired provider, the hospital that knew of the impairment bears some liability.[46] But if an employee knows that seeking help for an addiction ends his or her career as a health care provider, he or she may avoid treatment. Taken a step further, does a patient have the right to know that his or her provider is in recovery? These issues are not only relevant in substance

Health care leadership competencies					
Health care foundations	**Self-management**	**Team management**	**Influence and communication**	**Systems-based practice**	**Executing toward a vision**
• Maintaining patient centeredness • Professionalism	• Serving selflessly • Achievement orientation/pursuing excellence • Emotional intelligence	• Relationship management • Developing new talent • Human resources	• Communicating effectively • Advocacy • Having challenging conversations • Navigating "politics"	• Knowledge of the health care environment • Business knowledge and skills	• Vision and strategy • Creating culture • Creating sustainable solutions

Fig. 8.2 Health care leadership competencies by domains of health care foundations, self-management, team management, influence and communication, systems-based practice, and executing toward a vision.

abuse contexts, but have been brought to the fore in times of emerging infectious diseases, such as AIDS. Do patients have the right to know that their nurse or physician has the condition? Leaders in health care contribute to the evaluation of these issues on both local and broader scales and must balance truth-telling (full disclosure) with fairness.

B. Self-Management

1. Serving Selflessly

Putting the interests of others first is important to the success of a leader. Behaving partially can undermine credibility, especially if favors flow to the leader's own unit. Medical professionals accept the need to serve selflessly when they work with infectious patients or stay and care for unstable patients despite their nominal workday ending. Altruism is a core tenet of physician behavior whose expression resonates powerfully.

2. Achievement Orientation/Pursuing Excellence

Guiding individuals and institutions to higher achievement is part of the leader's job. Part of a leader's role requires creating a culture that enables and rewards achievement, clearing barriers to the pursuit of excellence, and garnering sufficient resources to facilitate success. Modeling these ideals for the community can propel organizations forward. As the concept of accountable care is increasingly operationalized, leaders will be called upon to set and meet intermediate goals that combine to achieve externally determined care targets.

3. Emotional Intelligence

Awareness of his or her own and others' emotions can transform an adequate leader into an exceptional one by enabling him or her to defuse conflict as well as motivate and empathize with others. At the most senior levels, it may be difficult to stay connected to large constituencies. Many leaders structure routine opportunities for interaction with their staff to remain attuned. On a smaller scale, contemplating the needs, fears, and motivations of those with whom one interacts can often help facilitate team building and the construction of mutually beneficial strategies.

C. Team Management

1. Relationship Management

Leaders rarely attain success solely through their own efforts. Tending to the aspirations and needs of colleagues and staff, fairly apportioning credit, and treating others with respect is necessary. Creating and sustaining good working relationships allows for an environment in which subordinates and peers can provide candid feedback and voice concerns. Receiving and learning from criticism is a mark of a mature leader, as is giving meaningful feedback to develop others.

2. Developing New Talent (Coaching, Mentoring, Sponsoring)

The talents and challenges that each individual brings to the work environment must be evaluated proactively.

Identifying ways to support, advance, and retain constructive and productive team members is part of the leader's role. Similarly, forging plans to re-engage and redirect disruptive or nonproductive workers is often a more difficult task. Jim Collins, writing in *Good to Great*, suggests that a key to successful organizations is "getting the right people on the bus, the wrong people off the bus, and the right people in the right seats."[47] Facilitating interactions, managing diverse personalities and work styles, and troubleshooting dysfunctional interactions can convert lackluster groups into energetic teams with the strength to tackle significant issues and the resilience to ride out setbacks.

3. Human Resources

Health care professionals without formal management training often have little knowledge about the role of human resources in complicated institutions. Many leaders, especially those with clinical backgrounds, have no experience performing basic management tasks such as running a meeting. Human resource skills include the ability to conduct effective interviews in order to hire based on values and qualities consistent with those of the organization. Equally important is the ability to direct the work of teams and incentivize individual performance through reward or recognition programs that honor the achievements of others. Other human resource skills include delegating responsibilities, holding others accountable, and deciding when to discipline or terminate an underperforming employee. While these skills are best learned through firsthand experience, health care professionals can enhance their leadership capacity by acknowledging their human resources skill gaps and preparing a plan for personal development.

D. Influence and Communication

1. Communicating Effectively

Leaders cannot accomplish anything without crafting and conveying compelling messages that inspire, educate, and motivate people. Communication is multidirectional. A leader must understand the perspective of those being led; to gain that knowledge, he or she must, through oral or written means, be receptive to opinions, concerns, and suggestions. Some choose to structure such communication through surveys or town halls; others rely on sporadic or spontaneous information. The term *affirmative listening* refers to the practice of listening with sincerity and with the intent to learn and act. Creating a **Just Culture** in which subordinates feel empowered to voice concerns without fear of reprisal is the responsibility of leadership.

Creating and implementing a vision is a critical task for leaders. Doing so requires sharing that vision with those impacted by change. This may include both employees and the broader community. As an example, if an institution chooses to close its emergency department due to high cost and low utilization, it would be important to share the rationale with staff who will need, in turn, to explain this to patients. Ideally, representatives of key stakeholders would have participated in making such decisions before they are solidified.

There is a delicate balance to be struck between sharing too much or too little information, releasing data too early or too late, and selecting how widely or narrowly to disseminate information. As the options for communication have expanded to include social media, in addition to more traditional streams, a savvy leader needs to construct communication strategies and policies for both himself and his unit. Both casual and formal, structured communication can be an effective tool to engage internal and external communities, can allow nimble and timely responses to the opportunities presented by events in real time, and can inspire confidence. Inartful use of media or angry, reactive e-mails can undo the best strategic endeavors. A successful leader is attentive to the messages he or she and his or her institution sends, and he or she practices self-awareness in communication. During times of crisis, leaders may have to be creative in their methods of communication. Following Hurricane Katrina in 2005, students, residents, fellows, faculty, and staff from the hospitals and medical schools of New Orleans were distributed across a multistate area. Main methods of communication were down. The power for the region was out, and there were many injured and dead.[48] Recognizing how critical it was to establish communication, the leadership of Tulane University School of Medicine and Louisiana State University School of Medicine were able to establish and maintain contact with their learners, and both institutions were able to resume classes within 4 weeks. One school communicated using a student listserv; the other rapidly established a website that was hosted by an institution in another state. This required an extraordinary level of proficiency in communication that allowed the schools to literally weather the storm.

2. Advocacy

Leaders advocate for specific people, programs, and ideas within their institutions and advocate for their institutions within the larger world. While the ability to fundraise is often used as a scorecard to measure effectiveness in this domain, there are many other arenas in which leaders serve as advocates. For example, intervening with legislators for approval for new programs or funding for facilities are common tasks for institutional leaders. Advocating for the adoption of health care practices ranging from hand washing to contraception to lifestyle changes is also responsibility of health care leaders.

3. Having Challenging Conversations

A successful leader manages conflict by rephrasing rants into heartfelt concerns and using fundamental values and motivations to redirect team members toward success. Clinicians are often adept at having difficult conversations with patients; having challenging conversations with colleagues and team members is equally as important. A white paper cosponsored by the American Association of Critical Care Nurses notes that "silence kills" and a majority of health care workers have sincere concerns about a coworker, usually regarding broken rules, mistakes, lack of support, incompetence, poor teamwork, disrespect, or micromanagement.[49] Reasons cited for avoiding difficult conversations include lack of ability, lack of "ownership" (belief it is not "their job"), low confidence that it will result in change, time constraints, and fear of retaliation. Leaders must create a culture of safety for holding these challenging conversations and must artfully address poor teamwork and team concerns.

4. Navigating Politics of a Situation or System

Health care systems are complex organizations complete with internal politics and competition. While individual health care professionals might share a common goal to improve patient care, many are part of larger coalitions with parochial beliefs and interests, each seeking various forms of power or access to finite resources. Consider a common scenario playing out in many academic medical centers today, where large multispecialty practice plans are replacing previously independent clinical departments or private physician groups. Politics is a central theme in the consolidation of these various provider groups into systems of care. Inevitable conflicts arise related to sharing risk, compensation, governance structure, transparency, and fundamentally—power. In this context, the term *politics* often evokes strong negative feelings, and it is easy to grow cynical when political agendas corrupt important decisions, especially in health care. To be effective, health care leaders must first realize that politics and leadership are universally intertwined. In limited-resource environments such as health care, leaders can navigate politics more constructively by identifying key stakeholders and seeking to understand the interests of both supporters and adversaries. Indeed, political effectiveness draws on many leadership competencies simultaneously: articulating a vision, negotiation skills, team building, and strategic planning. Through practice and preparation, health care leaders can use political skill constructively to create more effective organizations.

CASE STUDY 2

After 5 years working as a physical therapist at a large community hospital, Mark was eager to go out on his own. When a retiring colleague offered to sell Mark his office practice, he jumped at the opportunity. As a new small-business owner, Mark soon realized he was in way over his head. The practice had an outdated computer system that led to delays in appointment scheduling, billing, and reimbursement. The front office employees he inherited were set in their ways. They resisted any change to the patient flow process as well as a proposed redesign of the clinic to maximize space and efficiency. Mark openly expressed his frustration over the group's skepticism and the slow pace of change. Within 3 months of taking over, a dissatisfied administrator and a well-liked physical therapist resigned and left Mark short-staffed. He began to wonder if he had the requisite skills and temperament to lead this practice. Every day he thought about returning to his hospital-based job without all the headaches.

What type of person is well-suited to serving in a leadership role? Do certain personality traits predict effective leadership? What leadership competencies are important for leading an office-based practice? What are the unique challenges in this health care environment?

E. Systems-Based Practice/Management

1. Knowledge of the Health Care Environment

To shepherd a health care institution through the maze of regulations, accreditations, financial challenges, and evolving medical care models takes dedication to staying knowledgeable. Participating in regional or national peer group organizations and pursuing degrees such as Masters in health care administration or Masters in public health are common strategies to keep abreast of the ever-changing health care marketplace. As elements of the Affordable Care Act come online, dramatic changes in health care reimbursement, auditing, and reporting requirements have necessitated fluidity in the management of most health care enterprises. The imperative to implement electronic health records (EHRs) and the requirement to meet successively higher targets for "meaningful use" with the EHR have dramatically changed clinical practice patterns and workflow, creating new challenges across the spectrum of individuals collaborating in the delivery of health care.

2. Business Knowledge and Skills

Guiding an institution through changes in delivery models, reimbursement, legislative support, and the impact of economic upswings and downturns requires an in-depth understanding of business methods. A leader must be able to absorb and evaluate the streams of financial, market, and operational data to steward resources and negotiate favorable conditions for his or her institution. Engaging in strategic planning to chart an institution's direction involves assigning priorities to different programs or missions and allocating resources accordingly.

A bare minimum for a leader is the ability to read and interpret financial reports and budgets. Understanding the revenue and expense streams for his or her unit is essential for a leader making decisions about operations or planning for the future. Emotional reactions are normal in the context of health care. Though such reactions can inspire, a leader must make decisions driven by analysis of data and contextualized by the organization's mission.

Clinics, hospitals, and health systems function within a dynamic universe. The development of new technology or the passage of new legislation are examples of common perturbations in health care environments. Mass-casualty events or epidemics call for immediate responses. In 2014, the Ebola epidemic in Africa led to changes in hospital practice around the world and required rapid development of new procedures and policies. The urgency of the situation overrode existing budgets and strategic plans. Downstream consequences included revision of priorities as hospitals scrambled to train staff and modify their physical environment. There was tremendous fear associated with these events, and health care leaders provided clear, calm, and transparent strategies.

Change in health care is not always emergent. Expanding or contracting clinical services, switching payment models to staff, responding to unionization of workers, or merging with other institutions are common examples. A leader must be sensitive to the fears and concerns of those impacted and provide information and opportunities for input. He or she must address each strata of employees, make the case for change, and foster a sense of ownership of the change. Where possible, a leader should incentivize joining the change. Assessing the organization's culture and directly addressing counterproductive elements are part of the strategy as the leader crafts his or her message.

F. Executing Toward a Vision

1. Visioning and Strategy

Identifying organizational goals and designing strategies to achieve them is one of the most important responsibilities of health care leaders. Depending on the strata occupied, the urgency of goals will dictate their breadth. The leader of a clinic will likely focus on improving the patient experience, operational efficiency, and financial viability. The head of a statewide health care system has the opportunity to change the health of the state and should set goals accordingly. It is difficult to motivate people to close operational budget gaps. President Kennedy inspired America by setting the goal of putting a man on the moon by the end of the 1960s and would likely have been less successful if seeking the same level of support for significant changes to the operating budget of the department of education. Health care organizations often seek to raise funds for new hospitals or facilities and research to cure diseases. Although replacing the hospital heating system may be just as necessary, it is difficult to fundraise for that.

2. Creating Culture

Creative solutions to challenging problems in health care can be stifled by poor leadership. In contrast, strong leaders can implement exciting approaches that improve care delivery, save money, and improve resource utilization. Innovative fixes work around red tape, standard operating procedure, and tradition. Strong leaders create space within an institution for such deviations from the norm. Oregon's health care system has targeted emergency department "frequent flyers" as individuals who may use resources inappropriately and disproportionately. Through the institution of **case management** and the provision of such items as shoes and sleeping bags not normally covered by health plans, these patients achieved higher satisfaction and better care, and the system benefited from a dramatic drop-off in emergency department visits.[50] Convincing the system to pilot this approach required clear and effective messaging by leaders who were able to frame the situation in patient-centered terms. Strong working relationships based on a track record of trustworthiness and accountability set the stage for this program to be accepted.

3. Creating Sustainable Solutions

Creativity and innovation are critical in solving health care problems, though innovative measures must be tailored, improved, and sustained for optimal benefit. Leaders can create sustainable solutions by employing the **Plan-Do-Study-Act (PDSA) cycle.** Like any other form of scientific problem solving, organizational solutions can be piloted, studied, implemented, analyzed, and revised over time. Lean management principles, such as PDSA and kaizen

Table 8.1 Suggestions for Leadership and Management Training by Specific Health Care Business Function

Business Function	Domain of Health Care Leadership	Training Required for Leadership/Management
Operations	Day-to-day patient care, quality and safety programs	Clinicians optimally positioned both informally and formally; Lean training; specific operations management training for chief operations officer (COO), chief quality officer (CQO), chief medical officer (CMO), chief nursing officer (CNO)
Marketing	Market analysis and positioning, needs assessment	Marketing-specific training; course-based and experiential; advanced training for chief marketing officer (also labeled CMO, often not existing in health care administration)
Finance	Financial decision-making, projections of volume, and revenue	Chief financial officer (CFO) requires advanced business-specific degree and experience; CEO requires accounting and finance training for understanding
Inbound patient flow logistics	Referrals, scheduling	Physicians and advanced practitioners optimally positioned to engage front-office staff to optimize patient intake; Lean training; functions report to COO
Outbound patient flow logistics	Coordination of patients leaving the site of care (clinic, hospital)	Nursing and social work teams optimally positioned to improve transitions of care; Lean training; functions report to COO
Accounting	Billing (receivable), budgeting and purchasing (payable)	Course-based accounting training; functions usually report up to CFO with advanced training
Human resources	Hiring, scheduling	Course-based management training, legal training, conflict resolution experience; human resources matters for faculty and professional staff often run through chief of staff and/or chief medical officer
Communications	Website, community presence	Communications training and experience; marketing experience and course-based training
Executive	Visioning, strategy, executive functioning	Advanced degree generally helpful for CEO; basic understanding of all business functions to oversee and coordinate; communications training

(continuous incremental improvement to create value while reducing waste), have been applied and studied in health care. At ThedaCare in northeast Wisconsin, application of Lean management has led to sustained improvement and value creation.[51] All ThedaCare staff members must participate in an event week in which they have dedicated time to improve their work. Event weeks incorporate three tenets for change, including respect for people, teaching through experience, and focus on world-class performance. Staff are asked to improve care through improving staff morale, improving quality (reducing error or defects), and improving productivity. Through event weeks and the overall change in culture, ThedaCare realized millions of dollars in savings, a decrease in accounts receivable (days to be paid for services), a 35 percent decrease in phone triage (hold) time, a 50 percent decrease in time to complete admission paperwork, and a decrease in medication distribution time to patients from 15 minutes to 8 minutes.

VIII. SPECIFIC ATTRIBUTES FOR HEALTH CARE LEADERS IN DIFFERENT SETTINGS

Leadership in health care takes place through formal administrative structures as well as in an *ad hoc* situational fashion. The balance between leadership-specific and management-specific skill sets may vary in the distinct domain of health care leadership. At the front line, the abilities to engage, motivate, and problem-solve in teams are most critical and embody transformational leadership attributes. This is true in clinical care, education, and research. In the formal administrative realm (whether in private practice, running one's own laboratory, departmental management, or system-level management), a leader must still possess self-management and core leadership traits, particularly the abilities to set a vision, communicate effectively to broad audiences, and influence individuals and organizations. Beyond this, additional management knowledge and skills augment the leader's ability to execute change.

Table 8.1 describes opportunities for impacting health care delivery and outcomes by business function. Further, specific knowledge and skills training that may be needed in formal and informal settings are described. Cross-cutting all of these functional areas are the foundations of patient-centeredness, professionalism, and the competencies of self-management, team management, influence and communication, and systems-based problem solving.

IX. PATHWAYS TO LEADERSHIP

Formal pathways to leadership generally are through hospital or health system administrative structures, professional societies, nongovernmental organizations, and governmental/policy or political affiliations. Within health systems, elected positions such as chief of staff (COS) or other positions within the COS office are common launch pads for physician leaders in a formal setting. Appointment as the chief medical officer (CMO), chief nursing officer (CNO), chief academic officer, or to a hospital or organizational board of directors allows the opportunity to gain experience and "big picture" understanding. CMOs, CNOs, and board members may be chief operations officers (COOs) or CEOs in training. Generally, formal training in organizational management is not required in the COS office or for board participation but is certainly highly valued. Networking is an important aspect for these positions, and management skills may be built on the job. Within academics, departmental administration is another pathway to formal leadership. Traditionally, academic chairs have come to positions of authority through the ability to obtain grants and publish, as well as through networking and departmental service. Although these principles for climbing the academic ladder are well-ingrained, there is a slow shift toward appointing chairs with more formal management and finance experience. From the chair position in academia, a further step may be dean or an institutional vice president for medical/health affairs.

Individuals with a pure business administration background tend to have little to no expertise in direct patient care. Physicians and other health care professionals without additional training generally have little to no expertise in business management (particularly human resources, logistics, strategy, accounting, and financial decision-making on a systems level). Thus, in the formal administrative setting, advanced training in management may be obtained through competency-directed courses (e.g., executive education programs at business schools or within faculty development programs) or degree programs such as Masters of business administration or Masters of health care service administration (often within public health programs). Private for-profit and not-for-profit entities, such as the AAPL or the American College of Medical Practice Executives, offer certification programs toward Certified Physician Executive (CPE) or Certified Medical Practice Executive (CMPE) designation. In general, there is a trend away from health care service administration Master's degrees with an increase in MBA degrees among physician executives. There are little data on certification programs and outcomes.

Organizational and specialty society leadership positions are other, more traditional pathways to formal health care leadership. Clinicians have the opportunity through organized medicine to be mentored by respected peers with advocacy, policy, and communication experience. Local and regional roles may allow for increasing experience and the development of the knowledge and skills required for specialty- or domain-specific leadership. These roles may lead to national interest and experience.

Informally, clinicians in all settings are seen as leaders and can greatly impact patient safety and quality initiatives and directly improve outcomes. Clinicians can bring a valuable perspective on operations management (the day-to-day functioning in a hospital or clinic). In 2005, the Canadian Medical Association conducted a series of focus groups and found that most physicians ended up in leadership roles unintentionally as "accidental leaders."[52] Because of professional commitments to patient welfare, education, and growth of knowledge, clinicians value improvement in health care and naturally end up leading transformation in health care. Once in these roles, additional training is often required. Through mentored problem-solving, clinicians may learn to respect the roles and expertise, as well as the motivations, of team members. This can lead to a culture of empowerment and openness to change. Lean training and other domain-specific training opportunities are regionally abundant and often financially and administratively supported by local hospitals and health care systems.

Other leadership positions may require clinicians to step out of their clinical care roles and step into public health, media, or policy roles. There is generally no formal path or training for this, and again, clinicians in these roles frequently cite feeling the need and unique opportunity to have an impact in these new roles.

X. CHAPTER SUMMARY

The ever-changing landscape of medicine has created an imperative that the health system do a better job of preparing the emerging health care workforce to manage new therapies, new health care reimbursement models, new technologies, and the changing expectations of patients. This groundwork includes education and skills development in the domains of management of both teams and one's self, and communicating and exerting influence. Significant preparation is necessary in practical management of both clinical operations and the business aspects of health care. One of the most challenging competencies to master is change management as it incorporates elements of the other competencies. Individuals who excel in these areas may exert influence informally or may pursue either elected or appointed formal positions of authority. As students and learners envision their careers, it would be prudent to invest some time and energy in mastering the key competencies outlined in this chapter as a starting point.

QUESTIONS FOR FURTHER THOUGHT

1. What mental models and high-impact behaviors, as described by the IHI, enable health care leaders to promote change?
2. How do the personal qualities rewarded during the traditional education of clinicians match with those necessary to successfully lead change in our health care systems?
3. What opportunities exist outside of a formal leadership role for a health professions student to exhibit leadership?
4. Although leadership models may vary in how they define essential leadership qualities, what are some of the competencies that emerge from these models that are important for effective leadership?
5. What opportunities exist for health care professionals to gain experience in leadership positions or acquire additional expertise in leadership competency areas?

Annotated Bibliography

Atchison TA, Bujak JS. *Leading Transformational Change: The Physician-Executive Partnership.* Chicago, IL: Health Administration Press; 2001.
This book suggests ways to build productive relationships between physicians and executives to implement change. It addresses the differences between physicians and administrators, the reasons why collaboration efforts fail, and the importance of leadership style.
Barker A. *Improve Your Communication Skills.* London: Kogan Page; 2006.
This short book describes the basics of persuasive communication in the context of leadership and management.
Collins JC. *Good to Great and the Social Sectors: Why Business Thinking Is Not the Answer: A Monograph to Accompany Good to Great: Why Some Companies Make the Leap—and Others Don't.* Boulder, CO: Harper-Business; 2005.
Collins published this following the success of his book Good to Great, *which sought to identify how companies achieve superior performance and enduring impact. The monograph describes how the* Good to Great *framework applies to social sector organizations, including nonprofits and the health care industry.*
Fisher R, Ury W, Patton B. *Getting to Yes: Negotiating Agreement Without Giving In.* New York: Penguin Books; 1991.
This book about conflict resolution and negotiation simplifies the process by separating people from problems, focusing on interests rather

than positions, inventing options for mutual gain, and using objective criteria.

HBR's *10 Must Reads on Leadership*. Boston, MA: Harvard Business Review Press; 2011.
A compendium of ten classic articles on the central theme of leadership taken from the Harvard Business Review. *Many of the articles are drawn from the business sector, but have broad application to leadership in other settings.*

Quinn RE. Moments of greatness: entering the fundamental state of leadership. *Harv Bus Rev.* 2005;83(7):74–83, 191.
This article describes the "fundamental state of leadership," the state of leading with one's deepest values and instincts that come out in times of crisis. Dr. Quinn is a pre-eminent expert in transformational leadership who describes the value of being results-centered, internally directed, other-focused, and externally open.

Swensen S, Pugh M, McMullan C, Kabcenell A. *High Impact Leadership: Improve the Health of Populations, and Reduce Costs.* IHI White Paper. Cambridge, MA: Institute for Healthcare Improvement; 2013.
This paper describes mental models, attributes, and behaviors of high-functioning leaders in health care. Exemplars of leadership traits are identified within the paper, and the behaviors and outcomes of these exemplars are described.

References

1. Robeznieks A. Hospitals hire more doctors as CEOs as focus on quality grows. *Modern Healthcare.* May 10, 2014. http://www.modernhealthcare.com/article/20140510/MAGAZINE/305109988. Accessed January 5, 2016.
2. Feeley D. Leading improvement in population health: focusing on population health requires a new leadership approach. *Healthcare Executive.* 2014;29(3):82, 84–85.
3. Swensen S, Pugh M, McMullan C, Kabcenell A. *High Impact Leadership: Improve the Health of Populations, and Reduce Costs.* IHI White Paper. Cambridge, MA: Institute for Healthcare Improvement; 2013.
4. Gabow P, Halvorson G, Kaplan G. Marshaling leadership for high-value health care: an Institute of Medicine discussion paper. *JAMA.* 2012;308(3):239–240.
5. Institute of Medicine. *Academic Health Centers: Leading Change in the 21st Century.* Washington, DC: National Academies Press; 2004.
6. Enders T, Conroy J. *Advancing the Academic Health System for the Future: A Report of the AAMC Health Advisory Panel.* Washington, DC: The Association of American Medical Colleges; 2014.
7. *Core Entrustable Professional Activities for Entering Residency: Curriculum Developer's Guide.* Washington, DC: The Association of American Medical Colleges; 2014.
8. The Accreditation Council for Graduate Medical Education. ACGME Common Program Requirements. 2013; p. 9. Requirement IV.A.5.d. (3). http://www.acgme.org/Portals/0/PFAssets/ProgramRequirements/CPRs_07012015.pdf. Accessed May 24, 2015.
9. American Association of Colleges of Nursing. *Competencies and Curricular Expectations for Clinical Nurse Leader Education and Practice.* http://www.aacn.nche.edu/cnl/CNL-Competencies-October-2013.pdf. Published October 2013. Accessed March 21, 2016.
10. Royal College of Physicians and Surgeons of Canada. CanMEDS: Better standards, better physicians, better care. http://www.royalcollege.ca/rcsite/canmeds/canmeds-framework-e. Accessed November 2, 2016.
11. Bennis W. *On Becoming a Leader.* Reading, MA: Addison-Wesley; 1989.
12. Broome B, Grote K, Scott J, Sutaria S, Urban P. *Clinical Operations Excellence: Unlocking a Hospital's True Potential.* New York: McKinsey & Company; May 2013.
13. Institute for Healthcare Improvement. IHI Leadership Alliance. http://www.ihi.org/Engage/collaboratives/LeadershipAlliance. Accessed November 15, 2015.
14. Berwick DM, Feeley D, Loehrer S. Change from the inside out: health care leaders taking the helm. *JAMA.* 2015;313(17):1707–1708.
15. Swensen S, Pugh M, McMullan C, Kabcenell A. *High-Impact Leadership: Improve Care, Improve the Health of Populations, and Reduce Costs.* IHI White Paper. Cambridge, MA: Institute for Healthcare Improvement; 2013.
16. National Center for Healthcare Leadership. www.nchl.org. Accessed November 15, 2015.
17. Flint doctor Mona Hanna-Attisha on how she fought gov't denials to expose poisoning of city's kids. *Democracy Now.* http://www.democracynow.org/2016/1/15/flint_doctor_mona_hanna_attisha_on. Published January 15, 2016. Accessed January 31, 2016.
18. Reinertsen J. Institute for Healthcare Improvement. Introduction to health care leadership. http://app.ihi.org/lms/coursedetailview.aspx?CourseGUID=c1164ba8-5af1-438b-8a1f-d409911a4948&CatalogGUID=4220266a-94a3-4940-a3ce-546b82fdae25. Accessed November 2, 2016.
19. Moghimi Y. The "PharmFree" Campaign: educating medical students about industry influence. *PLoS Med.* 2006;3(1):PMC1360625. http://journals.plos.org/plosmedicine/article?id=10.1371/journal.pmed.0030030. Published January 31, 2006. Accessed February 1, 2016.
20. American Medical Study Association. AMSA PharmFree Campaign. http://www.pharmfree.org/campaign?id=0004. Accessed February 1, 2016.
21. Angood P, Birk S. The value of physician leadership. *Physician Exec.* May 2014. http://csms.org/wp-content/uploads/2015/04/The-Value-of-Physician-Leadership.pdf. Accessed November 2, 2016.
22. Day CS, Tabrizi S, Kramer J, Yule AC, Ahn BS. Effectiveness of the AAOS leadership fellows program for orthopaedic surgeons. *J Bone Joint Surg Am.* 2010;92(16):2700–2708.
23. Straus SE, Soobiah C, Levinson W. The impact of leadership training programs on physicians in academic medical centers: a systematic review. *Acad Med.* 2013;88(5):710–723.
24. Storey J, Holti R. *Towards a New Model of Leadership for the NHS.* National Health System (NHS) Leadership Academy. http://oro.open.ac.uk/37996/1/Towards-a-New-Model-of-Leadership-2013%20online.pdf. Published 2013.
25. Webb AM, Tsipis NE, McClellan TR, et al. A first step toward understanding best practices in leadership training in undergraduate medical education: a systematic review. *Acad Med.* 2014;89(11):1563–1570.
26. McKenna M, Gartland M. Development of physician leadership competencies. *J Health Admin Educ.* 2004;21:343–354.
27. Taylor CA, Taylor JC, Stoller JK. Exploring leadership competencies in established and aspiring physician leaders: an interview-based study. *J Gen Intern Med.* 2008;23(6):748–754.
28. Varkey P, Peloquin J, Reed D, Lindor K, Harris I. Leadership curriculum in undergraduate medical education: a study of student and faculty perspectives. *Med Teach.* 2009;31(3):244–250.
29. Stoller JK. Recommendations and remaining questions for health care leadership training programs. *Acad Med.* 2013;88(1):12–15.
30. Boyle M, Mullin T, Neumann J, Tsipsis N, Webb AB, Yerxa J. The Feagin Medical Leadership Model. Duke Institute for Health Innovation. http://www.dihi.org/sites/default/files/ldrmedmodel1.pdf. Accessed January 6, 2016.
31. Calhoun JG, Dollett L, Sinioris ME, et al. Development of an interprofessional competency model for healthcare leadership. *J Healthc Manag.* 2008;53(6):375–391.
32. Traynor AP, Boyle CJ, Janke KK. Guiding principles for student leadership development in the doctor of pharmacy program to assist administrators and faculty members in implementing or refining curricula. *Am J Pharm Educ.* 2013;77(10):1–10.
33. Korschun HW, Redding D, Teal GL, et al. Realizing the vision of leadership development in an academic health center: the Woodruff Leadership Academy. *Acad Med.* 2007;82(3):264–271.
34. Abraham PJ. Developing nurse leaders: a program enhancing staff nurse leadership skills and professionalism. *Nurs Admin Q.* 2011;35(4):306–312.
35. Omoike O, Stratton KM, Brooks BA, et al. Advancing nursing leadership: a model for program implementation and measurement. *Nurs Admin Q.* 2011;35(4):323–332.
36. Decker M. Competency integration in health management education. National Center for Healthcare Leadership. http://www.nchl.org/documents/ctrl_hyperlink/doccopy5755_uid892012228502.pdf. Accessed February 1, 2016.

37. NHS Leadership Academy. *Healthcare Leadership Model*, version 1.0. http://www.leadershipacademy.nhs.uk/wp-content/uploads/dlm_uploads/2014/10/NHSLeadership-LeadershipModel-colour.pdf. Accessed February 1, 2016.

38. Academy of Medical Royal Colleges. NHS Institute for Innovation and Improvement. *Medical Leadership Competency Framework: Enhancing Engagement in Medical Leadership*. http://www.leadershipacademy.nhs.uk/wp-content/uploads/2012/11/NHSLeadership-Leadership-Framework-Medical-Leadership-Competency-Framework-3rd-ed.pdf. Published July 2010. Accessed February 1, 2016.

39. Al-Touby SS. Functional results-oriented healthcare leadership: a novel leadership model. *Oman Med J*. 2012;27(2):104–107.

40. Shook J. *Managing to Learn: Using the A3 Management Process to Solve Problems, Gain Agreement, Mentor and Lead*. Cambridge, MA: Lean Enterprise Institute; 2008.

41. Bloche GM. Scandal as a sentinel event—recognizing hidden cost-quality trade-offs. *N Engl J Med*. 374(11):1001–1003.

42. Bass BM, Avolio B. *Improving Organizational Effectiveness Through Transformational Leadership*. Thousand Oaks, NJ: Sage Publications; 1994.

43. Quinn RE. Moments of greatness: entering the fundamental state of leadership. *Harv Bus Rev*. 2005;83(7):74–83, 191.

44. Hersey P, Blanchard K. *Management of Organizational Behavior: Utilizing Human Resources*. 6th ed. Englewood Cliffs, NJ: Prentice Hall; 1993.

45. Greenleaf RK. *Servant Leadership: A Journey into the Nature of Legitimate Power and Greatness*. Mahwah, NJ: Paulist Press; 1977.

46. Liang BA, Connelly NR, Raghunathan K. To tell the truth: potential liability for concealing physician impairment. *J Clin Anesth*. 2007;19(8):638–641.

47. Collins J. *Good to Great*. New York: Fast Company; October 2001.

48. Krane NK, DiCarlo RP, Kahn MJ. Medical education in post-Katrina New Orleans: a story of survival and renewal. *JAMA*. 2007;298(9):1052–1055.

49. Association of Critical Care Nurses. *Silence Kills: The Seven Crucial Conversations in Healthcare*. http://www.silenttreatmentstudy.com/silencekills/SilenceKills.pdf. Accessed February 7, 2016.

50. Foden-Vencil K. *How Oregon Is Getting "Frequent Flyers" Out of Hospital ERs*. Oregon Public Broadcasting; July 10, 2013.

51. Institute for Healthcare Improvement. Going Lean in health care. http://www.ihi.org/resources/pages/ihiwhitepapers/goingleaninhealthcare.aspx. Published 2005. Accessed February 7, 2016.

52. Collins-Nakai R. Leadership in medicine. *Mcgill J Med*. 2006;9(1):68–73.

9

Clinical Informatics

William Hersh, MD, and Jesse M. Ehrenfeld, MD

This chapter begins by describing the importance and relevance of health information technology and clinical informatics to safe and effective patient care. Applications of clinical informatics, particularly the electronic health record (EHR), are discussed. The value of the EHR in supporting high-quality patient care and the importance of EHR interoperability are emphasized. Next, the use of data analytics to support various information needs of health care providers and health systems are elucidated. Challenges and opportunities related to the use of EHRs and informatics are presented. Lastly, the authors highlight recently developed competencies in clinical informatics and briefly reflect on future directions in this increasingly important area in health care and medical education. Throughout the chapter, key terms and concepts are defined and described.

The optimal delivery of health care requires information. The discipline devoted to the efficient storage, acquisition, and use of information in health care is called *biomedical and health informatics*.[1] The area within the discipline of informatics focused on health care delivery is known as *clinical informatics*. This chapter focuses on how clinical informatics can be used to improve the quality, safety, and efficiency of health care delivery.

I. RATIONALE AND TERMINOLOGY OF CLINICAL INFORMATICS

The importance of clinical informatics in health care delivery began to emerge in the latter part of the 20th century. A series of seminal reports from the Institute of Medicine (IOM) documented significant problems in health care delivery and led to proposed solutions based on best information technology (IT) and evidence supporting its use. The first IOM report documented the harms resulting from incomplete and illegible paper-based medical records.[2] Probably the most high-profile of these reports focused on errors in hospitals estimated to result in up to 96,000 deaths per year.[3] Another IOM report noted a "chasm" of deficiencies in the quality of health care between the known, evidence-based best practices and their actual use in the health care system. Constraints on exploiting the revolution in information technology was named as one of the underlying reasons for inadequate quality of care, and increasing the use of information technology was cited as a means of improving quality of care.[4]

A number of studies supported the conclusions of these reports. In 1995, Bates and colleagues documented error rates of 6.5 adverse drug events (ADEs) per 100 hospitalized patients.[5] Quality problems were quantified more clearly in 2003 by McGlynn and coworkers, who assessed the records of 6259 patients in 12 metropolitan areas and found that only 54.9 percent of care delivered was consistent with evidence-based known best practices.[6] Paper-based medical information was associated with clinical decisions being made with incomplete information, as Smith and colleagues showed that information was missing and impacted up to 44 percent of patients in primary care settings.[7]

A. Value of Clinical Informatics in Improving the Quality, Safety, and Efficiency of Health Care

Additionally, there was emerging evidence for the value of health IT. In 1993, Tierney and colleagues documented that **computerized provider order entry (CPOE)** in hospitals was associated with a 12.7 percent decrease in total charges and a 0.9-day shorter length of stay.[8] In 1998, Bates and colleagues showed that CPOE reduced serious medication errors by 55 percent, with adverse drug events reduced by 17 percent.[9] Other studies showed that CPOE led to a reduction in redundant laboratory tests[10] and increased prescribing of equally efficacious but less costly medications.[11] Much of this early work was summarized in a systematic review of 257 studies of health IT documenting its association with increased adherence to guideline-based care, enhanced surveillance and monitoring, and decreased medical errors.[12]

Modeling studies were also being published demonstrating return on investment for electronic health records (EHRs) as well as **health information exchange (HIE),** the exchange of information across the boundaries of health care organizations.[13] Johnston and colleagues assessed the potential benefit of CPOE in ambulatory settings and noted savings of up to $28,000 per year, although most of the savings went to laboratories and insurance companies, and not the physician practices making the investment.[14] Another modeling study by Hillestad and coworkers applied results of known research in an attempt to scale to the entire US health care system, finding that HIE could potentially result in savings of $81 billion per year above costs and a reduction of 200,000 ADEs per year.[15]

B. ARRA, HITECH, and Adoption of Electronic Health Records

When these problems were considered in the context of an ongoing economic recession and a new president whose priorities included health care reform, the time was ripe for a substantial national investment in EHR adoption. One of the first acts of President Barack Obama's tenure was the passage of the American Recovery and Reinvestment Act (ARRA), a $787 billion economic stimulus that included the Health Information Technology for Economic and Clinical Health (HITECH) Act, which allocated approximately $30 billion for investment in the adoption of EHRs.[16] Such an investment was the type of "shovel ready" project needed for the stimulus, and there was additional evidence that such an investment could create tens of thousands of jobs in the health IT sector.[17] There already existed a template for the concept of "meaningful use" to measure adoption for incentive purposes that had been put forth earlier by Congressman Pete Stark.[18]

Since its inception in 2010, the HITECH Act has led to substantial growth of EHR adoption, with nearly all hospitals (96 percent)[19] and over four-fifths of office-based physicians (83 percent)[20] now using them. However, many challenges have emerged with the introduction of EHRs into health care, such as disruption in workflow, increased time required for patient documentation, and distraction by the computer in the examination room,[21] providing further imperative for the optimal understanding and application of clinical informatics.

C. Definitions of Informatics and Related Terms

A critical aspect of informatics is its focus on information and not technology. While IT infrastructure (i.e., the networks, devices, and software) is essential for effective application of informatics, the larger goal is the benefit that information provides to health care and optimal health of individuals and populations.[1,22,23] Friedman has defined the "fundamental theorem" of informatics, which states that informatics is more about using technology to help people perform their work better than about building systems to mimic or replace human expertise.[24] He has also described what informatics is (information sciences applied in a biomedical application domain with the aim of helping people) and is not (any use of IT or data analysis in health care).[25]

While informatics is a relatively new discipline compared to others in medicine, it has accumulated a history over a half-century that has evolved with advances in IT.[26] The various areas within biomedical and health informatics are depicted in Fig. 9.1. Sometimes narrower words appear in front of informatics. *Clinical informatics* generally refers to informatics applied in health care settings.[27] Sometimes *medical informatics* is used to describe this application as well. Other uses of informatics in biomedical and health-related areas include the following:

- *Bioinformatics*—the application of informatics in cellular and molecular biology, often with a focus on genomics[28]
- *Imaging informatics*—informatics with a focus on imaging, including the use of systems to store and retrieve images in health care settings[29]
- The application of informatics focused on specific health care disciplines, such as nursing *(nursing informatics),*[30] dentistry *(dental informatics),* pathology *(pathology informatics),*[31] and so on
- *Consumer health informatics*—the field devoted to informatics from a consumer view[32]
- *Clinical research informatics*—the use of informatics to facilitate clinical research, with increasing emphasis on translational research that aims to accelerate research findings into clinical practice[33]
- *Public health informatics*—the application of informatics in areas of public health, including surveillance, reporting, and health promotion[34]

D. Subspecialty Certification in Clinical Informatics

Even though not limited to the work of physicians, clinical informatics is now recognized as a medical subspecialty[27] and has been defined by the Accreditation Council for Graduate Medical Education (ACGME) as the field that "transforms health care by analyzing, designing, implementing, and evaluating information and communication systems to improve patient care, enhance access to care, advance individual and population health outcomes, and strengthen the

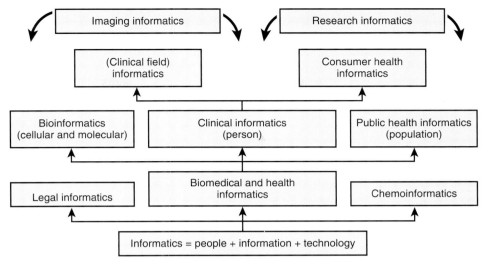

Fig. 9.1 Areas within biomedical and health informatics, including clinical informatics. (Adapted from Hersh W. A stimulus to define informatics and health information technology. *BMC Med Inform Decis Mak.* 2009;9:24. http://www.biomedcentral.com/1472-6947/9/24/.)

clinician-patient relationship."[35] Since 2013, physicians who have worked in the field or completed a fellowship in informatics and have a primary board certification in their specialty have been eligible to become board certified in clinical informatics. That subspecialty certification is available to physician specialists who are certified by any of the 24 member boards of the American Board of Medical Specialties, which endorses the broad clinical relevance of expertise in clinical informatics.[27] Since the first certification examination was offered in 2013, over 1100 physicians have become board-certified.

II. USE OF CLINICAL INFORMATICS IN HEALTH CARE DELIVERY

There are many applications of clinical informatics, with the EHR occupying a central role. The EHR serves several key functions, not only in documenting data and information of care delivery, but also providing access to other participants in the system, most importantly the patient, and it functions to improve care delivery.

A. Electronic Health Records

Probably the most central application of clinical informatics is the EHR. In the past, the term electronic medical record (EMR) was more commonly used, but EHR implies a broader and more longitudinal collection of information about the patient. There is also increasing use of the term personal health record (PHR). This usually refers to the patient-controlled aspect of the health record and may or may not be tethered to one or more EHRs from health care delivery organizations. There are a growing number of cloud-based PHR products available in which patients are able to manage their own health record.

The EHR is not meant to be a mere replacement for the paper-based record, but rather it should ideally serve as a tool to transform and improve health care delivery. One major component of the EHR is **clinical decision support (CDS),** which allows detection of errors and adverse events and can

facilitate improved care delivery and quality.[36] As the most critical time for intervention is when the physician is entering patient orders, the function of the CPOE is the optimal time to make CDS readily available. Related to CPOE is electronic prescribing (e-prescribing), which focuses more narrowly on the electronic ordering of medications. The major categories of CDS include the following:

- Information display—showing general or patient-specific information in context of the current clinical situation
- Reminder systems—reminding clinicians to perform actions, such as preventive measures, when they are due
- Alerts—alerting to critical clinical situations (e.g., interacting drugs, abnormal laboratory values that may negatively impact patient safety and health outcomes)
- Clinical practice guidelines—guiding treatment to provide consistent care based on best evidence

An exemplar EHR is the Veterans Health Information Systems and Technology Architecture (VistA) system (http://www.ehealth.va.gov/vista.asp), which is used in 1800 locations across the world including all Department of Veterans Affairs medical centers as well as by the national health systems of Finland, Egypt, and Jordan. Fig. 9.2 shows the cover page of the EHR, which provides an overview of the patient, including his or her active problems and medications as well as recent results. This page also shows an example of CDS, listing all clinical reminders. The tabs at the bottom of the screen allow the user to drill down into more details on specific aspects of the patient's care, such as medications and laboratory results. Many of these screens feature additional CDS, such as drug-drug interactions.

As the use of EHRs has grown, it has become apparent that information must seamlessly flow among health care providers, and it must flow across different health care organizations. This has led to growing advocacy for HIE, which is the exchange of health information for patient care across traditional business boundaries in health care. Even many health care organizations that have exemplary HIT systems have difficulty providing their patient information to other entities where the patient may receive care. An increasingly mobile population also needs to have "data following the patient" as patients move in, out, and across health care systems.

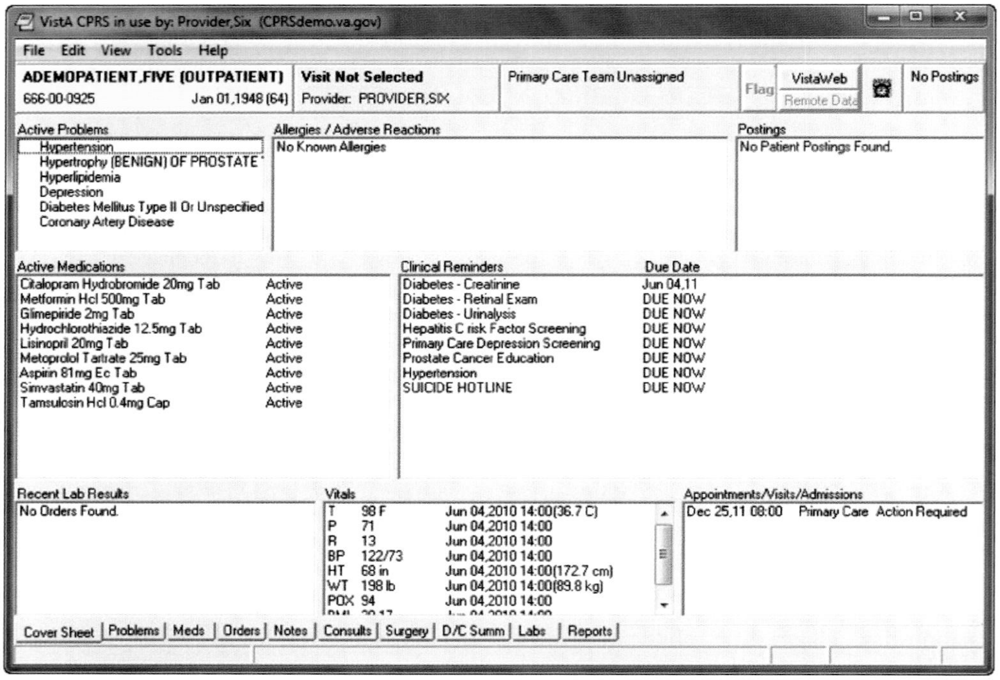

Fig. 9.2 **Cover page of the Veterans Health Information Systems and Technology Architecture system.** (VistA, http://www.ehealth.va.gov/vista.asp.)

B. Electronic Health Record Interoperability

One of the impediments to HIE has been suboptimal **interoperability** of EHR systems, with systems unable to seamlessly exchange data. Optimal interoperability requires adoption and adherence to standards to define data structures and formats. Although many standards exist for exchange of information and consistent use of terminology, they have not been applied for a variety of reasons.[37] The major categories of standards include the following:

- Identifiers—of patients, clinicians, health plans, insurance companies, and so on
- Transactions—eligibility, enrollment, payments, and so on
- Message exchange—transmission of data, images, documents, and so on
- Terminology—standard descriptions of diagnoses, tests, treatments, and so on

The presence of standardized interoperable data and systems not only leads to improved direct care of patients but also to secondary use or re-use of clinical data, where data from clinical settings is used for other applications, such as quality measurement and improvement, clinical and translational research, and public health.[38] All of these systems come together in the concept advanced by the IOM of the **learning health system.**[39,40]

C. Beyond the Electronic Health Record

Clinical informatics is not limited to EHRs. Another vital component for optimal patient care is access to information and knowledge. The field devoted to indexing and retrieval of knowledge-based information is called information retrieval or search.[41] Searching is a basic skill in the practice of **evidence-based medicine** (EBM), a skill set that includes the proper phrasing of clinical questions, seeking the best evidence to answer such questions, critically appraising what was retrieved, and applying such evidence to patient care. One recent textbook of EBM notes, "Searching for current best evidence in the medical literature has become a central skill in clinical practice. On average, clinicians have 5 to 8 questions about individual patients per daily shift… Some now even consider that 'the use of search engines is as essential as the stethoscope.'"[42]

Additional important applications of clinical informatics are telemedicine and telehealth.[43] **Telemedicine** is the delivery of health care when the participants are separated by time and/or distance, while telehealth has a larger aspect of all telecommunications applications devoted to health. As with informatics, the "tele-" terms sometimes reflect medical specialties in which they are applied (e.g., teleradiology, telepathology). A variety of practice models embracing telehealth have now emerged, including e-ICU and telestroke services that are commonly employed to deliver expertise to a broader population.

Table 9.1 lists some of the other chapters and their titles in this book and the role that informatics plays within them.

III. RE-USE OF CLINICAL DATA

One of the promises of the growing critical mass of clinical data accumulating in the EHR is secondary use (or re-use) of the data for other purposes, such as quality improvement, operations management, and clinical research.[38] There has also been substantial growth in other kinds of health-related data, most notably through efforts to sequence genomes and other biological structures and functions. The analysis of this data is usually called analytics or **data analytics.**[44]

Table 9.1 Role of Clinical Informatics in Topics Covered in Other Select Chapters

Chapter	Title	Role of Clinical Informatics
3	The Health Care Delivery System	Documenting and improving care
4	Value in Health Care	Providing decision support to achieve value
5	Patient Safety	Early detection and action upon safety issues
6	Quality Improvement	Measurement and improvement of quality
7	Principles of Teamwork and Team Science	Facilitating care coordination among teams
8	Leadership in Health Care	Allowing leaders to make better decisions
10	Population Health	Management and surveillance of populations
11	Socio-Ecologic Determinants of Health	Determination and action to reduce disparities
12	Health Care Policy and Economics	More informed policy decisions
13	Application Foundational Skills to Health Systems Science	Access to evidence-based information
14	The Use of Assessment to Support Learning and Improvement in Health Systems Science	Access to quality data and clinical evidence to improve delivery of care

A. Data Analytics

The terminology surrounding the use of large and varied types of data in health care is evolving, but the term analytics is achieving wide use both in and out of health care. A long-time leader in the field defines analytics as "the extensive use of data, statistical and quantitative analysis, explanatory and predictive models, and fact-based management to drive decisions and actions."[45] The company IBM defines analytics as "the systematic use of data and related business insights developed through applied analytical disciplines (e.g., statistical, contextual, quantitative, predictive, cognitive, other [including emerging] models) to drive fact-based decision making for planning, management, measurement and learning. Analytics may be descriptive, predictive or prescriptive."[46]

Adams and Klein have authored a primer on analytics in health care that defines different levels and their attributes of the application of analytics.[47] They noted three levels of analytics, each with increasing functionality and value:

- Descriptive—standard types of reporting that describe current situations and problems (e.g., reports of patients with certain diagnoses or outlier test results)
- Predictive—simulation and modeling techniques that identify trends and portend outcomes of actions taken (e.g., lists of patients who may be at risk for poor outcomes or repeated admissions to the hospital)
- Prescriptive—optimizing clinical, financial, and other outcomes (e.g., recommendations for patients to maintain health or to prevent poor outcomes)

Much work is focusing now on **predictive analytics,** especially in clinical settings attempting to optimize health and financial outcomes, including in clinical practice.[48]

There are a number of terms related to data analytics. A core methodology in data analytics is machine learning, which is the area of computer science that aims to build systems and algorithms that learn from data.[49] One of the major techniques of machine learning is data mining, which is defined as the processing and modeling of large amounts of data to discover previously unknown patterns or relationships.[50] A sub-area of data mining is text mining, which applies data mining techniques to mostly unstructured textual data.[51] Another close but more recent term in the vernacular is big data, which describes large and ever-increasing volumes of data that adhere to the following attributes:[52]

- Volume—ever-increasing amounts
- Velocity—quickly generated
- Variety—many different types
- Veracity—from sources whose trustworthiness can be known

B. Making Use of Data

Hospitals and other health care organizations are generating an exploding amount of data. Clinical data takes a variety of forms, from structured (e.g., images, laboratory results) to unstructured (e.g., textual notes including clinical narratives, reports, and other types of documents). Additionally, health care organizations capture and generate additional data as a byproduct of the care delivery process. This can include billing, quality, management, and other financial data, which are increasingly important in the optimization of health care delivery. Kaiser Permanente estimated in 2013 that its data store for its 9+ million members exceeds 30 petabytes of data.[53] Other organizations are planning for a data-intensive future. For example, the American Society for Clinical Oncology (ASCO) has been developing its Cancer Learning Intelligence Network for Quality (CancerLinQ).[54] CancerLinQ will provide a comprehensive system for clinicians and researchers consisting of EHR data collection, application of CDS, data mining and visualization, and quality measurement for improvement.

The world's growing base of scientific literature and its underlying data that are increasingly published with journal and other articles is another source of data and can be linked with EHR and other patient data aiming to improve outcomes of care. One approach to this problem that has generated attention is the IBM Watson project, which was made famous by winning at the television game show *Jeopardy!*[55] One of the areas where IBM and its partners have been applying Watson is in the health care arena.[56]

The growing quantity of data requires that its users have a good understanding of its provenance, which is where the data originated and how trustworthy it is for large-scale processing and analysis.[57] A number of researchers and thought leaders have started to specify the path that will be required for big data to be applied in health care and biomedicine.[58-60] Bates and colleagues elucidated a number of use cases in which big data methods might lead to improved outcomes[61]:

- High-cost patients—looking for ways to intervene early
- Re-admissions—prevention
- Triage—appropriate level of care
- Decompensation—when a patient's condition worsens
- Adverse events—awareness
- Treatment optimization—especially for diseases affecting multiple organ systems

Patients are also increasingly interested in seeing more than just basic transactional information (i.e., a test result or a notice of an overdue payment). They want summarized information along with recommendations for care that is personalized to them. Similarly, payers, providers, and health care institutions are all increasingly seeking information that can help them predict how to better serve their customers, clients, and patients.

A more peripheral but related term is business intelligence, which in health care refers to the "processes and technologies used to obtain timely, valuable insights into business and clinical data."[47] Another relevant term is the notion promoted by the IOM of the learning health system.[39,40] Advocates of this approach note that routinely collected data can be used for continuous learning to allow the health care system to better carry out disease surveillance and response, targeting of health care services, improving decision-making, managing misinformation, reducing harm, avoiding costly errors, and advancing clinical research.[62]

Another set of related terms come from the call for new and much more data-intensive approaches for diagnosis and treatment of disease, originally called personalized medicine[63] but now labeled precision medicine (i.e., identifying which approaches will be effective for which patients based on genetic, environmental, and lifestyle factors).[64] Pharmacogenomics is a subset of precision medicine that studies how genetics affect a person's response to particular drugs. The US government has recently committed a substantial investment in research around precision medicine.[65] But probably the major motivator for data-driven decision making in health care is the move from volume-driven reimbursement (e.g., fee for service) to value-driven reimbursement (in which health systems and providers share risk).[66]

As clinical data accumulate, so does the amount of metadata (or data about data). **Metadata** can be defined as data points used to identify data (e.g., who authored a particular clinical note) or how data are linked together (e.g., vital signs from multiple records that represent a single patient) or how data have been utilized (e.g., data access and audit logs). Analysis of metadata, rather than the underlying clinical data itself, can be informative. In the United States, since 1996, the Health Insurance Portability and Accountability Act (HIPAA) requires that hospitals maintain audit trails for 6 years. Metadata have been used by many researchers to understand health care processes in support of quality improvement. For example, one research team utilized audit log metadata to evaluate the composition of medical teams. They found that 25 percent of clinicians in their hospital had at least one contact with an obstetric patient over the course of 1 year representing over 300 clinicians. Another common place where metadata are used is in the process of understanding clinical workflows. A study of residents using EHR audit metadata revealed that they tended to view computed tomography scans themselves,

while relying on the attending radiologist's chest radiograph film reports. The study also found that more senior residents viewed images more frequently than junior residents, who also viewed images more often than medical students.[67]

Case Study 1

One Saturday evening, an elderly patient who lives in a suburb of Indianapolis develops sharp abdominal pain while visiting her sister in northern Indiana. The patient, who has difficulty keeping track of her medicines, decides to go to the local emergency department. During the triage process, the patient is asked to provide information about her medical history and a current list of medications. She is unable to provide much information given her limited capacity. Given that her regular doctor's office is closed and she is at a hospital she has never visited, what steps can the treating team use to provide the best patient-centered care for this patient? Is there a way that technology can help fill in the gaps?

The *Indiana Network for Patient Care* (INPC) is part of the Indiana Health Information Exchange (IHIE, www.ihie.org), which is one of the largest and original health information exchange (HIE) efforts in the world. The IHIE allows over 100 hospitals and 22,000 physicians, along with long-term care facilities, laboratories, and public health organizations to share data for patient care, research, public health, and other purposes.[68] The INPC is the data repository that enables the IHIE, with over 11 million patients and 4 billion structured observations. The emergency departments of all hospitals can access the records of patients who have received care at any IHIE-connected hospital, with the physicians able to query laboratory, radiology, and other reports of all patients in the INPC repository.

The INPC facilitates a number of best practices to use for improving patient care. A few examples include when patients present in the following situations[115]:

- Emergency department—accessing recent care activity and results from other care settings to reduce unnecessary redundant testing, facilitate medication reconciliation, and help clinicians identify patients who are at risk for medication abuse and "doctor shopping"; the HIE is particularly helpful when patients present after hours for urgent conditions
- Inpatient—providing a more complete picture of the patient at admission and facilitating medication reconciliation
- Case management—allowing better coordination of care and reducing redundant testing
- Radiology departments and centers—providing results for comparative assessment and reducing cost and radiation exposure
- Outpatient—preparing the chart prior to patient arrival and providing information about past visits to develop a more informed care plan
- Quality and performance improvement—accessing data for quality measures
- Accountable Care Organization (ACO) managers—facilitating access to information about the patient's care, including outside the ACO
- Long-term care—improving transitions of care and providing information when the patient needs to visit the emergency department or outpatient settings

C. Formulating Questions

The true utility of clinical data and metadata can only be realized when one is able to use these resources to answer relevant questions. Formulating such a question begins with a problem statement and an understanding of the underlying data that are available to help provide an answer. Treatment of the data and selecting an appropriate analytical approach should be the final step. For example, one might ask, "How often do medical students participate in vaginal deliveries?" or "How often are surgical cases canceled the morning of surgery?" Depending on the data available in the EHR, these types of questions might be easily answered by relatively simple case log queries. More complex questions such as "How often are dialysis patients re-admitted within 30 days after AV-fistula creation due to a surgical complication" pose more challenges, depending on how the underlying data are stored. In the latter example, most EHRs can provide admission and re-admission data, but fewer store the data on the reason for a re-admission in a structured fashion. Depending on what data are available in a particular system, the question about re-admissions from surgical complications may or may not be able to be answered using data queried from an EHR.

D. Clinical Data Warehousing, Registries, and Quality Reporting

Clinical data warehouses are central repositories of data where information is integrated together from disparate sources. They are typically maintained at the institutional level (i.e., within a hospital or health care system). **Clinical data registries** are collections of data about patients with a similar disease or therapeutic process. For example, the Cancer Genetics Network collects data about patients with cancer, and the Society of Thoracic Surgeons Database collects data from 1100 hospitals about patients who have undergone cardiothoracic surgery. The Multicenter Perioperative Outcomes Groups (MPOG) is a consortium of 47 medical centers that share anesthesia and surgical outcomes data. In 2014, the federal government created a standardized approach reporting clinical data registries through the Qualified Clinical Data Registry (QCDR) reporting mechanism. This was an attempt to motivate physicians to collect clinical data to foster quality improvement and to penalize those who did not through a system of reimbursement incentives and penalties.

The case study in this chapter describes the Indiana Network for Patient Care (INPC), an HIE implementation that covers most of Indiana and provides data that facilitate care in hospitals, emergency departments, outpatient settings, long-term care facilities, and public health agencies.[68] Data from the INPC not only improve access to data for direct care but also facilitate population health management and calculation of quality measures. Although HIE efforts have been challenging to generalize, they have been associated with improved quality and efficiency of care.[69]

E. Challenges for Data Analytics

A concern for more intensive use of data is that data generated in the routine care of patients may be limited for analytical purposes.[70] For example, such data may be inaccurate or incomplete. It may be transformed in ways that undermine its meaning (e.g., coding for billing priorities). For example, services or diagnoses that are highly reimbursed may be coded more reliably than other entities. It may exhibit the well-known statistical phenomenon of *censoring*, for example, the first instance of disease in record may not be when it was first manifested (left censoring) or the data source may not cover a sufficiently long time interval (right censoring). Data may also incompletely adhere to well-known standards, which makes combining it from different sources more difficult.

There is an emerging base of research that demonstrates how data from operational clinical systems can be used to identify critical situations or patients whose costs are outliers. There is less research, however, demonstrating how these data can be put to use to actually improve clinical outcomes or reduce costs. Studies using EHR data for clinical prediction have been proliferating. One common area of focus has been the use of data analytics to identify patients at risk for hospital re-admission within 30 days of discharge. The importance of this factor stems from the US Centers for Medicare and Medicaid Services (CMS) Readmissions Reduction Program that penalizes hospitals for excessive rates of re-admissions.[71] This has led several researchers to assess EHR data in its value to predict patients at risk for re-admission.[72-74]

IV. OUTCOMES AND IMPLICATIONS OF CLINICAL INFORMATICS

With the massive adoption of EHRs in the United States driven by the HITECH Act, there has been a dichotomy between focused research describing specific benefits and general dissatisfaction with current systems and their impact on medical practice. Following the original systematic review in 2006, three subsequent reviews using a similar methodology published in 2009,[75] 2011,[76] and 2014[77] have shown persistent benefits for health IT.

A. Adverse Effects of Electronic Health Records

At the same time, there have been great concerns about the adverse impact of EHR use in health care delivery. A number of surveys have documented substantial dissatisfaction among EHR users[78] and identified EHRs as a major source of physician dissatisfaction in medical practice.[79] It is unknown whether this is a temporary transitional problem to better systems or will result in ongoing problems with their use in medical practice.[21]

Among the problems of EHRs emerging include excess focus on the computer over the patient,[80,81] the demise of traditional communications such as radiology rounds,[82] and problems with documentation such as losing the patient's story through use of documentation templates[83] and inappropriate use of "copy and paste."[84]

Although EHRs have been touted to improve patient safety, there are also growing concerns that some aspects of their use may introduce new safety problems.[85] Two recent high-profile mishaps included massive overdosing of a common antibiotic[86] and accidental discharge of a patient who was infected with the Ebola virus.[87] There are also growing concerns over the security of health information.[88] The year 2015 saw several massive security breaches, leading to exposure of records of over 100 million Americans.[89–91] The black market value of a medical record has been estimated to be 10 times that of a credit card number.[92]

Nonetheless, there are many who believe that we should continue to improve EHRs and leverage their benefits to improve health care delivery. Two high-profile professional organizations have issued white papers specifying improvements in the EHR[93] and patient documentation.[94] The American Medical Association has laid out the following set of principles for improved usability and interoperability:[95]

- Enhance physicians' ability to provide high-quality patient care
- Support team-based care
- Promote care coordination
- Offer product modularity and configurability
- Reduce cognitive workload
- Promote data liquidity
- Facilitate digital and mobile patient engagement
- Expedite user input into product design and post-implementation feedback

B. Benefits of Electronic Health Records

In balance, a (mostly) positive evidence base continues to accumulate on EHR use. Evidence in support of the value of EHRs shows that they detect and help overcome delays in cancer diagnosis,[96,97] reduce risk of hospital re-admission,[98,99] and improve identification of postoperative complications.[100] EHRs have also been shown to enhance patient-provider communication[101] and facilitate research through extracting phenotype information about patients.[102,103] Within the surgical patients, EHRs have been shown to improve care in a number of ways by reducing postoperative nausea and vomiting, surgical site infections, and wrong-sided surgeries.[104] There are even emerging models for more optimal examination room use of EHRs.[105] Optimists continue to note other benefits, such as the "data dividend" of EHR adoption from the HITECH Act.[106] Others note that problems with diagnostic[107] and therapeutic[108] errors in health care continue.

C. Clinical Informatics Research: Challenges and Opportunities

Informatics has a tremendous potential to facilitate both high-quality outcomes research and quality improvement efforts. EHRs, data warehouses, and clinical registries are all tools that have become ubiquitous across health care. New approaches to data storage, management, and analysis are enabling a growing number of end-users the ability to turn data into information with greater ease. These tools, when taken together, can be used to identify patients or processes of interests, obtain data, and study interventions in ways that have been impossible heretofore. Additionally, clinical data that is re-used for these purposes often come

at a fraction of the price of data that have to be manually extracted or collected by research personnel. The success of these efforts, however, is dependent on data quality, standards, and availability. Additionally, overcoming the regulatory challenges associated with data sharing and privacy concerns remains a significant issue. Finally, none of this work is possible without expert informaticians who are able to lead these efforts.

V. COMPETENCIES OF CLINICAL INFORMATICS

Health care providers, including physicians and medical students, have been using health IT for decades. During this time, the role of health IT has changed dramatically from a useful tool for data access and occasional information retrieval to a ubiquitous presence that permeates health care and medical practice in many ways. But 21st-century clinicians face a clinical world that is quite different from that of their predecessors. The quantity of biomedical knowledge continues to expand, with an attendant increase in the primary scientific literature.[109] Secondary sources that summarize this information proliferate as well, not only for use by clinicians but also by patients and those who are healthy but consuming health-related information. The accelerated adoption of EHRs under the HITECH Act requires competency in their use, including for secondary uses as discussed earlier. Patients want to interact with the health care system the same way they interact with airlines, banks, and retailers, that is, through digital means using technologies such as the PHR.[110] Patients, payers, and purchasers demand more accountability in health care quality, safety, and cost,[111] leading to an expectation of measurement and reporting of quality of care as a routine part of participation in new delivery mechanisms such as primary care medical homes and accountable care organizations. These trends emphasize the need for health care professionals to develop and maintain the knowledge and skills necessary to use clinical informatics optimally in delivering safe and effective patient care. Table 9.2 lists competencies developed for medical education but has application for physicians beyond medical school and other health care professionals.[112]

While all physicians need basic competence in clinical informatics, there is also a need for a modest-sized cadre of experts in the area. Growing numbers of physicians assume roles in health care settings under titles such as Chief Medical Informatics Officer (CMIO).[113] There are also opportunities in industry, government, and other settings. These opportunities have led to the designation of a new medical subspecialty (of all medical specialties) of clinical informatics.[27] Since 2013, over 1100 physicians practicing clinical informatics have been able to become board-certified in this new subspecialty. In addition, fellowship programs accredited by the ACGME are starting to be established.[114] This underscores the need for introduction of the concepts and competencies of clinical informatics as part of medical training.

Table 9.2   Competencies in Clinical Informatics for Health Care Professionals[112]

1. Find, search, and apply knowledge-based information to patient care and other clinical tasks
   a. Information retrieval/search: Choose correct source for specific task, search using advanced features, apply results
   b. Evaluate information resources (e.g., literature, databases) for their quality, funding sources, biases
   c. Identify tools to assess patient safety (e.g., medication interactions)
   d. Utilize knowledge-based tools to answer clinical questions at the point of care (e.g., text resources, calculators)
   e. Formulate an answerable clinical question
   f. Determine the costs/charges of medications and tests
   g. Identify deviations from normal (laboratory tests/radiographs/results), and develop a list of causes of the deviation

2. Effectively read and write from the electronic health record for patient care and other clinical activities
   a. Graph, display, and trend vital signs and laboratory values over time
   b. Adopt a uniform method of reviewing a patient record
   c. Create and maintain an accurate problem list
   d. Recognize medical safety issues related to poor chart maintenance
   e. Identify a normal range of results for a specific patient
   f. Access and compare radiographs over time
   g. Identify inaccuracies in the problem list/history/medication list/allergies
   h. Create useable notes
   i. Write orders and prescriptions
   j. List common errors with data entry (e.g., drop-down lists, copy and paste)

3. Use and guide implementation of clinical decision support (CDS)
   a. Recognize different types of CDS
   b. Be able to use different types of CDS
   c. Work with clinical and informatics colleagues to guide CDS use in clinical settings

4. Provide care using population health management approaches
   a. Utilize patient record (data collection and data entry) to assist with disease management
   b. Create reports for populations in different health care delivery systems
   c. Use and apply data in accountable care, care coordination, and the primary care medical home settings

5. Protect patient privacy and security
   a. Use security features of information systems
   b. Adhere to HIPAA privacy and security regulations
   c. Describe and manage ethical issues in privacy and security

6. Use information technology to improve patient safety
   a. Perform a root-cause analysis to uncover patient safety problems
   b. Become familiar with safety issues
   c. Use resources to solve safety issues

7. Engage in quality measurement selection and improvement
   a. Recognize the types and limitations of different types of quality measures
   b. Determine the pros and cons of a quality measure, how to measure it, and how to use it to change care

8. Use health information exchange (HIE) to identify and access patient information across clinical settings
   a. Recognize issues of dispersed patient information across clinical locations
   b. Participate in the use of the HIE to improve clinical care

9. Engage patients to improve their health and care delivery though personal health records and patient portals
   a. Instruct patients in the proper use of a personal health record (PHR)
   b. Write an e-mail to a patient using a patient portal
   c. Demonstrate appropriate written communication with all members of the health care team
   d. Integrate technology into patient education (e.g., decision-making tools, diagrams, patient education)
   e. Educate patients to discern quality of online medical resources (e.g., websites, apps, patient support groups, social media)
   f. Maintain patient engagement while using an EHR (e.g., eye contact, body language)

10. Maintain professionalism through use of information technology tools
    a. Describe and manage ethics of media use (cloud storage issues, texting, cell phones, social media professionalism)

11. Provide clinical care via telemedicine, and refer those for whom it is necessary
    a. Be able to function clinically in telemedicine/telehealth environments

12. Apply personalized/precision medicine
    a. Recognize the growing role of genomics and personalized medicine in care
    b. Identify resources enabling access to actionable information related to precision medicine

13. Participate in practice-based clinical and translational research
    a. Use EHR alerts and other tools to identify patients and populations for offering clinical trial participation
    b. Participate in practice-based research to advance medical knowledge

VI. CHAPTER SUMMARY

Across health care, major changes have been spawned by innovation, regulatory efforts, and consumer demands. All three are likely to play a role in shaping the future of clinical informatics. We will undoubtedly see continued innovation, as technology evolves and continues to permeate our health care delivery systems. The government, through its purchasing power, regulatory requirements, and incentive programs, is also likely to shape the use of clinical informatics. What is less clear is what role consumers will play. Some predict that consumer demand for access to health care information will drive changes to EHRs, interoperability, information exchange, and the use of personal health records. Others predict that today's EHRs will be replaced entirely by cloud-based approaches to managing health IT. Regardless of what the future holds, clinical informatics will be an important tool in optimizing the care we deliver to our patients.

One of the ongoing challenges facing our health care system is the need for astute clinicians who understand how information systems work and can provide leadership in the design and redesign of our medical systems. Many challenges arise when information systems are either developed or implemented without a clear understanding of the clinical workflow or how end-users (i.e. clinicians) intend to use them. While many EHR vendors employ clinicians in a variety of advisory capacities, even well-designed systems can fail if not implemented in a way that matches the local workflow of a given clinical environment. For example, a nursing flow sheet that is optimized for an intensive care unit may not work for an outpatient clinic. Hence the increased adoption, reliance, and importance of EHRs is creating more demand for informaticians.

QUESTIONS FOR FURTHER THOUGHT

1. What forms of clinical decision support (CDS) are available for use in association with electronic health records (EHRs), and how might they help enhance the safety and quality of health care?
2. What are the three types of data analytics, and how can each one help in managing or improving the value of care provided to a population of patients?
3. What are some of the areas in which the use of big data can potentially lead to improved health outcomes?
4. Why have EHRs not obtained uniform support within the patient and physician communities?
5. Which of the clinical informatics competencies do you feel least comfortable with, and how can you target your learning activities and clinical experiences to improve your knowledge and skills in these areas?

Annotated Bibliography

Detmer DE, Shortliffe EH. Clinical informatics: prospects for a new medical subspecialty. *JAMA*. 2014;311(20):2067–2068.
   An overview of the clinical informatics subspecialty.
Hersh W. A stimulus to define informatics and health information technology. *BMC Med Inform Decis Mak*. 2009;9:24. http://www.biomedcentral.com/1472-6947/9/24/.
   A discussion of the definitions in the biomedical and health informatics field.
Hoyt RE, Yoshihashi A, eds. *Health Informatics: Practical Guide for Healthcare and Information Technology Professionals*. 6th ed. Pensacola, FL: Lulu.com; 2014.
   An introductory applied textbook.
Kulikowski CA, Shortliffe EH, Currie LM, et al. AMIA Board white paper: definition of biomedical informatics and specification of core competencies for graduate education in the discipline. *J Am Med Inform Assoc*. 2012;19(6):931–938.
   A discussion of the core competencies in the biomedical informatics field.
Shortliffe EH, Cimino JJ, eds. *Biomedical Informatics: Computer Applications in Health Care and Biomedicine*. 4th ed. London, England: Springer; 2014.
   An introductory academic textbook.

References

1. Hersh W. A stimulus to define informatics and health information technology. *BMC Med Inform Decis Mak*. 2009;9:24. http://www.biomedcentral.com/1472-6947/9/24/.
2. Dick RS, Steen EB, Detmer DE, eds. *The Computer-Based Patient Record: an Essential Technology for Health Care*. Revised Edition. Washington, DC: National Academies Press; 1997.
3. Kohn LT, Corrigan JM, Donaldson MS, eds. *To Err Is Human: Building a Safer Health System*. Washington, DC: National Academies Press; 2000.
4. Anonymous. *Crossing the Quality Chasm: A New Health System for the 21st Century*. Washington, DC: National Academies Press; 2001.
5. Bates DW, Cullen DJ, Laird N, et al. Incidence of adverse drug events and potential adverse drug events. Implications for prevention. ADE Prevention Study Group. *JAMA*. 1995;274:29–34.
6. McGlynn EA, Asch SM, Adams J, et al. The quality of health care delivered to adults in the United States. *N Engl J Med*. 2003;348(26):2635–2645.
7. Smith PC, Araya-Guerra R, Bublitz C, et al. Missing clinical information during primary care visits. *JAMA*. 2005;293(5):565–571.
8. Tierney WM, Miller ME, Overhage JM, McDonald CJ. Physician inpatient order writing on microcomputer workstations: effects on resource utilization. *JAMA*. 1993;269(3):379–383.
9. Bates DW, Leape LL, Cullen DJ, et al. Effect of computerized physician order entry and a team intervention on prevention of serious medication errors. *JAMA*. 1998;280(15):1311–1316.
10. Bates DW, Kuperman GJ, Rittenberg E, et al. A randomized trial of a computer-based intervention to reduce utilization of redundant laboratory tests. *Am J Med*. 1999;106(2):144–150.
11. Teich JM, Merchia PR, Schmiz JL, Kuperman GJ, Spurr CD, Bates DW. Effects of computerized physician order entry on prescribing practices. *Arch Intern Med*. 2000;160(18):2741–2747.
12. Chaudhry B, Wang J, Wu S, et al. Systematic review: impact of health information technology on quality, efficiency, and costs of medical care. *Ann Intern Med*. 2006;144(10):742–752.
13. Williams C, Mostashari F, Mertz K, Hogin E, Atwal P. From the Office of the National Coordinator: the strategy for advancing the exchange of health information. *Health Aff*. 2012;31(3):527–536.
14. Johnston D, Pan E, Walker J, Bates DW, Middleton B. *The Value of Computerized Provider Order Entry in Ambulatory Settings*. Boston, MA: Center for Information Technology Leadership; 2003.
15. Hillestad R, Bigelow J, Bower A, et al. Can electronic medical record systems transform health care? *Health Aff (Millwood)*. 2005;24(5):1103–1117.
16. Blumenthal D. Launching HITECH. *N Engl J Med*. 2010;362(5):382–385.
17. Hersh WR, Wright A. *What Workforce Is Needed to Implement the Health Information Technology Agenda? An Analysis from the HIMSS Analytics™ Database*. AMIA Annual Symposium Proceedings. Washington, DC: American Medical Informatics Association; 2008:303–307.
18. Stark P. Congressional intent for the HITECH Act. *Am J Manag Care*. 2010;16(12 suppl HIT):SP24–SP28.
19. Charles D, Gabriel M, Searcy T. *Adoption of Electronic Health Record Systems among U.S. Non-Federal Acute Care Hospitals: 2008–2014*. Washington, DC: Department of Health and Human Services; 2015. http://www.healthit.gov/sites/default/files/data-brief/2014HospitalAdoptionDataBrief.pdf.
20. DesRoches CM, Painter MW, Jha AK. *Health Information Technology in the United States 2015: Transition to a Post-HITECH World*. Princeton, NJ: Robert Wood Johnson Foundation; 2015. http://www.rwjf.org/en/library/research/2015/09/health-information-technology-in-the-united-states-2015.html.
21. Rosenbaum L. Transitional chaos or enduring harm? The EHR and the disruption of medicine. *N Engl J Med*. 2015;373(17):1585–1588.
22. Kulikowski CA, Shortliffe EH, Currie LM, et al. AMIA Board white paper: definition of biomedical informatics and specification of core competencies for graduate education in the discipline. *J Am Med Inform Assoc*. 2012;19(6):931–938.

23. Shortliffe EH, Cimino JJ, eds. *Biomedical Informatics: Computer Applications in Health Care and Biomedicine*. 4th ed. London, England: Springer; 2014.

24. Friedman CP. A "fundamental theorem" of biomedical informatics. *J Am Med Inform Assoc*. 2009;16(2):169–170.

25. Friedman CP. What informatics is and isn't. *J Am Med Inform Assoc*. 2012;20(2):224–226.

26. Collen MF, Ball MJ, eds. *The History of Medical Informatics in the United States*. New York, NY: Springer; 2015.

27. Detmer DE, Shortliffe EH. Clinical informatics: prospects for a new medical subspecialty. *JAMA*. 2014;311(20):2067–2068.

28. Lesk A. *Introduction to Bioinformatics*. 4th ed. Oxford, England: Oxford University Press; 2014.

29. Bui AAT, Taira RK, eds. *Medical Imaging Informatics*. New York, NY: Springer; 2010.

30. Ball MJ, Douglas JV, Hinton-Walker P, et al, eds. *Nursing Informatics: Where Technology and Caring Meet*. 4th ed. New York, NY: Springer; 2011.

31. Pantanowitz L, Tuthill JM, Balis UGJ, eds. *Pathology Informatics: Theory and Practice*. Chicago, IL: American Society for Clinical Pathology; 2011.

32. Wetter T. *Consumer Health Informatics: New Services, Roles, and Responsibilities*. New York, NY: Springer; 2016.

33. Richesson RL, Andrews JE, eds. *Clinical Research Informatics*. New York, NY: Springer; 2012.

34. Magnuson JA, Fu PC, eds. *Public Health Informatics and Information Systems*. New York, NY: Springer; 2014.

35. Anonymous. *ACGME Program Requirements for Graduate Medical Education in Clinical Informatics*. Chicago, IL: Accreditation Council for Graduate Medical Education; 2014.

36. Greenes R. *Clinical Decision Support: The Road to Broad Adoption*. 2nd ed. Amsterdam, Netherlands: Elsevier; 2014.

37. Anonymous. *Connecting Health and Care for the Nation: a Shared Nationwide Interoperability Roadmap Version 1.0 (Roadmap)*. Washington, DC: Department of Health and Human Services; 2015. https://www.healthit.gov/sites/default/files/hie-interoperability/natio nwide-interoperability-roadmap-final-version-1.0.pdf.

38. Safran C, Bloomrosen M, Hammond WE, et al. Toward a national framework for the secondary use of health data: an American Medical Informatics Association white paper. *J Am Med Inform Assoc*. 2007;14(1):1–9.

39. Friedman CP, Wong AK, Blumenthal D. Achieving a nationwide learning health system. *Sci Transl Med*. 2010;2(57): 57cm29. http://stm.sciencemag.org/content/2/57/57cm29.full.

40. Smith M, Saunders R, Stuckhardt L, McGinnis JM. *Best Care at Lower Cost: The Path to Continuously Learning Health Care in America*. Washington, DC: National Academies Press; 2012.

41. Hersh WR. *Information Retrieval: A Health and Biomedical Perspective*. 3rd ed. New York, NY: Springer; 2009.

42. Guyatt G, Rennie D, Meade MO, Cook DJ, eds. *Users' Guides to the Medical Literature: A Manual for Evidence-Based Clinical Practice*. 3rd ed. New York, NY: McGraw-Hill; 2014.

43. van Dyk L. A review of telehealth service implementation frameworks. *Int J Environ Res Public Health*. 2014;11(2):1279–1298.

44. Hersh WR. *Healthcare Data Analytics*. In: Hoyt RE, Yoshihashi A, eds. *Health Informatics: Practical Guide for Healthcare and Information Technology Professionals*. 6th ed. Pensacola, FL: Lulu.com; 2014:62–75.

45. Davenport TH, Harris JG. *Competing on Analytics: the New Science of Winning*. Cambridge, MA: Harvard Business School Press; 2007.

46. Anonymous. *The Value of Analytics in Healthcare: From Insights to Outcomes*. Somers, NY: IBM Global Services; 2012. http://www-935. ibm.com/services/us/gbs/thoughtleadership/ibv-healthcare-analytic s.html.

47. Adams J, Klein J. *Business Intelligence and Analytics in Health Care: a Primer*. Washington, DC: The Advisory Board Company; 2011. http://www.advisory.com/Research/IT-Strategy-Council/Research-Notes/2011/Business-Intelligence-and-Analytics-in-Health-Care.

48. Sniderman AD, D'Agostino RB, Pencina MJ. The role of physicians in the era of predictive analytics. *JAMA*. 2015;314(1):25–26.

49. Mohri M, Rostamizadeh A, Talwalkar A. *Foundations of Machine Learning*. Cambridge, MA: MIT Press; 2012.

50. Bellazzi R, Zupan B. Predictive data mining in clinical medicine: current issues and guidelines. *Int J Med Inform*. 2008;77(2):81–97.

51. Cohen AM, Hersh WR. A survey of current work in biomedical text mining. *Brief Bioinform*. 2005;6(1):57–71.

52. Zikopoulos P, Eaton C, deRoos D, Deutsch T, Lapis G. *Understanding Big Data: Analytics for Enterprise Class Hadoop and Streaming Data*. New York, NY: McGraw-Hill; 2011.

53. Gardner E. The HIT approach to big data. *Health Data Manag*. 2013; 21(3):4.

54. Sledge GW, Miller RS, Hauser R. CancerLinQ and the future of cancer care. *ASCO Educational Book*; 2013:430–434. http://meetinglib rary.asco.org/content/58-132.

55. Ferrucci D, Brown E, Chu-Carroll J, et al. Building Watson: an overview of the DeepQA Project. *AI Magazine*. 2010;31(3):59–79. http://w ww.aaai.org/ojs/index.php/aimagazine/article/view/2303.

56. Ferrucci D, Levas A, Bagchi S, Gondek D, Mueller E. Watson: beyond Jeopardy! *Artif Intell*. 2013;199:93–105.

57. Buneman P, Davidson SB. *Data Provenance—The Foundation of Data Quality*. Pittsburgh, PA: Carnegie Mellon University Software Engineering Institute; 2010. http://www.sei.cmu.edu/measurement/re search/upload/Davidson.pdf.

58. Minelli M, Chambers M, Dhiraj A. *Big Data, Big Analytics: Emerging Business Intelligence and Analytic Trends for Today's Businesses*. Hoboken, NJ: Wiley; 2013.

59. Murdoch TB, Detsky AS. The inevitable application of big data to health care. *JAMA*. 2013;309(13):1351–1352.

60. Groves, Kayyali B, Knott D, VanKuiken S. The big-data revolution in US health care: accelerating value and innovation. McKinsey Global Institute; 2013. http://www.mckinsey.com/insights/health_systems_a nd_services/the_big-data_revolution_in_us_health_care.

61. Bates DW, Saria S, Ohno-Machado L, Shah A, Escobar G. Big data in health care: using analytics to identify and manage high-risk and high-cost patients. *Health Aff*. 2014;33(7):1123–1131.

62. Okun S, McGraw D, Stang P, et al. *Making the Case for Continuous Learning from Routinely Collected Data*. Washington, DC: Institute of Medicine; 2013. https://nam.edu/perspectives-2013-making-the-case-for-continuous-learning-from-routinely-collected-data/. Accessed November 2, 2016.

63. Hamburg MA, Collins FS. The path to personalized medicine. *N Engl J Med*. 2010;363(4):301–304.

64. Anonymous. *Toward Precision Medicine: Building a Knowledge Network for Biomedical Research and a New Taxonomy of Disease*. Washington, DC: National Academies Press; 2011.

65. Collins FS, Varmus H. A new initiative on precision medicine. *N Engl J Med*. 2015;372(9):793–795.

66. Burwell SM. Setting value-based payment goals—HHS efforts to improve U.S. health care. *N Engl J Med*. 2015;372(10):897–899.

67. McLean TR, Burton L, Haller CC, McLean PB. Electronic medical record metadata: uses and liability. *J Am Coll Surg*. 2008;206(3):405–411.

68. Overhage JM. Case study 1: the Indiana Health Information Exchange. In: Dixon B, ed. *Health Information Exchange: Navigating and Managing a Network of Health Information Systems*. Amsterdam, Netherlands: Elsevier; 2016. In press.

69. Hersh WR, Totten AM, Eden K, et al. Outcomes from health information exchange: systematic review and future research needs. *JMIR Med Inform*. 2015;3(4):e39. http://medinform.jmir.org/2015/ 4/e39/.

70. Hersh WR, Weiner MG, Embi PJ, et al. Caveats for the use of operational electronic health record data in comparative effectiveness research. *Med Care*. 2013;51(suppl 3):S30–S37.

71. Anonymous. *Readmissions Reduction Program (HRRP)*. Washington, DC: Center for Medicare and Medicaid Services; 2013. http://www.c ms.gov/Medicare/Medicare-Fee-for-Service-Payment/AcuteInpatient PPS/Readmissions-Reduction-Program.html.

72. Amarasingham R, Moore BJ, Tabak YP, et al. An automated model to identify heart failure patients at risk for 30-day readmission or death using electronic medical record data. *Med Care.* 2010;48(11):981–988.

73. Donzé J, Aujesky D, Williams D, Schnipper JL. Potentially avoidable 30-day hospital readmissions in medical patients: derivation and validation of a prediction model. *JAMA Intern Med.* 2013;173(8):632–638.

74. Gildersleeve R, Cooper P. Development of an automated, real time surveillance tool for predicting readmissions at a community hospital. *Appl Clin Inform.* 2013;4(2):153–169.

75. Goldzweig CL, Towfigh A, Maglione M, Shekelle PG. Costs and benefits of health information technology: new trends from the literature. *Health Aff (Millwood).* 2009;28(2):w282–w293.

76. Buntin MB, Burke MF, Hoaglin MC, Blumenthal D. The benefits of health information technology: a review of the recent literature shows predominantly positive results. *Health Aff (Millwood).* 2011;30(3):464–471.

77. Jones SS, Rudin RS, Perry T, Shekelle PG. Health information technology: an updated systematic review with a focus on meaningful use. *Ann Intern Med.* 2014;160(1):48–54.

78. Martineau M, Brookstone A, Stringham T, Hodgkins M. *Physicians Use of EHR Systems 2014.* Vancouver, BC: AmericanEHR; 2014. http://www.americanehr.com/research/reports/Physicians-Use-of-EHR-Systems-2014.aspx.

79. Friedberg MW, Chen PG, VanBusum KR, et al. *Factors Affecting Physician Professional Satisfaction and Their Implications for Patient Care, Health Systems, and Health Policy.* Santa Monica, CA: RAND Corporation; 2013. http://www.rand.org/pubs/research_reports/RR439.html.

80. Toll E. The cost of technology. *JAMA.* 2012;307(23):2497–2498.

81. Patel JJ. Writing the wrong. *JAMA.* 2015;314(7):671–672.

82. Jersild S. The Cause of—and Solution to—Radiology's Problems. *Diagnostic Imaging*; November 27, 2012. http://www.diagnosticimaging.com/pac-and-informatics/informatics-cause-%E2%80%94-and-solution-%E2%80%94-radiology%E2%80%99s-problems.

83. Lewis S. Brave new EMR. *Ann Intern Med.* 2011;154(5):368–369.

84. O'Reilly KB. EHRs: "Sloppy and paste" endures despite patient safety risk. *American Medical News;* February 4, 2013. http://www.ama-assn.org/amednews/2013/02/04/prl20204.htm.

85. Anonymous. *Health IT and Patient Safety: Building Safer Systems for Better Care.* Washington, DC: National Academies Press; 2012.

86. Wachter R. *The Digital Doctor: Hope, Hype, and Harm at the Dawn of Medicine's Computer Age.* New York, NY: McGraw-Hill; 2015.

87. Cortese D, Abbott P, Chassin M, Lyon GM, Riley WJ. *The Expert Panel Report to Texas Health Resources Leadership on the 2014 Ebola Events.* Arlington, TX: Texas Health Resources; 2015. https://www.texashealth.org/Documents/System/Public_Relations/Expert_Panel_Report_to_THR_on_EVD_response.pdf.

88. Perakslis ED. Cybersecurity in health care. *N Engl J Med.* 2014;371(5):395–397.

89. Rubenfire A. Hackers breach Anthem; 80M exposed. *Modern Healthcare.* February 4, 2015. http://www.modernhealthcare.com/article/20150204/NEWS/302049928/hackers-breach-anthem-80m-exposed.

90. Rubenfire A. Cyberattack on New York Blues plan Excellus affects 10 million. *Modern Healthcare.* September 9, 2015. http://www.modernhealthcare.com/article/20150909/NEWS/150909880/cyberattack-on-new-york-blues-plan-excellus-affects-10-million.

91. Vinton K. Premera Blue Cross breach may have exposed 11 million customers' medical and financial data. *Forbes.* March 17, 2015. http://www.forbes.com/sites/katevinton/2015/03/17/11-million-customers-medical-and-financial-data-may-have-been-exposed-in-premera-blue-cross-breach/.

92. Humer C, Finkle J. Your medical record is worth more to hackers than your credit card. *Reuters.* September 24, 2014. http://www.reuters.com/article/us-cybersecurity-hospitals-idUSKCN0HJ21I20140924.

93. Payne TH, Corley S, Cullen TA, et al. Report of the AMIA EHR-2020 Task Force on the status and future direction of EHRs. *J Am Med Inform Assoc.* 2015;22(5):1102–1110.

94. Kuhn T, Basch P, Barr M, Yackel T. Clinical documentation in the 21st century: executive summary of a policy position paper from the American College of Physicians. *Ann Intern Med.* 2015;162(4):301–303.

95. Anonymous. *Improving Care: Priorities to Improve Electronic Health Record Usability.* Chicago, IL: American Medical Association; 2014. https://www.aace.com/files/ehr-priorities.pdf.

96. Murphy DR, Laxmisan A, Reis BA, et al. Electronic health record-based triggers to detect potential delays in cancer diagnosis. *BMJ Qual Saf.* 2014;23(1):8–16.

97. Murphy DR, Wu L, Thomas EJ, Forjuoh SN, Meyer AND, Singh H. Electronic trigger-based intervention to reduce delays in diagnostic evaluation for cancer: a cluster randomized controlled trial. *J Clin Oncol.* 2015;33(31):3560–3567.

98. Amarasingham R, Patel PC, Toto K, et al. Allocating scarce resources in real-time to reduce heart failure readmissions: a prospective, controlled study. *BMJ Qual Saf.* 2013;22(12):998–1005.

99. Hebert C, Shivade C, Foraker R, et al. Diagnosis-specific readmission risk prediction using electronic health data: a retrospective cohort study. *BMC Med Inform Decis Mak.* 2014;14:65. http://www.biomedcentral.com/1472-6947/14/65.

100. Menendez ME, Janssen SJ, Ring D. Electronic health record-based triggers to detect adverse events after outpatient orthopaedic surgery. *BMJ Qual Saf.* 2016;25:25–30.

101. Berry DL, Blumenstein BA, Halpenny B, et al. Enhancing patient-provider communication with the electronic self-report assessment for cancer: a randomized trial. *J Clin Oncol.* 2011;29(8):1029–1035.

102. Denny JC, Bastarache L, Ritchie MD, et al. Systematic comparison of phenome-wide association study of electronic medical record data and genome-wide association study data. *Nat Biotechnol.* 2013;31(12):1102–1110.

103. Wei WQ, Denny JC. Extracting research-quality phenotypes from electronic health records to support precision medicine. *Genome Med.* 2015;7(1):41. http://www.genomemedicine.com/content/7/1/41.

104. Kooij FO, Vos N, Siebenga P, Klok T, Hollmann MW, Kal JE. Automated reminders decrease postoperative nausea and vomiting incidence in a general surgical population. *Br J Anaesthesiol.* 2012;108(6):961–965.

105. Duke P, Frankel RM, Reis S. How to integrate the electronic health record and patient-centered communication into the medical visit: a skills-based approach. *Teach Learn Med.* 2013;25(4):358–365.

106. Walsh B. Endless possibilities for the digital infrastructure's data dividend. *Clinical Innovation & Technology.* August 11, 2015. http://www.clinical-innovation.com/partner-voice/nuance/endless-possibilities-digital-infrastructure-s-data-dividend.

107. Anonymous. *Improving Diagnosis in Healthcare.* Washington, DC: Institute of Medicine; 2015. http://iom.nationalacademies.org/Reports/2015/Improving-Diagnosis-in-Healthcare.aspx.

108. James JT. A new, evidence-based estimate of patient harms associated with hospital care. *J Patient Saf.* 2013;9(3):122–128.

109. Bastian H, Glasziou P, Chalmers I. Seventy-five trials and eleven systematic reviews a day: how will we ever keep up? *PLoS Med.* 2010;7(9):e1000326.

110. Miller HD, Yasnoff WA, Burde HA. *Personal Health Records: the Essential Missing Element in 21st Century Healthcare.* Chicago, IL: Healthcare Information and Management Systems Society; 2009.

111. Berwick DM, Nolan TW, Whittington J. The triple aim: care, health, and cost. *Health Aff.* 2008;27(3):759–769.

112. Hersh WR, Gorman PN, Biagioli FE, Mohan V, Gold JA, Mejicano GC. Beyond information retrieval and electronic health record use: competencies in clinical informatics for medical education. *Adv Med Educ Pract.* 2014;5:205–212.

113. Hersh W. The health information technology workforce: estimations of demands and a framework for requirements. *Appl Clin Inform.* 2010;1(2):197–212.

114. Longhurst CA, Pageler NM, Palma JP, et al. Early experiences of accredited clinical informatics fellowships. *J Am Med Inform Assoc.* 2016;23(4):829–834.

115. Anonymous. *Best Practice and Use Cases.* Indianapolis, IN: Indiana Health Information Exchange; 2013. http://az480170.vo.msecnd.net/bd985247-f489-435f-a7b4-49df92ec868e/docs/2db74d60-73f6-4f85-aa9c-d88d9f0c6c26/careweb14bestpractices.pdf.

10

Population Health

Natalia Wilson, MD, MPH, Paul George, MD, MHPE, and
Jill M. Huber, MD

LEARNING OBJECTIVES

1. Describe population health.
2. Compare and contrast population health, public health, and population medicine.
3. Summarize how population health is being implemented in medical care.
4. Analyze the contributions of integrated health care delivery, public health, prevention and health promotion, community engagement and resources, and health policy efforts to improve population health.

This chapter focuses on the dynamic and evolving area of population health, a topic that has attracted increasing attention in the United States over the past decade. Population health, public health, and population medicine are defined and compared. The role of population health in health care delivery is examined, including new models of care, alternative payment models, new technology, and new, evolving roles for health care workers. Examples of population health initiatives bridging medical care, public health, and the community are provided to help illustrate the core principles of population health. The chapter concludes with a focus on the future of population health including new directions in health professions education.

I. INTRODUCTION

The changing landscape of health and health care in the United States has fueled an expansion in focus from solely individual care toward population health management. This shift is driven by many factors, including greater attention to quality of patient care, patient safety, and the rapidly increasing cost of health care. Increased awareness of the limitations of US health care, including less than ideal national health outcomes and a growing consensus that the status quo in US health care is unsustainable, has helped expand the conversation from the health of individuals to the health of populations. Many key health issues facing the United States—chronic disease, obesity, disability, and behavioral health issues—are particularly well addressed through a population health focus. Finally, there is growing recognition of the acute need to address the many determinants of population health that fall outside of the health care arena.

Population health adopts a broader perspective than traditional medical care in that it extends the traditional 1:1 individual focus of medical care to a group, community, or population and encompasses health care delivery, public health, prevention, wellness and health promotion efforts, community engagement and resources, and health policy efforts. Population health, both as a concept and a field of study, is undergoing considerable evolution and growth and is garnering increased attention from the traditional health care delivery sectors in the United States. Several factors have contributed to this new focus, including shifting health care reimbursement to alternative payment models, from volume care (fee-for-service) to value-based care, and heightened attention given to measuring quality outcomes in health. Factors reinforcing the increased focus include the Institute for Healthcare Improvement's Triple Aim goals of improved patient experience of care, improved health of populations, and reduced per capita cost of health care[1,2] and the movement toward new models of care delivery, such as those supported by implementation of the Affordable Care Act (ACA).

The increased emphasis on population health is supporting a growing number of initiatives focused on collaborative efforts among health care delivery, public health, and the community. Greater attention is being given to the impact of social and behavioral determinants on population health, and medical schools are beginning to include population health content in the curriculum for their medical students.

II. WHAT IS POPULATION HEALTH?

A. Definition and Characteristics

Population health is most commonly defined as "the health outcomes of a group of individuals, including the distribution of health outcomes within the group."[3] The National Academy of Medicine Roundtable on Population Health Improvement further elaborates on this definition: "while not part of the definition itself, it is understood that such population health outcomes are the product of multiple determinants of health."[4] Population health extends beyond the individual patient focus of traditional medical care and encompasses health outcomes of groups, communities, or populations of individuals. Individuals are members of a variety of populations, communities, or groups, and collectively individual health constitutes the health of populations. US population health is the health of the nation as a whole, including members of various subpopulations, communities, and groups.

Populations may be defined in multiple ways. Examples of defined populations include individuals in a specific geographic area or community, patient panels in an accountable care organization (ACO) or patient-centered medical home (PCMH), individuals with a certain ethnicity, patients with a specific medical condition such as diabetes mellitus or cardiovascular disease in a medical practice, employees of a certain organization, or individuals in a certain health insurance plan. Populations may be viewed and designated from the perspectives of many different stakeholders including physicians, other members of the clinical team, hospitals, public health workers or organizations, community liaisons, administrators, employers, and insurers. Public health, which is discussed further later in the chapter, has traditionally defined populations within communities and specific geographic areas. Physicians and others in the health care setting may typically define populations within a designated clinical setting or as members of an alternative payment model such as an ACO.

Population health is composed of four major pillars: chronic care management, quality and safety, public health, and health policy.[5] Population health encompasses a broad set of initiatives including the engagement of multiple stakeholders in the areas of prevention and health promotion, health care delivery, medical intervention, public health, and policy. Population health is strongly focused on analysis of outcomes to drive process change and new policy.[5] Chronic care management, quality, and safety are activities that have historically been primarily delivered within health care settings but increasingly extend into community locations. Public health has traditionally focused on the community setting. Health policy efforts work to influence change in both health care delivery and community settings.

The overall measure of the health of populations results from the interplay of **determinants of health,** which are the multiple factors that influence an individual's health and health of populations. Determinants can be characterized as behavior, genetics, social circumstances, environmental exposures, and health care categories, as indicated in Fig. 10.1.[6,7]

Historically, initiatives and programs provided through the US public health system have been designed to address behavioral, social, and environmental determinants of

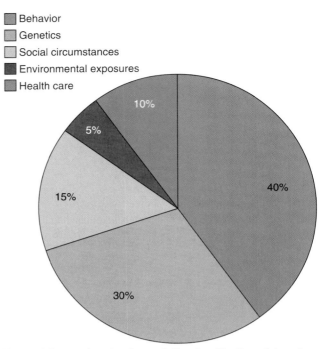

■ Behavior
□ Genetics
□ Social circumstances
■ Environmental exposures
■ Health care

Fig. 10.1 Determinants of population health. (From Schroeder SA. Shattuck Lecture. We can do better—improving the health of the American people. *N Engl J Med.* 2007;357(12):1221–1228. Adapted from McGinnis JM, Williams-Russo P, Knickman JR. The case for more active policy attention to health promotion. Health Aff [Millwood]. 2002;21[2]:78–93.)

health. The health care system has concentrated on providing disease-based diagnosis, care, and treatment, and while it has also worked to address the other determinants of health, its historic focus on these areas has generally not been robust. It is noteworthy that only 10 percent of the determinants of population health are attributed to medical care, yet medical care is the predominant focus in the health arena in the United States. The vast majority of population health determinants fall into the realm of behavior or lifestyle choices, social circumstances, and environmental exposures. Improving US population health will necessitate broad, prolonged, and determined change and collaboration across multiple stakeholders.

B. Determinants of Population Health

As discussed earlier, the multiple factors that influence an individual's health and the health of populations are collectively called the *determinants of health* and include the following: behavior, genetics (also called biologic), social, environmental, and health care.[7] Examples of genetic or biologic determinants are age, gender, and inherited health conditions. Behavioral determinants of health include smoking, risk-taking behaviors, exercise, and nutrition. Social determinants include income, social support, and education. Physical and environmental determinants include the natural environment, such as green spaces, as well as the built environment, housing quality, conditions, and exposures. Health care determinants include the availability of quality health care, access, and health insurance. Health outcomes are a complex interplay between the varied health determinants at the individual and population levels.

A significant focus on social determinants of health and their influence on population health has followed the recognition that health begins where people live, work, play, and age.[8–10] The social environment, physical environment, and health care services all contribute to "the social patterning of health, disease, and illness."[9] They are recognized to interact with and influence behavior and contribute substantially to differences in health outcomes between groups of people.[9] More detailed information on social determinants of health is provided in Chapter 11.

Healthy People 2020, a national initiative focused on promoting health for all, has identified five key areas to target improved health. These include economic stability; education; social and community context; health and health care; and the neighborhood and built environment.[9] Examples of unique determinants in these categories, outlined by Healthy People 2020 include the following:

1. Economic stability: poverty, food security, employment
2. Education: quality of education, rate of high school graduation, secondary education, early childhood education and development
3. Social and community context: civic participation and sense of community, perceptions of discrimination and equity, incarceration
4. Health and health care: access to health care and insurance, health literacy, prescription coverage
5. Neighborhood and built environment: access to healthy foods and areas to exercise, quality of housing, crime and violence

Historically, the health care system has focused on those determinants that are associated with disease processes and with activities that are influenced by systems of care. As discussed earlier, this is a relatively small portion of all determinants that influence population health, accounting for only 10 percent of overall health.[7] Population health recognizes that an individual's health status is linked to his or her home, work, school, and other environments, and not just determined by his or her interactions with the health care system. New strategies are needed to improve the health of populations, working beyond the health care setting, with enhanced collaboration with community organizations and public health initiatives. For example, immunization programs in the schools help to avoid challenges with health care access, transportation, or the ability to take time away from work for appointments. The goal is to work collaboratively to support positive change in the places in which people live, work, and learn, thereby promoting the ability to live healthy lives.

As an example, consider a 21-year-old woman with insulin-dependent diabetes mellitus. She has been hospitalized six times in the preceding 6 weeks with diabetic ketoacidosis (markedly elevated blood sugars causing acid buildup in the blood). The patient is homeless, cannot afford her food or insulin, and has no transportation to get her to regularly scheduled health care appointments. Without addressing the social determinants—her lack of housing, her food insecurity, and her lack of transportation—her diabetes cannot be treated adequately.

C. Public Health

Public health is defined as "What we as a society do collectively to assure the conditions in which people can be healthy."[11] Public health is a long-standing discipline that has focused on the health of entire populations, communities, states, countries, and even regions of the world. Public health agencies exist at the federal, state, local, and tribal levels, although primary responsibility rests at the state and local levels. Important public health fundamentals include prevention of disease, promotion of health, protection against environmental hazards, disaster preparedness, and assurance of health care quality and accessibility.[12] Public health traditionally has not been focused on individual medical care and private sector health care delivery.

Public health has three core functions and ten essential services (Fig. 10.2). In its assessment function, public health agencies monitor health status to identify and solve community health problems and diagnose and investigate health problems and hazards in the community. An example is the use of the Behavioral Risk Factor Surveillance System (BRFSS) data to determine state-based prevalence of chronic disease.[13] Another example is the investigation of community infectious disease outbreaks such as measles. In its policy development function, public health informs, educates, and empowers individuals about health and health issues; mobilizes community partnerships to identify and solve community health challenges; and develops policies and plans in support of individual and community health efforts. Examples include media campaigns and community outreach targeted at disease prevention and health promotion opportunities such as tobacco use, immunizations, chronic disease, and involvement in policy development for mandatory reporting of certain disease conditions or smoke-free environments. In its assurance function, public health enforces laws and regulations that protect health; links individuals to health services when otherwise unavailable; and evaluates effectiveness, accessibility, and quality of person- and population-based health services. An example is the provision of health care services for vulnerable populations such as immunization or infant formula programs. Research is a central component of public health that allows the study and development of innovative solutions to health problems.[12]

The five core disciplines of public health are: 1) epidemiology and 2) biostatistics, both of which provide the basis for the assessment function of public health; 3) environmental health sciences and 4) social and behavioral sciences, both of which help inform the assessment and policy development functions of public health; and 5) health policy and management, which integrates with the assurance function of public health. Public health is additionally dependent on the biomedical sciences to apply fundamental concepts to public health issues such as chronic disease and prevention.[14]

Public health systems exist to safeguard the health and well-being of the community. Federal, state, and local governments assume many responsibilities needed to protect public health. The network of public health agencies is extensive and includes public, private, and voluntary entities[12,14] (Fig. 10.3).

Important data sources are available for information on community health including the BRFSS[13] and County Health Rankings and Roadmaps[15] as well as individual state and county-level public health data. In addition, state and county health assessment and improvement plans, hospital and county **community health needs assessments (CHNAs),**

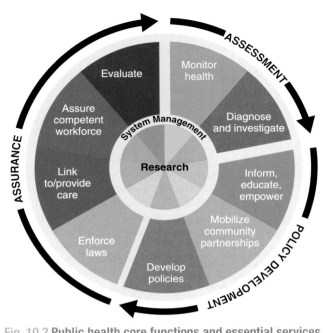

Fig. 10.2 **Public health core functions and essential services.** (From Centers for Disease Control and Prevention. Office for State, Local, Tribal, and Territorial Support. NPHPS Overview.)

and the Healthy People 2020 objectives and progress tracker all provide measures of public health.

D. Population Health, Public Health, and Population Medicine

Population health is built on important public health fundamentals, particularly disease prevention and health promotion. *Public health* is one of the four pillars of population health,[5] and the core disciplines and competencies of public health are important elements of population health management.

Public health actively monitors community health status, investigates health problems, develops programs and initiatives focused on health, develops policy, and engages in research for better community health. Public health is programmatically focused on health promotion and disease prevention and is primarily community-based.[12,14] The public health system involves "all public, private, and voluntary entities that contribute to the delivery of essential public health services within a jurisdiction."[12]

Population health reaches more broadly into the delivery arena and encompasses health promotion, disease prevention, and engagement of multiple stakeholders in the areas of prevention, health care delivery, medical intervention, public health, and policy.[5] In addition, population health is less directly connected to government health departments.[16]

With advancement of new models of care and reimbursement, population health in hospitals, clinics, and other health care delivery sites is increasingly focused on designated populations of patients. Increased use of data, process change, and extended interdisciplinary clinical teams characterize a new population focus. An emerging term in the area of population health is *population medicine,* defined as "the design, delivery, coordination, and payment of high-quality health care services to manage the Triple Aim for a population using the best resources we have available within

the health care system."[17] While population health is emphasized in this chapter, knowledge and understanding of the terms *population health, public health,* and *population medicine* will be important in a rapidly evolving health care system (Table 10.1).

The approach to a medical condition such as diabetes mellitus helps to portray the differences but also the synergies within population health, public health, and population medicine. In a medical clinic, broader use of information technology and an extended health care team help support a population medicine focus. Data for a panel of diabetic patients including pertinent laboratory results (e.g., Hemoglobin A1c), frequency of routine office visits, visits to the emergency department or hospitalization, and maintenance of preventive care can be aggregated and analyzed. In an effort to improve population health of the (patient) panel, these data can be used to risk-stratify patients into high/medium/low risk, to highlight needed process change in the clinic (if applicable), and to assign higher-risk patients to care management professionals.

From a public health perspective, county, state, and federal data is assessed and used by public health officers to establish the prevalence of chronic diseases, including diabetes, in a community. Diabetes mellitus is an example of a prevalent chronic disease that has been a top health priority for public health.[9,18] Public health performs many activities including the following:

- Routine collection of epidemiologic data on diabetes mellitus
- Creation of workgroups in the community to assess needs and barriers
- Development of community initiatives and events focused on wellness, nutrition, and physical activity
- Provision of community resources for diabetes education and services
- Development of guidelines and toolkits for school and worksite wellness and nutrition
- Provision of health services for vulnerable populations
- Establishment of goals to reduce the disease burden of diabetes mellitus[18–20]

Health of populations and overall US population health are the result of outcomes and initiatives across health care delivery and public health through prevention and promotion efforts, a focus on broad determinants of health, a reduction of disparities and inequity, and, ultimately, engagement of individuals and patients themselves. Many opportunities exist for integration of health care delivery and public health efforts to support robust improvement in the health of designated populations and overall US population health. As evidenced by Fig. 10.3, public health has an extensive network and many developed and long-standing relationships at the community level. As discussed in the example earlier in the chapter, public health performs significant activities in the community. Greater connection between medical care and community resources and available data provides the opportunity for support of individual patient needs and population health. This connection also provides the opportunity for more tailored focus utilizing expertise from both medical and public health arenas. Examples of ongoing initiatives bridging medical care, public health, and the community for improved population health include Camden Coalition of Healthcare Providers,[21] Homeless Patient Aligned Care Teams,[22] and Million Hearts,[23] which will be further elaborated upon later in the chapter.

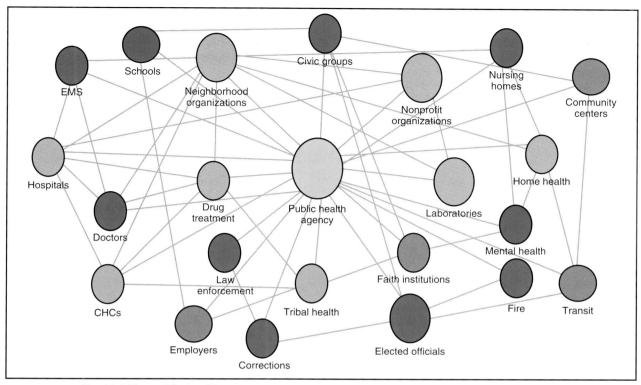

Fig. 10.3 **The public health system.** (From Centers for Disease Control and Prevention. Office for State, Local, Tribal and Territorial Support. NPHPS Overview.)

III. WHY A FOCUS ON POPULATION HEALTH?

A. Limitations in US Health and Health Care

A number of significant limitations in US health care must be overcome in order to achieve improved population health. These include the following:

A focus on sick care over prevention and wellness. Clinical training has traditionally emphasized acute illness and chronic disease care over prevention and wellness. The fee-for-service reimbursement system has been more heavily based on acute care and procedures.[24] Prevention, chronic disease management, nutrition, and behavioral health have been traditionally undervalued and reimbursed at a rate less than acute care. Preventive services for patients are also generally more difficult than access to acute care in the United States, with some speculating that one contributing reason may be more medical school graduates entering specialties rather than primary care.[25] In addition, the public health sector with its focus on prevention and health promotion has been relatively underfunded when compared with acute care reimbursement[26] and has not been well integrated with medical care.[27]

Siloed and fragmented efforts for health and health care. Health care is often organized and prioritized around the health care delivery system rather than the patient. Patients typically must initiate contact and access many different points in order to receive their health care. Lack of coordination, integration, and communication between different points of a patient's care all contribute to fragmentation of the health care system. Frequent changes in a patient's insurance coverage or changes in provider networks for insurance companies can also contribute to fragmentation, as patients may need to access new health care providers based on requirement of their current insurance coverage.[28] Connections between medical care, public health, and community resources for patients to support their health and health care have been limited.[16]

Inadequate assimilation and use of data. Communication and sharing information between the various parties involved in care of a patient is often limited. Barriers to greater communication and coordination of care include interoperability of electronic health records (EHRs) and limitation in capability for health information exchange.[29] For data that are available, clear delineation of information needed, goals for data analysis, and data analysis itself is often inadequate and inconsistent. Medical care and public health data sources are not well connected.

Suboptimal patient engagement. Lack of defined teams for patient care, lack of tools, and time constraints on an individual provider impact the achievement of greater patient engagement in their health care. Patient-centeredness and shared decision making, as well as the methods to operationalize these concepts in a busy clinical practice, have typically not been robust areas of emphasis in clinical training. Patient education resources and tools are often inadequate.

Inequality and inequity in health and health outcomes. Where people live; their socioeconomic status; and their race, ethnicity, gender, age, sexual orientation, and disability status have historically impacted health and health outcomes.[30] Comprehensive solutions to address the impact of the social determinants of health on health outcomes have been difficult to develop. Root causes are often

Table 10.1 Comparison of Population Health, Public Health, and Population Medicine

	Definition	Core Elements
Population health	"The health outcomes of a group of individuals, including the distribution of such outcomes within the group"[3]	• Public health • Population medicine • Prevention and health promotion • Community engagement and resources • Health policy
Public health	"What we as a society do collectively to assure the conditions in which people can be healthy"[11]	Assessment • Monitor community health status • Diagnose and investigate community health problems and hazards Policy development • Inform, educate, and empower community about health and health issues • Mobilize community partnerships to identify and solve health issues • Develop policies focused on health Assurance • Enforce laws and regulations that protect health • Link individuals to health services • Ensure a competent public health workforce • Evaluate community public health services[12]
Population medicine	"The design, delivery, coordination, and payment of high-quality health care services to manage the Triple Aim for a population using the best resources we have available within the health care system"[17]	• Health care delivery • New models of care and alternative payment models • Extended care teams • Health information technology

complex, and policy, funding, and support targeted at these areas has not been robust.[31]

Reimbursement systems, incentives, education, and culture that support the status quo. A fee-for-service reimbursement system often reinforces fragmented efforts as individual providers are paid separately for their part of a patient's care. Accountability, reimbursement based on quality, and care coordination have not characterized traditional fee-for-service systems. Finally, as discussed earlier, incentives are often misaligned in health care as acute care and procedures are reimbursed at a greater rate than preventive care. This is accentuated by the training of medical students, residents, and other health care professionals in hospitals where sick care is most often provided.

Outcomes of these limitations are significant from a clinical, cost, and population health perspective. Among other challenges, there is a significant prevalence of chronic disease (including diabetes, hypertension, and cardiovascular disease), obesity, an aging population, and dysfunction in behavioral health care with high cost and comparatively poor overall population health as compared to almost all developed countries.

Chronic diseases, long-lasting conditions that can be controlled but not cured, are the most common health conditions and the most costly. Fifty percent of US adults have one or more chronic diseases, increasing to 80 percent for those older than 65 years of age.[32] Nine out of 10 of the leading causes of death in 2010 were due to a chronic disease or generally associated with patients with chronic disease.[33]

The growing obesity epidemic in the United States is an important factor in health status. Thirty-eight percent of adults in the United States are obese. Seventeen percent of children and adolescents are obese.[34] Obesity is associated with significant comorbidities including cardiovascular disease, hypertension, Type II diabetes mellitus, and cancer.[35] Evidence is accumulating of cardiovascular damage in obese children.[36]

An aging population also presents the United States with significant health issues, including chronic disease, falls, polypharmacy, diminished quality of life, dependency, and disability.[14] Fifty percent of those older than 65 years of age have two or more chronic diseases.[19] Falls are a significant cause of morbidity, dependency, and diminished quality of life.[37] By 2030, one in five individuals in the United States will be an older adult.[38]

The impact of mental health on physical health has received increased attention.[39,40] Twenty-five percent of adults in the United States experience mental illness, with 1 in 17 having a serious mental illness. Mood disorders are the third leading cause of hospitalization in those 18 to 44 years of age. Those with serious mental illness are at increased risk for chronic disease.[41]

National health care expenditures were 17.9 percent of the gross domestic product (GDP) in 2011. The breakdown of expenditures included 31.5 percent spent on hospital care, 20 percent on physician and clinical services, and 9.7 percent on prescription medications.[42] Eighty-six percent of health care costs are attributed to treating chronic disease.[43] In a global comparison, the United States spends the highest percentage of GDP on health care by far. However, in comparison to countries of similar income, the United States lags on key outcome measures including life expectancy and prevalence of chronic disease.[44,45]

Optimal disease management necessitates coordinated care along with use and exchange of data and patient engagement. In addition, health care providers must have greater knowledge of and connection with the resources outside of the health care system, including those resources in the public health sector and the community where individuals spend the majority of their time. Finally, in order to optimize the health of a population, there needs to be a much greater focus on and support for prevention. All of these areas are limitations in the current US health care system. The overall impact is relatively poor population health in the United States, and comparatively poor population health in relation to countries of similar income globally.

CASE STUDY 1

Mr. Reed is a 66-year-old African-American male with Type II diabetes mellitus whose blood sugar control has not been optimal. Additionally, he is overweight and is not physically active. His primary care physician (PCP) has had multiple discussions with Mr. Reed about the importance of good blood sugar control, optimal weight, and regular exercise. The PCP has discussed concerns about the development of comorbidities, particularly coronary artery disease. Mr. Reed has been referred to the dietician at the local hospital, but the PCP has had to alter Mr. Reed's diabetes medication multiple times as his diabetes markers continue to show inadequate glycemic control.

Mr. Reed's PCP recently became part of an accountable care organization (ACO) and is evaluating and optimizing support for the population of diabetic patients including Mr. Reed. Steps taken include the following:

- Obtaining data from the electronic health record on all of the diabetic patients for the past 2 years including Hemoglobin A1c, number of emergency department visits, number of hospitalizations, and compliance with routine office visits
- Risk-stratifying diabetic patients into high-risk, medium-risk, and low-risk categories based on these data
- Developing a process for follow-up with high-risk and medium-risk patients to assure that they are taking their medications, keeping routine office visits, staying up-to-date with their preventive care, and do not have problems or barriers to controlling their diabetes. A nurse care manager in the PCP's office has been designated with this job
- Creating a patient portal where patients can access their laboratory results, send e-mails to the PCP or his or her nurse, make office appointments, and access resources including transportation options listed with contact information
- Providing patient education brochures and materials to be made available in the waiting room and examination rooms as well as health educators to help patients gain an understanding of their medical conditions and gain skills in self-management
- Providing support for diabetic patients to optimize their diet and physical activity. After investigation by the PCP's office staff, the PCP becomes aware of a number of resources available in the community. These include diabetes self-management classes, nutrition classes where patients are taught how to shop, cook, and make choices while eating out, and exercise programs at both the local YMCA and senior center. The PCP is able to get a list of locations, dates/times, and contact information for these classes to provide to patients in the office and through the patient portal. Additionally, a local supermarket chain offers reduced prices for fruit and vegetables with a physician's prescription "coupon"
- The local hospital's Community Health Needs Assessment and the county's Health Improvement Plan both indicate diabetes as a high-priority condition and a number of planned targeted initiatives at the community level. The local hospital is now offering a sustainability program for seniors.

Mr. Reed presents to the emergency department with a complaint of weakness. Workup in the emergency department is significant for elevated blood pressure and elevated nonfasting blood sugar. In light of Mr. Reed's complaint and medical history, he is admitted to the hospitalist service at the hospital to rule out a cardiac event. During his hospitalization, his blood pressure is controlled and his blood sugar improves with a diabetic diet and rest. A myocardial infarction is ruled out. Mr. Reed is discharged home on a new medication for blood pressure.

In the past, Mr. Reed (and other patients in the practice) would receive discharge instructions and a new prescription, and would be instructed to schedule a follow-up appointment with their PCP. Mr. Reed did not always do this. The hospital discharge summary may have arrived in the PCP's office several days later or may have to be requested when Mr. Reed has his next appointment and says he was hospitalized.

Since both the PCP and the hospital are part of the same ACO, new changes instituted to support Mr. Reed are as follows:

- Upon discharge, Mr. Reed is assigned a nurse care manager to oversee his transition from the hospital to home.
- His care manager is tasked with assuring that his PCP receives discharge paperwork, contacting Mr. Reed by phone within 48 hours of his hospital discharge and helping facilitate a follow-up primary care appointment.
- Mr. Reed will also receive a visit from a community nurse within 30 days of discharge through a hospital program. The hospital is working to optimize support for the population of patients in the ACO.

B. Health Disparities

A fundamental health care question is "Why are some Americans healthier than others?" The answer is complex. Differences in health and health outcomes between groups of people are considered **health disparities.** There are a number of proposed definitions for *health disparities* or *health inequalities,* terms often used interchangeably, and the definition applied is often related to the context in which it is used.[46] Additional discussion of these concepts and terms is provided in Chapter 11.

Healthy People 2020 defines a health disparity as "a particular type of health difference that is closely linked with social, economic, and/or environmental disadvantage. Health disparities adversely affect groups of people who have systematically experienced greater obstacles to health based on their racial or ethnic group; religion; socioeconomic status; gender; age; mental health; cognitive, sensory, or physical disability; sexual orientation or gender identity; geographic location; or other characteristics historically linked to discrimination or exclusion."[47] These differences are significantly influenced by social determinants of health at the individual and population levels and the associated differences in the allocation of resources. These differences are often considered avoidable, unjust, or unfair and sometimes referred to as *health inequities.*[46]

Sadly, there are innumerable examples of health disparities in the United States. In Chicago, Illinois, the difference in life expectancy is 16 years when comparing the

Washington Park neighborhood on the South Side, which is predominantly African-American, and the Loop in the city center just 5 miles away, which is predominantly white.[48] Nationally, infant mortality remains highest for non-Hispanic black women.[49] Diabetes prevalence is highest among males, individuals 65 years of age and older, non-Hispanic blacks and those of mixed race, Hispanics, individuals with less than a high school education, those who are poor, and those with a disability.[49] These disparities often relate to complex interactions of social, economic, environmental, and systemic factors, making it difficult to design readily applicable solutions.

In addition, the absence of disease does not necessarily denote health. For example, there remain differences in an individual's ability to lead a healthy lifestyle and avoid disease. In 2011, 30 percent of people did not have close access to stores with healthy foods.[49] The combined cost of health inequalities and premature deaths in the United States between 2003 and 2006 was estimated to be $1.24 trillion.[50]

Ultimately, health and health care efforts aim to achieve health equity (or the state in which all individuals achieve their full health potential). As the cause for health disparities is complex, the solution to eliminate avoidable disparities is also complex. This requires a collaborative effort with policy makers, national initiatives focused on health promotion, research on health outcomes and disparities, the health care system, public health, social services, and community programs.

Population health can play an important role in analyzing these disparities and associated social determinants of health at the local, community, and national level to identify trends and associated solutions. In addition, contributing to ongoing population health research efforts, including community engagement designs such as translational research and community-based participatory research, is important.

Health care organizations can collaborate with community residents and organizations to define health priorities for communities through CHNAs. A CHNA is a "process that uses quantitative and qualitative methods to systematically collect and analyze data to understand health within a specific community. The data can inform community decision making, the prioritization of health problems, and the development, implementation, and evaluation of community health improvement plans."[51]

Innovative health care delivery models focusing on value, using enhanced technology, and incorporating team-based approaches are key new initiatives with promise to improve population health. National initiatives, such as Healthy People 2020, the National Partnership for Action to End Health Disparities sponsored by the Office of Minority Health within the US Department of Health and Human Services, and the National Institutes of Health Centers for Population Health and Health Disparities are important because they further inform health policy and legislation designed to eliminate health disparities and lead to improved population health.

C. Health Care Delivery

Prior to the passage of the ACA in 2010, health care delivery focused primarily on the care of individual patients. With recent implementation of new payment and delivery models, such as accountable care organizations, physicians and other health care providers are expected to manage individual patients, but are also increasingly responsible for managing populations of patients.[52]

In earlier times, when a physician saw a patient with diabetes mellitus, several things may have occurred. They would likely prescribe medication to control the patient's blood sugar, ensure that the patient had influenza and pneumonia vaccines, ensure that the patient saw an ophthalmologist for eye care and a podiatrist for foot care, and check laboratory values, such as Hemoglobin A1c, every 3 to 6 months. The physician was likely focused solely on ensuring that the individual patient received the recommended care.

Increasingly, in this new era of being accountable for patient populations, physicians and health care professionals would still perform the activities listed in the previous paragraph. However, a team of health care providers, potentially including physicians and/or nurse practitioners, physician assistants, nurse care managers, patient navigators, and pharmacists, would analyze the team's patient panel (the "population") to ensure that all those on the panel were receiving this care; that Hemoglobin A1c values are at goal; that all are seeing an ophthalmologist; and that all are getting influenza vaccines. In addition to helping the individual patients, these teams might also institute system changes that would better serve the panel, such as checklists, new protocols, and outreach via new types of health care team members. As previously defined, population health is "the health outcomes of a group of individuals, including the distribution of such outcomes within the group."[3,53] In the first example, only individual medical care was considered the responsibility of the provider and the health care system. Drawing on Kindig's population health definition, another fundamental change in health care delivery in the era of population health is focusing on the nonbiologic determinants that affect health and managing those as well. These nonbiologic determinants are diverse and may include an individual's or population's access to health care, their behaviors, the social environment, and the physical environment.

Following our early example, a patient with diabetes mellitus may present to a physician's office with a Hemoglobin A1c that is markedly elevated. That same patient may not have seen an ophthalmologist for 2 or 3 years. In the health care system of the past, the patient would likely have had his or her diabetic medications increased and been counseled on the importance of having an eye examination. Those same things may occur today in the new era of population health. However, in addition, a physician or health care professional may also inquire about a patient's access to healthy food ("Does the patient live in a food desert?"); his or her ability to exercise ("Are there safe areas for a patient to exercise?" "Are there parks around the patient's home?"); and his or her access to transportation for an eye examination.

Optimizing population health means moving beyond traditional thinking and the confines of medical practice to address the other factors that influence health, and consider solutions and resources in order to effectively manage the health of individual patients and populations.

IV. SOLUTIONS TO IMPROVE POPULATION HEALTH

A. Regulation and Legislation Driving Change

The Triple Aim of improved patient experience, improved health of populations, and lowered per capita cost has focused attention on key outcome goals for US health care delivery. The ACA-instituted new models of care, and alternative payment models are focused on and responsive to these goals. Through these models, the 1:1 medical care focus is being broadened to include a population health focus that includes population health management.

Increased access, insurance regulation, cost-containment, quality improvement, improvement in public health and prevention, and research support are all components of the ACA and are areas intended to enhance US health and health care. New models of care, alternative payment models, and programs that impact traditional fee-for-service reimbursement fall in the realm of cost-containment and quality improvement. These include ACOs, PCMHs, bundled payments, value-based purchasing, the Hospital Readmission Reduction Program, and the Hospital Acquired Condition Reduction Program. Although not a new model or program that directly impacts care or reimbursement, the ACA requirement for a CHNA is included because of its contribution to broadening the population health focus.

An ACO is an integrated system of health care professionals/organizations in a formal agreement with a payer to care for a defined patient population. The ACO is accountable for quality, cost, and outcomes of its population of patients.[54] This accountability has prompted ACOs to focus on a number of areas including process improvement, judicious use of data, transitions of care, and optimal patient follow-up. Thirty-three ACO quality metrics exist for Medicare inclusive of metrics for at-risk populations.[55] Financial risk differs among different models of ACOs, with the Pioneer ACOs at higher risk than Medicare Shared Savings Plans (MSSPs). ACOs may be accountable for losses and repayment to Medicare if patient care expenditures exceed set benchmarks.[56] With higher risk comes greater accountability and attention to improving the health and health outcomes for individual patients and the patient population. Recent Centers for Medicare & Medicaid Services data from 2014 indicate improved quality and lowered costs for the MSSPs and Pioneer ACOs.[57]

The PCMH is a model of primary care that provides comprehensive, team-based, patient-centered, coordinated, accessible care that is focused on quality and patient safety. PCMHs are additionally focused on patient engagement in self-management, utilization of community support and resources, and population health management.[58] PCMHs may undergo accreditation through various accrediting bodies. PCMHs may be part of shared savings models. Patient-centered specialty practices have received recent recognition, although implementation and support has been slow.[59,60] The patient-centered medical neighborhood (Fig. 10.4) is a framework to further enhance PCMHs by linking primary care, specialty care, health care delivery sites, public health, and community resources. However, challenges exist with reimbursement, robust health information technology, and the overall fragmentation of the health care system.[61]

Bundled payments are set payments for services rendered during a patient's episode of care (course of treatment for a certain medical condition or illness). The clinicians and hospital are accountable for the quality and cost, encouraging care coordination.[62] An example of an episode of care that may fall under a bundled payment arrangement is a total knee arthroplasty. It is important to consider that process improvement, greater care coordination, and enhanced quality impact not only the individual patient, but also the population of patients that may experience the particular episode of care.

In value-based purchasing, hospitals are eligible for a value-based incentive payment, measured by clinical processes of care, patient experience, and outcomes.[63] Value-based purchasing has forced hospitals to analyze their processes, patient satisfaction with their care experience, and overall quality and outcomes. Hospital performance data has been made publicly available on the *Hospital Compare* website.[64] Enhancing these outcome measures not only benefits the individual patient but also the population of patients that access care in the hospital.

The Hospital Readmission Reduction Program penalizes hospitals for relatively higher Medicare re-admissions. Fiscal year 2015 penalties applied to acute myocardial infarction, heart failure, pneumonia, chronic obstructive pulmonary disease, and hip/knee arthroplasty.[65,66] Hospitals have had to analyze process, quality, and transitions of care as part of their efforts to reduce re-admission penalties. These improvements not only benefit the individual patient but also the population of patients that may be hospitalized for these clinical conditions.

The Hospital Acquired Condition Reduction Program reduces Medicare payment to the poorest performing hospitals. Included has been assessment of central-line–associated blood stream infections and catheter-associated urinary tract infections.[67,68] Hospitals have adopted the best evidence for prevention and focused on quality improvement in efforts to reduce hospital-acquired condition penalties. Again, these improvements not only benefit the individual patient but also the population of patients that may experience these procedures as part of their hospitalization.

Not-for-profit hospitals are required to perform a CHNA and develop an implementation plan every 3 years in order to keep their 501(c)(3) status.[54] This requirement is an additional change that has introduced a population health focus into the medical care arena. Some hospitals are working collaboratively with local public health agencies on CHNAs and solutions.

New models of care and alternative payment models have made a significant contribution to the paradigm shift toward population health. Data collection, analysis, and research on the success of these programs are ongoing to determine the most effective interventions to improve population health.

B. New Tools Supporting Population Health

In addition to new models of care and alternative payment models, new technology is also being introduced to

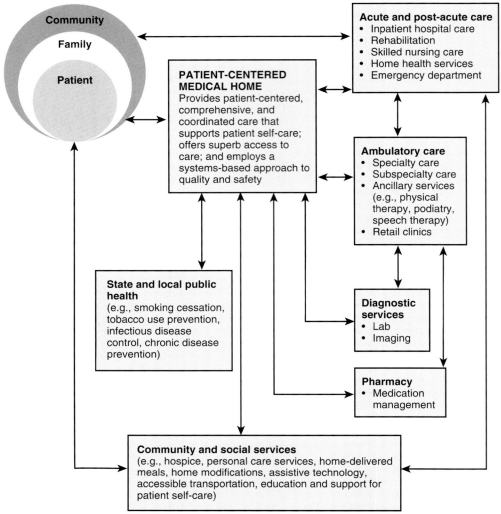

Fig. 10.4 The patient-centered medical neighborhood. (From Taylor EF, Lake T, Nysenbaum J, Peterson G, Meyers D. *Coordinating Care in the Medical Neighborhood: Critical Components and Available Mechanisms.* AHRQ Publication No. 11-0064. Rockville, MD: Agency for Healthcare Research and Quality. June 2011.)

help manage a population's health. These tools include the following:

- EHRs
- Analytic software
- Patient portals
- Wearable devices and biosensors
- Telemedicine

1. Electronic Health Records

According to the US Department of Health and Human Services, EHRs "are built to go beyond standard clinical data collected in a provider's office and are inclusive of a broader view of a patient's care. EHRs contain information from all the clinicians involved in a patient's care, and all authorized clinicians involved in a patient's care can access the information to provide care to that patient. EHRs also share information with other health care providers, such as laboratories and specialists. EHRs follow patients—to the specialist, the hospital, the nursing home, or even across the country."[69]

An EHR potentially allows timely, efficient access to large sets of population data, such as Hemoglobin A1c readings for populations of diabetic patients; blood pressure readings for populations of hypertensive patients; and cholesterol data for populations of patients with lipid disorders. Access to this data allows individual providers, medical practices, and health care systems to analyze how well clinicians are managing both acute and chronic disease processes.

While an EHR allows for timely and efficient access to data, there are limitations. Many EHR systems do not communicate with each other, limiting the generalizability of data to settings outside of the population the EHR is serving. In addition, EHRs may not contain retrievable data on the nonbiologic determinants that affect health (such as socioeconomic status), and thus a complete picture of a population's health status may not be achievable solely through use of an EHR.

2. Analytic Software

The use of analytics to manage populations of patients is becoming increasingly prevalent. In order to use analytics effectively to manage populations, systems must have access to data that do the following:

1. Integrate data from multiple health sources, across the continuum of care, including from EHRs, but also from mobile applications, wearable technology, and other data sources from which a patient may interact.
2. Develop and then integrate clinical risk algorithms into the care of patients and populations to ensure that those who need treatment receive it and those who do not need treatment are not overtreated.
3. Deliver the analysis of data to those who must act on it, such as health care administrators, who must allocate resources based on population need; providers, who must act on their data to improve the clinical care of patients and populations; and individual members within the population, who can use the data to advocate for their own health care needs.

3. Patient Portals

A patient portal is "a secure website that can interface with an EHR. It serves as a 24/7 access point for patients and can provide two-way communications between patients and practices, including providers, care teams, and administrative staff."[70] Patients can typically access the following through a portal:

- Summaries of recent physician visits
- Hospital discharge summaries
- Medications
- Immunizations
- Allergies
- Laboratory results

Depending on the patient portal, patients may also be able to schedule physician visits, e-mail their physician with nonurgent questions about their health, and request prescription refills.[71]

Patient portals may benefit both health care providers and patients. Health care providers and patients may e-mail each other with nonurgent questions, decreasing the need for phone calls. Patients have access to their health care record and can check to ensure that medications and refills are correct. In addition, patient portals have the potential to improve population health. Portals are designed to allow easier, more direct communication between the patient and provider. For example, if a medicine needs to be adjusted for better diabetes or blood pressure control, a provider may simply e-mail a patient through the portal, instead of trying to track down the patient by phone or making the patient come in for an office visit.

4. Wearable Devices and Biosensors

Wearable technology can be defined as "mobile electronic devices that can be unobtrusively embedded in the user's outfit as part of the clothing or an accessory."[72] Wearable technology allows for monitoring of factors influencing an individual's health including monitoring of vital signs (such as heart rate and blood pressure) and number of steps an individual has taken. The information gathered from this wearable technology then can be integrated with other health care data to manage the health of an individual or a population more effectively.

One recent example of wearable technology is Google Glass, which currently may affect patient care more through its adoption by providers than by patients. Google Glass is wearable technology, placed on an individual's face as a set of eyeglasses would be. Google Glass is voice-control enabled to record both audio and video. Among its different functionalities, Google Glass allows surgeons to record their surgery from a first-person perspective, allowing for the teaching of a procedure to a multitude of learners. Google Glass also allows for remote consultations (e.g., by transmitting an image of a rash to a remote dermatologist).[73]

There are other examples of how population health may be improved by wearable technology. Patients may be encouraged to reduce their salt intake and have their blood pressure measured by a wearable, with the results automatically transmitted to the patient's primary health care professional. Wearables may also be employed to measure patients' weight, blood pressure, and pulse to assess the effectiveness of population health campaigns to encourage exercise.

5. Telemedicine

According to the American Academy of Family Physicians, "Telemedicine is the use of medical information that is exchanged from one site to another through electronic communications. It includes varying types of processes and services intended to enrich the delivery of medical care and improve the health status of patients."[74]

Examples of telemedicine include the following:

- A dermatologist in a remote setting providing care to a patient in a rural setting through an internet connection to examine a newly developed rash; or the broader use of telemedicine for dermatological screenings of populations of farmers with a history of sun exposure
- A patient admitted to an intensive care unit at a rural hospital being monitored remotely by a team of physicians and nurses
- A panel of diabetic patients monitoring their blood sugars at home and uploading their blood sugars to an endocrinologist, who will then adjust insulin doses to improve Hemoglobin A1c values across a population

Telemedicine is expected to expand exponentially in the next several decades as technology improves, populations age, and the prevalence of chronic disease increases.

C. New Types of Health Care Workers

The health care system of the 21st century still requires the knowledge and skills of traditional health care providers, including physicians, nurses, and pharmacists. However, as health care becomes increasingly complex and health care providers are asked to manage both individual patients and populations, other interdisciplinary health care providers with new knowledge and skills are required. These new types of health care professionals include the following:

- Nurse care managers
- Community health workers
- Patient navigators

1. Nurse Care Managers

Nurse care managers coordinate and organize clinical care around individual patients as well as populations of patients.[75] Nurse care managers may perform some or all of the following tasks:

- Act as a conduit between the patient and physician.
- Answer patient questions.
- Assist in managing chronic medical conditions.
- Facilitate the transfer of information among a patient's providers, including specialty physicians.
- Conduct home or hospital visits.

Nurse care managers often serve as a bridge between patients and their physicians and health care professionals in primary care or specialty practice. For example, in a busy primary care practice, a primary care provider may have only 15 minutes to spend with a patient who has multiple chronic medical issues, such as diabetes mellitus, chronic obstructive pulmonary disease (COPD), and hypertension. A nurse care manager may reach out in between office visits to ensure that this patient's blood sugars are controlled, that the patient has oxygen for his or her COPD, and that the patient is taking blood pressure medications.

2. Community Health Workers

The American Public Health Association defines a *community health worker* as "a frontline public health worker who is a trusted member of and/or has an unusually close understanding of the community served."[76] Community health workers are located not only in the United States, but also worldwide. Their role is typically adapted to the needs of the community they serve. For example, a community health worker in an urban location in the United States may provide counseling around sexually transmitted diseases or provide directly observed therapy for tuberculosis. The role of community health workers is expanding to integration into hospital and clinic health care teams.[77]

3. Patient Navigators

A *patient navigator* is defined as "a member of the health care team who helps patients 'navigate' the health care system and get timely care. Navigators help coordinate patient care, connect patients with resources, and help patients understand the health care system."[78] Patient navigators are often found in physician offices and help navigate patients through one or more chronic health care conditions, such as diabetes or cancer. Some medical schools now train early medical students to serve as patient navigators to gain an understanding of the health care system prior to taking care of patients.[79]

The roles of a patient navigator and a community health worker overlap to some extent. However, for the purposes of this text, a patient navigator does not necessarily need to be a trusted member of the community in order to serve a population.

There are many other types of health care providers who contribute to the care of individual patients and populations, including physicians, nurses, nurse practitioners, physician assistants, diabetic educators, pharmacists, dentists, social workers, and medical assistants. These health care professionals and others are discussed in Chapter 7.

D. Population Health Initiatives

1. Camden Coalition of Healthcare Providers

Camden, New Jersey, is a city located across from Philadelphia, Pennsylvania, and the Delaware River runs between the two very different cities. Camden has the highest rate of crime of any city in the United States[80] and is one of the poorest cities in the United States, with over one-third of its population living below the poverty line. The Camden Coalition of Healthcare Providers is a prime example of a local organization integrating public health, clinical medicine, and the community in a poor, urban area.

The Camden Coalition of Healthcare Providers led by Jeffrey Brenner, MD, is a nonprofit "citywide coalition of hospitals, primary care providers, and community representatives that collaborate to deliver better health care to the most vulnerable citizens."[21]

At the center of the Coalition's work is "hotspotting."[81] This is a data-driven process in which the highest utilizers of health care resources are identified (for example, in many communities, as few as 10 percent of hospital patients account for 75 percent of health care spending). The Coalition uses insurance data to identify these high health care utilizers. Once these patients are identified, resources are mobilized. These resources include a care management team, composed of multiple health care professionals, including social workers, nurses, community health workers, and others who visit the patient both while in the hospital and once discharged, to help reduce re-admissions to the hospital[82] and maximize health.

2. Homeless Patient Aligned Care Teams

An example of a national initiative integrating population health into clinical medicine is the Homeless Patient Aligned Care Teams (H-PACTs). H-PACTs are being implemented nationally at Veterans Administration (VA) medical centers. The goal of the H-PACTs is to end veteran homelessness in this high-risk population.

H-PACTs are located on the campus of VA medical centers. H-PACTs integrate many health care professionals including physicians, nurses, social workers, behavioral health specialists, and substance abuse counselors. This team provides services to homeless veterans, including helping find permanent housing. Patients can also receive medical care through H-PACTs as well as a warm shower and clean clothes if needed. One of H-PACTs' main tenets is that improving health goes beyond medical care. H-PACTs espouse the idea that providing safe, stable housing is providing health care.

While the data analyzing H-PACT outcomes are pending, preliminary results demonstrate that patients enrolled in an H-PACT are hospitalized and use the emergency department less than patients who are not enrolled. This decrease in hospital utilization translates to a savings for the VA system of about $5 million per year.[22]

3. Million Hearts

The goal of the Million Hearts initiative is to prevent 1 million heart attacks and strokes by 2017. The targeted focus is to optimize medical care in delivery sites through aspirin use, blood pressure control, cholesterol management, and smoking cessation within a framework of health technology and tools and innovation in health care delivery. The targeted focus is also on changing the environment for smoking, sodium intake, and trans fat intake.[83]

Million Hearts has extensive partners from the public and private health care sectors, inclusive of federal agencies, state departments of health, national specialty- and disease-focused associations, health care systems, physician groups, local associations, and payers. The partnership has extended to 100 Congregations for Million Hearts. This faith-based program includes congregations that have committed to strengthen relationships with community resources including community health centers and community health workers for their members.[84]

Through Million Hearts, a significant number of protocols, guides, and tools have been made available for clinicians, patients, public health workers, and employers to focus on control of hypertension and cardiovascular health. Collaborations are bringing together public health and medical care surrounding cardiovascular health and prevention.[23,83]

V. THE FUTURE OF POPULATION HEALTH

Population health is growing and evolving. A number of new initiatives set the tone for this growth to accelerate and to continue to impact medical care. The US Department of Health and Human Services has been increasingly focused on payment for quality over quantity. Goals have been set to tie certain percentages of traditional payments from Medicare to new payment models such as ACOs or bundled payments and tie all Medicare payments to quality or value through value-based purchasing or the Hospital Readmission Reduction Program.[85] The Health Care Payment Learning and Action Network was created to bring together public and private payers to delineate best practices in this arena.[86] Hospital providers in an industry consortium, the Health Care Transformation Task Force, have committed to 75 percent of their business operating in value-based payment arrangements by 2020.[87] A next-generation ACO model that is higher risk than any current ACO is in the pilot stages.[88] For the first time, mandatory bundled payments are required for hip and knee replacement surgeries in certain geographic areas.[89] Increased accountability and financial risk are accelerating focus in medical care on optimizing quality, cost, outcomes, and health for individual patients and populations of patients.

Significant work is ongoing through the State Innovation Models (SIM) initiative to test state-led multipayer health care delivery and payment models. This is inclusive of work focused on collaborative efforts between primary care, public health, community organizations, and social services.[90] Maryland's all-payer global budget model has shown early success. This model provides a framework for movement forward toward integration of local health care delivery and public health initiatives.[91]

The American College of Cardiology has created a population health committee. Their goals include focus on primary prevention, health promotion, greater collaboration with primary care, and greater attention to the behavioral and social determinants of health. This is a significant paradigm shift for a specialty group that has been historically procedure-based rather than focused on prevention and population health.[92]

From the community perspective, Accountable Communities for Health are being tested. Particular focus is being paid to determinants of population health and integration of health care, public health, and social services.[93]

Significant opportunity exists for collaborative efforts between medical care and public health activities. The siloed nature of these disciplines as well as different sources of funding and reimbursement have been barriers. However, ongoing initiatives such as the Camden Coalition of Healthcare Providers, Homeless Patient Aligned Care Teams, and Million Hearts are bridging health care delivery, public health, and the community. The ACA has supported assessment and connection to community resources through new models of care and other requirements. Outcomes of SIMs are expected to provide insight into ways to support health care delivery–public health collaborations.

Despite these encouraging efforts, there is still much work to do. A population health focus in medical care needs to expand to all specialties and sites of care. As noted earlier, health care is deemed responsible for only 10 percent of the determinants of population health, yet health care garners the most attention and financial support. The health care delivery–public health collaboration needs to become much more comprehensive so resources, attention to prevention, and health promotion, and data are shared more effectively. Attention and action to address the determinants of population health and their root causes, particularly behavior, social circumstances, and environmental exposures, needs to be much more robust. Population health will face greatest improvement in the future with the broad acceptance of responsibility beyond one sector or one determinant, and with multi-stakeholder engagement and collaboration.

A. Education Initiatives in Population Health

Realizing that physicians must possess the knowledge and skills related to population health in a rapidly evolving health care system, medical schools across the United States are responding by integrating population health content into curriculum. The following are examples of schools integrating population health content:

The Warren Alpert Medical School of Brown University (AMS): The AMS created a dual-degree program in which students receive a medical degree and a Master of Science in population medicine in 4 years. A proportion of all of their students will enter this program each year. Students will take courses directly related to population health, including courses on health disparities, social determinants of health, leadership, health systems, biostatistics and epidemiology, and the intersection of population health with clinical medicine.

Mayo Medical School (MMS): The MMS in collaboration with Arizona State University's School for the Science of Healthcare Delivery has developed a required certificate in the science of health care delivery for their medical students. Both online and classroom teaching are delivered throughout the 4 years of medical school in the areas of population-centered care, high-value care, team-based care, leadership, person-centered care, and health policy, economics, and technology. Students have the option to complete a Master of Science in the Science of Healthcare Delivery through Arizona State University.

Penn State College of Medicine: Penn State created a new longitudinal course that all students will take directly related to population health. This course will intertwine content on evidence-based medicine, teamwork, and leadership. In addition, all students at Penn State will become patient navigators, in which they help patients navigate through the different facets of the health care system.

Other examples of schools responding to the need to integrate population health into their curriculum include Case Western University, which is introducing a patient navigator program into their curriculum; Florida International University, which is integrating the social determinants of health into its curriculum; and Rutgers Robert Wood Johnson Medical School, which is training its medical students in care coordination. The American Medical Association's Accelerating Change in Medical Education grant initiative has provided support for these innovative changes in medical school education.[94]

VI. CHAPTER SUMMARY

Population health as a concept and field is gaining significant momentum due to policy, regulatory change, research funding, and multi-stakeholder engagement through collaborative initiatives at the national, state, community, public health, and medical care levels. The population health agenda is aligned with the goals of the Triple Aim, new models of care, and alternative payment models with a population health focus. National and local population health initiatives and the Center for Medicare and Medicaid Innovation funding are establishing new models that can be disseminated and emulated more broadly. Integration of population health content into health professions curriculum is producing a new generation of health care professionals ready to employ the principles of population health to improve the health of our communities.

Much work still remains, but current efforts are creating a foundation for both a focus on population health and a means for improvement of population health in the United States.

QUESTIONS FOR FURTHER THOUGHT

1. What are drivers of the population health focus in the United States?
2. What is the difference between population health, public health, and population medicine?
3. What is setting the tone for the future of population health?
4. How is a population health focus being operationalized in the medical care setting?

Annotated Bibliography

Bodenheimer T, Grumbach K. *Understanding Health Policy.* 7th ed. New York, NY: McGraw-Hill; 2016.
   This textbook on health policy, now in its 7th edition, is edited by two leading health policy experts, Dr. Bodenheimer and Dr. Grumbach, both from the Department of Family Medicine, University of California–San Francisco School of Medicine. The text focuses on multiple aspects of medicine related to population health including access to and paying for health care; the organization of health care including primary, secondary, and tertiary care; costs of care, including how to control costs; and other health care systems. Throughout the text, examples of the Triple Aim and population health are emphasized, including quality health care, controlling costs, and enhancing the patient experience.

Healthy People 2020. Washington, DC: U.S. Department of Health and Human Services, Office of Disease Prevention and Health Promotion. http://www.healthypeople.gov.
   Healthy People 2020 is managed by the Office of Disease Prevention and Health Promotion (ODPHP) within the US Department of Health and Human Services (HHS), but is a collaboration with other federal agencies as well as local community organizations. This initiative is a nationwide program to improve the health of all through a focus on disease prevention and health promotion. The original health goals were issued in 1979. Updates were subsequently made with new goals for improved health over 10 years by 2000, 2010, and now 2020. Current goals are to attain high-quality, longer lives free of preventable disease, disability, injury, and premature death; achieve health equity, eliminate disparities, and improve the health of all groups; create social and physical environments that promote good health for all; and promote quality of life, healthy development, and healthy behaviors across all life stages.

Kindig D, Stoddart G. What is population health? *Am J Public Health.* 2003;93(3):380–383.
   This is a seminal article on population health. Dr. Kindig from the Department of Population Health Sciences, University of Wisconsin–Madison School of Medicine and Dr. Stoddard from the Department of Clinical Epidemiology and Biostatistics, McMaster University Health Science Centre, very thoughtfully consider the meaning of population health based on prior definitions and considerations. They discuss population health as a concept of health that most appropriately involves health outcomes, determinants of health, and policy. In the article, they put forth a definition of population health, to provide some consensus for the field. Their definition "the health outcomes of a group of individuals, including the distribution of such outcomes within the group" is now widely used and respected. The authors further discuss the concern of population health with interactions between determinants of population health and the importance for multi-stakeholder "attention and action" for improved population health. Lastly, they put forth population health as a framework to consider health outcomes and their distribution, and to assess the determinants of population health, forcing broad responsibility for population health beyond one sector or one determinant.

McGinnis JM, Williams-Russo P, Knickman JR. The case for more active policy attention to health promotion. *Health Aff (Millwood).* 2002;21(2):78–93.
   This article, authored by a group from the Robert Wood Johnson Foundation, provides a comprehensive review of the determinants of health, genetics, social circumstances, environmental conditions, behavioral choices, and medical care, to emphasize the importance of supporting policy and funding of health promotion initiatives to meaningfully improve population health. Included is a review on factors limiting these initiatives and recommendations for further progress.

Nash DB, Fabius RJ, Skoufalos A, Clarke JL, Horowitz MR, eds. *Population Health: Creating a Culture of Wellness.* 2nd ed. Burlington, MA: Jones & Bartlett Learning; 2016.
   This textbook on population health, now in its 2nd edition, is edited by a group of educators including Founding Dean David Nash from the Jefferson School of Population Health. Particularly aimed at those training and working in health care delivery sites, the book focuses both on key aspects of population health management and strategy for creation of a culture of wellness in the United States. The impact of the Affordable Care Act on population health is woven throughout the book. The book is organized into five sections that highlight key concepts of population health; the role of the consumer in a health care system characterized by population health; consideration of the continuum of care; population health and the business case for a value-driven health care delivery system; and future

directions in research. Put forth are four pillars of population health inclusive of chronic care management, quality and safety, public health, and health policy. Discussed is the broad set of initiatives that defines population health, including health promotion, disease prevention, and engagement of multiple stakeholders in the areas of prevention, health care delivery, medical intervention, public health, and policy. Lastly, emphasized is the strong focus of population health on analysis of outcomes to drive process change and new policy.

References

1. Berwick DM, Nolan TW, Whittington J. The Triple Aim: care, health and cost. *Health Aff (Millwood)*. 2008;27(3):759–769.

2. Institute for Healthcare Improvement. IHI Triple Aim initiative. http://www.ihi.org/engage/initiatives/tripleaim/Pages/default.aspx. Accessed January 3, 2016.

3. Kindig D, Stoddart G. What is population health? *Am J Public Health*. 2003;93(3):380–383.

4. The National Academies of Science, Engineering, and Medicine. Institute of Medicine. Vision, mission, and definition of the roundtable on population health improvement. http://www.nationalacademies.org/hmd/Activities/PublicHealth/PopulationHealthImprovementRT/VisionMission. Published 2015. Accessed October 12, 2015.

5. Nash DB, Fabius RJ, Skoufalos A, Clarke JL, Horowitz MR, eds. *Population Health: Creating a Culture of Wellness*. 2nd ed. Burlington, MA: Jones & Bartlett Learning; 2016.

6. Centers for Disease Control and Prevention. National Center for HIV/AIDS, Viral Hepatitis, STD, and TB Prevention social determinants of health. http://www.cdc.gov/nchhstp/socialdeterminants/definitions.html. Updated March 21, 2014. Accessed February 20, 2016.

7. McGinnis JM, Williams-Russo P, Knickman JR. The case for more active policy attention to health promotion. *Health Aff (Millwood)*. 2002;21(2):78–93.

8. Commission on Social Determinants of Health (CSDH). *Closing the gap in a generation: health equity through action on the social determinants of health. Final report of the Commission on Social Determinants of Health*. Geneva, Switzerland: World Health Organization; 2008.

9. Healthy People 2020. Social determinants of health. http://www.healthypeople.gov/2020/topics-objectives/topic/social-determinants-health. Accessed November 30, 2015.

10. U.S. Department of Health and Human Services. Healthy People 2020: an opportunity to address the societal determinants of health in the United States. http://www.healthypeople.gov/2010/hp2020/advisory/SocietalDeterminantsHealth.htm. Updated July 26, 2010. Accessed November 30, 2015.

11. Institute of Medicine. *The Future of Public Health*. Washington, DC: National Academies Press; 1988.

12. Centers for Disease Control and Prevention. National Public Health Performance Standards. The public health system and the 10 essential public health services. http://www.cdc.gov/nphpsp/essentialservices.html. Updated May 29, 2014. Accessed November 13, 2015.

13. Centers for Disease Control and Prevention. Behavioral Risk Factor Surveillance System. http://www.cdc.gov/brfss/. Updated September 15, 2015. Accessed November 13, 2015.

14. Schneider M-J. *Introduction to Public Health*. 4th ed. Burlington, MA: Jones & Bartlett Learning; 2014.

15. County Health Rankings and Roadmaps. http://www.countyhealthrankings.org/. Accessed November 13, 2015.

16. Stoto MA. Population health in the Affordable Care Act era. *Academy Health*. February 21, 2013.

17. Lewis N. Populations, population health, and the evolution of population management: making sense of the terminology in US healthcare today. Institute for Healthcare Improvement Leadership Blog. http://www.ihi.org/communities/blogs/_layouts/ihi/community/blog/itemview.aspx?List=81ca4a47-4ccd-4e9e-89d9-14d88ec59e8d&ID=50. Accessed June 5, 2015.

18. Centers for Disease Control and Prevention. Diabetes home. http://www.cdc.gov/diabetes/home/. Updated November 4, 2015. Accessed January 8, 2016.

19. Centers for Disease Control and Prevention. Chronic Disease Prevention and Health Promotion. http://www.cdc.gov/chronicdisease/about/state-public-health-actions.htm. Updated September 28, 2015. Accessed January 8, 2016.

20. Maricopa Department of Public Health. Community Health Improvement Plan, Maricopa County 2012–2017.

21. Camden Coalition of Healthcare Providers. https://www.camdenhealth.org/. Accessed November 1, 2015.

22. US Department of Veteran's Affairs. Homeless veterans. http://www.va.gov/homeless/h_pact.asp. Accessed November 17, 2015.

23. Million Hearts. http://millionhearts.hhs.gov/. Accessed November 1, 2015.

24. Marvasti FF, Stafford RS. From sick care to health care—reengineering prevention into the U.S. system. *N Engl J Med*. 2012;367(10):889–891.

25. DesRoches CM, Buerhaus P, Dittus RS, Donelan K. Primary care workforce shortages and career recommendations from practicing clinicians. *Acad Med*. 2015;90(5):671–677.

26. Levi J, Segal LM, Gougelet R, St. Laurent R. *Investing in America's Health 2015*. Princeton, NJ: Robert Wood Johnson Foundation; April 2015.

27. Bauer UE, Briss PA, Goodman RA, Bowman BA. Prevention of chronic disease in the 21st century: elimination of the leading preventable causes of premature death and disability in the USA. *Lancet*. 2014;384(9937):45–52.

28. Pizer SD, Gardner JA. Is fragmented financing bad for your health? *Inquiry*. 2011;48(2):109–122.

29. Bendix J. Meaningful use 2: 2013's interoperability challenge. Connectivity barriers remain as physicians move from EHR implementation to data exchange, communication. *Med Econ*. 2013;90(6):18–19, 24–27.

30. Braveman P, Egerter S. *Overcoming Obstacles to Health in 2013 and Beyond. RWJF Commission to Build a Healthier America*. Princeton, NJ: Robert Wood Johnson Foundation; 2013.

31. Woolf SH, Braveman P. Where health disparities begin: the role of social and economic determinants—and why current policies may make matters worse. *Health Aff (Millwood)*. 2011;30(10):1852–1859.

32. Centers for Disease Control and Prevention. Chronic Disease Prevention and Health Promotion. http://www.cdc.gov/chronicdisease/overview/index.htm. Updated August 26, 2015. Accessed October 12, 2015.

33. Heron M. Deaths: leading causes for 2010. *Natl Vital Stat Rep*. 2013;62(6):1–96.

34. Ogden CL, Carroll MD, Fryar CD, Flegal KM. Prevalence of obesity among adults and youth: United States, 2011–2014. *NCHS Data Brief*. 2015;(219):1–8.

35. National Institutes of Health, National Heart, Lung, and Blood Institute. *Clinical Guidelines on the Identification, Evaluation, and Treatment of Overweight and Obesity in Adults*, NIH Publication No. 98-4083; September 1998.

36. Cote AT, Harris KC, Panagiotopoulos C, Sandor GG, Devlin AM. Childhood obesity and cardiovascular dysfunction. *J Am Coll Cardiol*. 2013;62(15):1309–1319.

37. OrthoInfo. Guidelines for preventing falls. http://orthoinfo.aaos.org/topic.cfm?topic=A00135. Reviewed October 2012. Accessed October 12, 2015.

38. Centers for Disease Control and Prevention. *The State of Aging & Health in America 2013*. Atlanta, GA: Centers for Disease Control and Prevention, U.S. Department of Health and Human Services; 2013.

39. Kuehn BM. AAP: toxic stress threatens kids' long-term health. *JAMA*. 2014;312(6):585–586.

40. Dicat L, Philipson LH, Anderson BJ. The mental health comorbidities of diabetes. *JAMA*. 2014;312(7):691–692.

41. National Alliance on Mental Illness. Mental health conditions. http://www.nami.org/Learn-More/Mental-Health-Conditions. Reviewed March 2013. Accessed November 3, 2016.

42. Centers for Medicare and Medicaid Services. Office of the Actuary Health Statistics Group, National Health Expenditure Accounts, National Health Expenditures Aggregate 1960–2011.

43. Gerteis J, Izrael D, Deitz D, et al. *Multiple Chronic Conditions Chartbook*. AHRQ Publications No. Q14–0038. Rockville, MD: Agency for Healthcare Research and Quality; April 2014.

44. OECD. OECD health statistics. http://www.oecd.org/unitedstates/Country-Note-UNITED%20STATES-OECD-Health-Statistics-2015.pdf. Published July 7, 2015. Accessed October 27, 2015.

45. Squires D, Anderson C. US healthcare from a global perspective: spending, use of services, prices and health in 13 countries. *Commonwealth Fund*. 2015;1819(15):1–15.

46. Braveman P. Health disparities and health equity: concepts and measurement. *Annu Rev Public Health*. 2006;27:167–194.

47. U.S. Department of Health and Human Services. The Secretary's Advisory Committee on National Health Promotion and Disease Prevention Objectives for 2020. Phase I Report: Recommendations for the Framework and Format of Healthy People 2020. http://www.healthypeople.gov/sites/default/files/PhaseI_0.pdf. Published October 28, 2008. Accessed November 30, 2015.

48. Robert Wood Johnson Foundation. Life expectancy map: Chicago. http://www.rwjf.org/en/library/infographics/life-expectancy-map–chicago.html?cq_ck=1430259368495. Published April 29, 2015. Accessed November 30, 2015.

49. Centers for Disease Control and Prevention. CDC Health Disparities and Inequalities Report—United States, 2013. *MMWR*. 2013;62(suppl 3):1–184.

50. LaVeist TA, Gaskin D, Richard P. Estimating the economic burden of racial health inequalities in the United States. *Int J Health Serv*. 2011;41(2):231–238.

51. National Association of County and City Health Officials. Definitions of community health assessments (CHA) and community health improvement plans (CHIPs). http://naccho.org/topics/infrastructure/community-health-assessment-and-improvement-planning/upload/Definitions.pdf. Accessed November 30, 2015.

52. Bodenheimer T, Grumbach K. *Understanding Health Policy*. 7th ed. New York, NY: McGraw-Hill; 2016.

53. Kindig DA. Understanding population health terminology. *Milbank Q*. 2007;85(1):139–161.

54. Kaiser Family Foundation. Health Reform. Summary of the Affordable Care Act. http://kff.org/health-reform/fact-sheet/summary-of-the-affordable-care-act/. Published April 25, 2013. Accessed November 17, 2015.

55. Accountable Care Organization 2015 Program Analysis Quality Performance Standards Narrative Measure Specifications. https://www.cms.gov/medicare/medicare-fee-for-service-payment/sharedsavingsprogram/downloads/ry2015-narrative-specifications.pdf. Published January 9, 2015.

56. Centers for Medicare & Medicaid Services. Pioneer ACO Model. https://innovation.cms.gov/initiatives/Pioneer-ACO-Model/. Updated December 7, 2015. Accessed January 3, 2016.

57. Centers for Medicare & Medicaid Services. Medicare ACOs provide improved care while slowing cost growth in 2014. https://www.cms.gov/Newsroom/MediaReleaseDatabase/Fact-sheets/2015-Fact-sheets-items/2015-08-25.html. Published August 25, 2015. Accessed November 17, 2015.

58. Agency for Healthcare Research and Quality. Patient Centered Medical Home Resource Center. https://pcmh.ahrq.gov/page/defining-pcmh. Accessed November 17, 2015.

59. National Committee for Quality Assurance. Patient-Centered Specialty Practice Recognition. http://www.ncqa.org/Programs/Recognition/Practices/PatientCenteredSpecialtyPracticePCSP.aspx. Accessed November 17, 2015.

60. Huang X, Rosenthal MB. Transforming specialty practice—the patient-centered medical neighborhood. *N Engl J Med*. 2014;370(15):1376–1379.

61. Agency for Healthcare Research and Quality. Coordinating Care in the Medical Neighborhood: Critical Components and Available Mechanisms. AHRQ Publication No. 11–0064. https://pcmh.ahrq.gov/page/coordinating-care-medical-neighborhood-critical-components-and-available-mechanisms. Published June 2011. Accessed November 20, 2015.

62. Centers for Medicare & Medicaid Services. Bundled Payments for Care Improvement Initiative. http://innovation.cms.gov/initiatives/bundled-payments/. Updated November 4, 2015. Accessed November 20, 2015.

63. Centers for Medicare & Medicaid Services. Hospital value-based purchasing. http://www.cms.gov/Medicare/Quality-Initiatives-Patient-Assessment-Instruments/hospital-value-based-purchasing/index.html. Updated October 30, 2015. Accessed November 20, 2015.

64. Medicare.gov. Hospital Compare. https://www.medicare.gov/hospitalcompare/search.html. Accessed November 20, 2015.

65. Kaiser Family Foundation. Aiming for fewer hospital U-turns: the Medicare Hospital Readmission Reduction Program. Issue Brief. http://kff.org/medicare/issue-brief/aiming-for-fewer-hospital-u-turns-the-medicare-hospital-readmission-reduction-program/. Published January 29, 2015. Accessed November 21, 2015.

66. Centers for Medicare & Medicaid Services. Readmissions Reduction Program. https://www.cms.gov/Medicare/medicare-fee-for-service-payment/acuteinpatientPPS/readmissions-reduction-program.html. Updated November 16, 2015. Accessed November 21, 2015.

67. Centers for Medicare & Medicaid Services. Hospital-Acquired Condition Reduction Program. https://www.cms.gov/Medicare/Medicare-Fee-for-Service-Payment/AcuteInpatientPPS/HAC-Reduction-Program.html. Updated December 18, 2014. Accessed November 20, 2015.

68. Health Policy Brief: Medicare's Hospital-Acquired Condition Reduction Program. *Health Aff (Millwood)*. http://www.healthaffairs.org/healthpolicybriefs/brief.php?brief_id=142. Accessed November 3, 2016.

69. HealthIT.gov. What are the differences between electronic medical records, electronic health records, and personal health records? https://www.healthit.gov/providers-professionals/faqs/what-are-differences-between-electronic-medical-records-electronic. Updated November 2, 2015. Accessed February 20, 2016.

70. Terry K. Patient portals: essential but underused by physicians. Medical Economics. http://medicaleconomics.modernmedicine.com/medical-economics/news/patient-portals-essential-under-used-physicians?page=full. Published April 29, 2015.

71. HealthIT.gov. What is a patient portal? https://www.healthit.gov/providers-professionals/faqs/what-patient-portal. Updated November 2, 2015.

72. Lukowicz P, Kirstein T, Tröster G. Wearable systems for health care applications. *Methods Inf Med*. 2004;43(3):232–238.

73. Aungst TD, Lewis TL. Potential uses of wearable technology in medicine: lessons learnt from Google Glass. *Int J Clinic Pract*. 2015;69(10):1179–1183.

74. AAFP. Telemedicine. http://www.aafp.org/about/policies/all/telemedicine.html. Accessed January 20, 2016.

75. DeJesus RS, Howell L, Williams M, Hathaway J, Vickers KS. Collaborative care management effectively promotes self-management: patient evaluation of care management for depression in primary care. *Postgrad Med*. 2014;126(2):141–146.

76. American Public Health Association. Community health workers. https://www.apha.org/apha-communities/member-sections/community-health-workers. Accessed January 20, 2016.

77. Allen CG, Escoffery C, Satsangi A, Brownstein JN. Strategies to improve the integration of community health workers into health care teams: "a little fish in a big pond." *Prev Chronic Dis*. 2015 Sep 17;12:E154.

78. Patient Navigator Training Collaborative. http://patientnavigatortraining.org/. Accessed January 20, 2016.

79. Gonzalo JD, Haidet P, Papp KK, et al. Educating for the 21st-century health care system: an interdependent framework of basic, clinical and systems sciences. *Acad Med*. October 16, 2015. [Epub ahead of print].

80. Federal Bureau of Investigation. Crime in the United States 2012: New Jersey offenses known to law enforcement by city. https://www.fbi.gov/about-us/cjis/ucr/crime-in-the-u.s/2012/crime-in-the-u.s.-2012/tables/8tabledatadecpdf/table-8-state-cuts/table_8_offenses_known_to_law_enforcement_by_new_jersey_by_city_2012.xls. Published 2012. Accessed December 20, 2015.

81. Robert Wood Johnson Foundation. A revolutionary approach to improving health care delivery. http://www.rwjf.org/en/library/articles-and-news/2014/02/improving-management-of-health-care-superutilizers.html. Accessed January 20, 2016.

82. Center for Health Care Strategies. Hotspotting: the driver behind the Camden Coalition's innovations. http://www.chcs.org/hotspotting-driver-behind-camden-coalitions-innovations/. Accessed January 20, 2016.

83. Million Hearts. Preventing 1 Million Heart Attacks and Strokes. A Turning Point for Impact; 2014. http://millionhearts.hhs.gov/files/MH_Mid-Course_Review.pdf.

84. Hearts Million. Partners and progress. http://millionhearts.hhs.gov/partners-progress/index.html. Accessed November 21, 2015.

85. Burwell SM. Setting value-based payment goals—HHS efforts to improve US health care. *N Engl J Med*. 2015;372(10):897–899.

86. Centers for Medicare & Medicaid Services. Healthcare Payment Learning and Action Network. http://innovation.cms.gov/initiatives/Health-Care-Payment-Learning-and-Action-Network. Updated November 3, 2015. Accessed November 23, 2015.

87. Health Care Transformation Task Force. About Health Care Transformation Task Force. http://www.hcttf.org/aboutus/. Accessed November 23, 2015.

88. Centers for Medicare and Medicaid Services. Next Generation ACO Model. http://innovation.cms.gov/initiatives/Next-Generation-ACO-Model/. Updated November 2, 2015. Accessed November 23, 2015.

89. Centers for Medicare and Medicaid Services. Comprehensive Care for Joint Replacement Model. http://innovation.cms.gov/initiatives/ccjr/. Updated January 4, 2016. Accessed January 8, 2016.

90. Kaiser Family Foundation. The State Innovation Models (SIM) program: an overview. http://kff.org/medicaid/fact-sheet/the-state-innovation-models-sim-program-an-overview/. Published December 9, 2014. Accessed November 23, 2015.

91. Patel A, Rajkumar R, Colmers JM, Dinzer D, Conway PH, Sharfstein JM. Maryland's global hospital budgets—preliminary results from an all-payer model. *N Engl J Med*. 2015;373(20):1899–1901.

92. Williams KA, Martin GR. New American College of Cardiology population health agenda to focus on primary prevention. *J Am Coll Cardiol*. 2015;66(14):1625–1626.

93. Tipirnene R, Vickery KD, Ehlinger EP. Accountable communities for health: moving from providing accountable care to creating health. *Ann Fam Med*. 2015;13(4):367–369.

94. American Medical Association. Creating the medical school of the future. http://www.ama-assn.org/ama/pub/about-ama/strategic-focus/accelerating-change-in-medical-education/innovations.page. Accessed January 3, 2016.

11

Socio-Ecologic Determinants of Health

Daniel Goldberg, JD, PhD, Elizabeth G. Baxley, MD, and
Tonya L. Fancher, MD, MPH

This chapter explains the evidence base regarding the social determinants of health and the significance of such determinants in health systems science. The social determinants of health are crucial both to overall population health and to the equitable distribution of health within a population. Understanding the reasons why social and economic conditions are so strongly correlated with health outcomes helps explain the wide health inequalities that exist in the United States and in many other places around the world. The chapter then turns to analysis of the ways that attention to the social determinants of health can be integrated into clinical practice and health systems in general.

I. INTRODUCTION

In a 2006 editorial, Stonington, Holmes, and the editors of the journal *PLoS Medicine* put it simply: "The stark fact is that most disease on the planet is a product of the social conditions in which people work and live."[1] Explaining how and why this is the case, as well as exploring the role that physicians can play in ameliorating this situation, are the central aims of this chapter. Exploring how social and economic conditions determine health outcomes requires an understanding of patterns of disease within and between different populations. This means that understanding the social determinants of health requires an understanding of the widespread differences in health status among demographic groups in the United States and across the globe.

Such differences are often referred to as *health disparities, health inequalities,* or *health inequities.* The authors prefer the second term, and in exploring the concept, adopt the World Health Organization's definition of health inequalities as "differences in health status or in the distribution of health determinants between different population groups."[2]

In the interest of beginning the analysis and introducing some key concepts, this chapter opens with a case study to frame the content regarding the social determinants of health.

CASE STUDY 1

You are seeing Mrs. H for the first time. She is 34 years of age and has arrived with her two young children. She has moderately controlled diabetes and hypertension. Both of her children have asthma. She took them out of school so they could all see you today. She is hoping you can refill their medications too. Mrs. H adds "They don't like school anyway. They are always getting in trouble." Her blood pressure today is 150/84. Her fingerstick blood glucose in the office is 254 mg/dL.

As you read through the chapter, think about the following questions:

1. What modifiable environmental or social factors might be contributing to the health of this family?
2. How might you ask about them?
3. Is there more to the story about her children having trouble in school?
4. What additional resources could you offer this family beyond medication management?

There will be more about this case later in the chapter.

II. HISTORY AND EPIDEMIOLOGY: THE SOCIAL DETERMINANTS OF HEALTH

In 1848, German physician and anthropologist Rudolf Virchow published a report entitled *On the Typhus Epidemic in Upper Silesia*.[3] This innocuous-sounding report would go on to become one of the most important documents in the modern history of public health. Understanding the reasons for this serves as a useful framework for thinking about socio-ecologic determinants of health. In 1848, Silesia was an economically depressed Prussian province (current-day Poland). When Virchow set out to analyze the typhus epidemic, he noticed that while outbreaks of typhus were unfortunately common in the region at the time, the epidemic affecting Silesia seemed to be unusually severe. In epidemiologic terms, Virchow was interested in differential patterns of disease. Why did people living in the specific communities he examined seem to get sicker and die more quickly than some of their counterparts?

Virchow found the answer by examining the social and economic conditions in which the Silesian people lived, worked, and played. He found significant poverty and material deprivation as well as oppressive social institutions that suppressed education and various other freedoms:

> *There cannot be any doubt that such a typhoid epidemic was only possible under these conditions and that ultimately they were the result of the poverty and underdevelopment in Upper Silesia.*[3]

What is especially interesting is what Virchow proposed as the appropriate intervention for the typhus epidemic in Upper Silesia: "education, with its daughters, liberty and prosperity." In other words, Virchow argued, improving the social and economic conditions in which the populace lived was the primary means of responding to the typhus epidemic. This does not mean that Virchow was unconcerned with taking care of sick people; he was a physician, after all. But, he was clear that the priority could not be the provision of medical services, that "it is no longer a question of treating one typhus patient or another by drugs."[3]

Virchow is remembered today as the father of modern cellular pathology. Yet he is also known as the father of social medicine. (Although there is no consensus definition of *social medicine*, the field revolves around three main points: social and economic conditions profoundly impact health, population health is a social concern, and society has an obligation to promote health through individual and social means).[4] Every medical school in the United States requires its students to pass courses in pathology in order to graduate. Fewer schools require students to receive training in social medicine. Virchow almost certainly would not have

approved of this discrepancy. Understanding the evidence behind Virchow's perspective and equipped with a better comprehension of the evidence base regarding the socio-ecologic determinants of health, physicians and other health care professionals can gain an appreciation of the place of interventions targeted at ameliorating adverse socioeconomic conditions within clinical practice.

Americans tend to see health as a function of access to health care services. Those who have access to health care services are healthy, and those who are unhealthy are so primarily because they lack such access. By most indices, the United States currently ranks near the bottom of the developed world in terms of overall health outcomes. For example, The Commonwealth Fund's 2014 report on the health care systems of 11 industrialized nations put the United States in last place—the same position it occupied in 2010, 2007, 2006, and 2004.[5] The Centers for Disease Control and Prevention's (CDC) 2014 international comparison of infant mortality—a key indicator of population health—ranked the United States the sixth worst in the group of 26 industrialized nations composing the Organisation for Economic Co-operation and Development (OECD),[6] prompting *The Washington Post* to term the ranking a "national embarrassment."[7] A common narrative among both laypeople and experts suggests that if the health status of the population is to be improved, the fact that millions of people lack access to basic health care services must be remedied. But here it is crucial to separate the moral claim from the factual claim. While some might well say that ensuring access to basic health care services is morally good, that ethical claim is not equivalent to an empirical prediction that if such access was provided, population health in the United States would substantially improve. In fact, there is surprisingly little evidence for the latter claim.

To understand why access to health care seems only a relatively minor determinant of population health, it is important to distinguish **population health** from **population medicine**. Kindig and Stoddart define population health as "the health outcomes of a group of individuals, including the distribution of such outcomes within the group."[8] But the term has increasingly been applied in clinical contexts, to describe the clinical (often chronic disease) outcomes of patients within a practice, a health system, a community, or even a group of people with similar insurance coverage. Also, many clinicians and medical managers have begun to use the terms *population health management* or *population medicine.*

Kindig argues that population health is not equivalent to population medicine precisely because the latter focuses its attention on clinical outcomes among a population of patients who have been able to engage with the health care system.[9] But if there is reason to believe that the health outcomes of populations, in general, are not primarily driven by access to health care services, it would make little sense to think of population health in terms of population medicine. These are two different concepts that arguably capture different dimensions of health and well-being.

While terminology related to health outcomes, inequalities, and populations may be used in different ways, the take-home point is simply this: *Health is not equivalent to health care.* As leading social epidemiologist Ichiro Kawachi puts it, the fact that aspirin treats fever does not imply that the cause of fever is lack of aspirin.[10] While health care services are important, even critical, for those patients with medical conditions, the epidemiologic evidence strongly supports Virchow's basic argument: If overall population health is to be improved and health inequalities are to be compressed, a country has to look beyond the provision of medical services. What follows next is a more detailed discussion of that evidence.

III. TYPES OF SOCIAL DETERMINANTS OF HEALTH

A. Evidence for Social Determinants of Health

What is the evidence supporting the claim that access to health care services is only a minor determinant of population health?

Consider the Whitehall Studies, which are generally acknowledged as some of the more important epidemiologic studies of the last 50 years. The Whitehall Studies are a longitudinal investigation of the health of British civil servants. Initiated in the 1950s, follow-up data collection and analysis is still going on in phase III of the project. The data are very high quality for an epidemiologic study, because the investigators were able to control for a number of confounders to evaluate the impact of different variables on the participants' health outcomes. For our purposes, what matters most is that given that the participants were all British citizens, they all enjoyed access to medical services through the United Kingdom's National Health Service. This means that if the study showed significant differences in health among different groups, those differences simply could not be attributable to differences in access to medical services. In fact, the research team led by Sir Michael Marmot—a physician and epidemiologist who remains one of the world's most prominent and vocal researchers and advocates on the social determinants of health—found stark differences in health outcomes in the study.

Differences in mortality rates closely tracked employment grade, which the Whitehall investigators used as a marker for social class. The lower a participant's status in his or her work hierarchy, the worse his or her health, and the higher a participant's status, the better his or her health. However, Whitehall showed something even more significant: the connection between class and health held at *every step* in the work hierarchy; not only was the highest social class far better off than the lowest social class, but the second-highest class had slightly better health than the third-highest class, the third-highest class had better health than the fourth-highest class, and so on, all the way down the class hierarchy.[11] This concept is known as the **social gradient of health,** and it stands for the proposition that health and wealth are typically correlated in a linear, stepwise fashion at all levels of income and class. The metaphor epidemiologists often use to explain this idea further is that of a ladder, with the rungs representing social class.

Several important points can be derived from the Whitehall Studies. First, a rigorous study documented significant health inequalities among a population who all enjoyed basic access to health care services. This buttresses the already-strong evidence that access to such services is likely not a prime determinant of health and its distribution. Second, the study also produces positive evidence linking social class to health outcomes. This suggests that social class itself is a significant determinant of health. An immense amount of evidence since the Whitehall Studies supports this claim.[12–14]

B. Social Class as a Primary Determinant of Population Health

Akin to the findings in the Whitehall Studies, abundant evidence suggests that one's position in the social hierarchy is the single best predictor of population health outcomes. However, substantial methodologic difficulties arise in trying to measure something like social status, or class. For example, what is the relationship between class and income? Is income equivalent to wealth? Which is a better indicator of class? To what extent is housing status a marker of class? Are indicators of class equivalent to criteria of class? Are the terms **socioeconomic status (SES)** or **socioeconomic position (SEP)** proxies for many other variables (e.g., housing, income, wealth, employment status, gender, race/ethnicity)? These methodologic challenges and many others are quite real when it comes to studying and understanding the impact of social determinants on health. Nevertheless, among most social epidemiologists, there is little doubt that social class, however this is operationalized, is one of the most powerful determinants of health.

One question at this point might be "how does social class determine health outcomes?" This is an important question that goes to one of the key issues relevant in discussing the evidence related to social determinants of health: Because the vast majority of studies in epidemiology are cohort-based, inferring causation is difficult. As such, most of the considerable evidence linking social class and health finds correlations rather than causation. So, causal mechanisms are needed to explain the correlation, that is, to explain how lower social class and lower SEP actually cause poorer health (and the inverse for higher social class). This will be discussed in the context of each of the social determinants of health presented in this chapter.

For now, the takeaway point is that the Whitehall Studies, along with a significant amount of additional evidence, support the idea that social class is a major determinant of population health. And yet, as suggested earlier in the chapter, it is undeniable that a number of social factors that go into SEP are also themselves independent determinants of health. That is, at the same time that factors such as housing, income, and employment status shape one's SEP, there is excellent evidence that these factors are also strongly and independently correlated with population health.

C. Some Significant Social Determinants of Health

The myriad social determinants of health that have been studied or suggested are numerous. The following discussion of several significant determinants is illustrative, and time and space preclude a detailed discussion of many other such determinants. An excellent and readable introduction to some of these factors can be found in the Final Report of the World Health Organization's (WHO) WHO's Commission on Social Determinants of Health, or in the award-winning documentary film *Unnatural Causes*.[10,12]

1. Educational Attainment

The evidence linking educational attainment to population health is robust.[12,15,16] Here, however, it is important to be precise about what is meant by the term *education*. There are many different types of education, and the evidence positioning education as a major determinant of health varies depending on the particular definition chosen. Many health professions students and clinicians often think of education in the context of patient counseling or, in public health contexts, as a component of health education and promotion. While a legitimate way to think about education, this is not what the best evidence supports as key to health outcomes over the lifespan. The evidence strongly suggests little impact of health education and promotion practices on population health. Rather, the evidence suggests that generalized education beginning in early childhood (birth to 8 years of age) and continuing into adolescence and young adulthood is the key to maximizing the impact of educational attainment on population health.[16] As Low and colleagues explain:

> [A]ppropriate stimulation and positive early experiences have profound impact not only on the development of the neural systems involved in cognitive, emotional, neuroendocrine and neuroimmune functions, but also on the expression of genetic factors that modify the effects of hormone receptors and influence an individual's response to stress throughout life.[15]

While there is traditionally strong public support for K–12 compulsory schooling and for postsecondary education as well, financial support and educational infrastructure is not equally distributed in the United States. Analysis of the social determinants of health requires a population-based understanding of the distribution of health and illness. Patterns of disease and health outcomes are strongly linked to patterns in the distribution of social and economic conditions. Educational attainment is linked with population health, and educational attainment is highly unequal in the United States. Therefore, inequalities in educational attainment are correlated with inequalities in health.[15,16] There are many reasons for educational inequalities, including but not limited to the reliance on local and municipal resources for funding public schools beyond that required and provided by the federal government. Because towns and communities have widely variable tax bases, poorer communities have fewer resources to support educational programs in and out of schools. These variable resources lead to widespread educational inequalities, which then correlate strongly with health inequalities.

Another key issue that often arises in discussing education and the social determinants of health is the manner in which education impacts population health. That is, as noted earlier, one of the key findings regarding the social gradient of health is that it is graded rather than bimodal. Increasing or decreasing social class is correlated with corresponding improvements or declinations in health at every step in the social hierarchy. However, this is not the case with regard to educational attainment. Rather, evidence suggests that after a certain level of education is reached, the health effects level off. Some have interpreted this finding to mean that educational attainment should not be considered a true root determinant of health, but is rather an intermediary for factors that continue to impact health at all levels such as SEP. The critics are undoubtedly correct that inequalities in education are strongly driven by inequalities in SEP. Although the linkage does go in the other direction as well—educational attainment can drive changes in SEP— it is neither as robust nor as enduring as the SEP-education relationship.

Nevertheless, education should be considered a major determinant of health.[15,16] As a population, educational attainment in the United States is not near the critical mass at which its impact on health begins to diminish substantially. Health care professionals should therefore consider advocating for policy that can overcome educational inequalities just as they might "advocate against smoking or in support of early childhood immunization."[16] Furthermore, the overlap between educational attainment and early childhood development is clearly connected, although formal education obviously occurs well after early childhood. The evidence is strong to show that the kind of education and environments that occur in early childhood are uniquely important in determining population health across the entire lifespan.

2. Early Childhood Development

The evidence linking early childhood development to health across the lifespan is so impressive it has given birth to an entire subfield of epidemiology, typically referred to as *life course epidemiology*.[17] At the core of the field is an emphasis on early childhood as an epidemiologically critical and sensitive period. A **critical period** is defined as "a limited time window in which an exposure can have adverse or protective effects on development and subsequent disease outcome."[17] Outside this window, this developmental mechanism for mediating exposure and disease risk is no longer available. A **sensitive period** is "a time period when an exposure has a stronger effect on development and hence disease risk than it would at other times."[17] Taken together, this means that experiences during early childhood have a disproportionately strong impact on health across the lifespan.

As a field, life course epidemiology began to take shape on the basis of the consistent evidence that social and economic conditions experienced during early childhood robustly predicted health outcomes many decades later (i.e., later in the participants' lives). The connection between such conditions and childhood is so strong that it can be demonstrated intergenerationally. Investigators measure the impact of adverse or beneficial socioeconomic conditions by examining the extent of the relationship between parental SEP during offspring's early childhood and longitudinal health outcomes of those offspring. However, epidemiologists have gone further, finding connections between the social conditions that the *parents* experienced in *their* early childhood and the longitudinal health outcomes of the offspring later in life.[17,18] One group of researchers even found an attenuated but statistically significant relationship between the social conditions that an individual's grandparents experienced during the grandparents' early childhood and the longitudinal health outcomes of the grandchildren later in the grandchildren's lives.[19]

A core tenet of life course epidemiology is that the social and economic conditions in which early childhood unfolds are powerful and intergenerational determinants of population health. The epidemiologic evidence supporting experiences of early childhood as a primary social determinant of health is so strong as to have resulted in consensus among social epidemiologists and pediatricians, as well as beyond the health professions. Nobel laureate economist James Heckman, for example, has been involved for many years in research on the social cost of investment in early childhood development. In an important longitudinal study known as

The Abecedarian Project, Heckman and colleagues documented stunning results: Every $1 invested in intensive early childhood development would return approximately $2.50.[20] Heckman and colleagues concluded that such investment would "prevent costly chronic diseases, increase productivity and potentially reduce health spending."[21] On the basis of this evidence, Heckman created the "Heckman Equation":

$$\text{Invest} + \text{Develop} + \text{Sustain} = \text{Gain}$$

where what is gained is a healthier, "more capable, productive and valuable workforce that pays dividends to America for generations to come."[22]

If intensive investment in early childhood can have such a positive impact on population health, one would predict that adverse conditions in early childhood can have a significant negative impact. And this is what the evidence suggests. A 1998 paradigm study led by the CDC and Kaiser Permanente investigated this question, assigning scores based on the accumulation of adverse childhood events (ACEs).[23] Such ACEs include, but are not limited to, childhood abuse, neglect, and household dysfunction, which are typically referred to as *traumatic stressors*. The study revealed a strong and graded correlation between the number of ACEs and myriad chronic illnesses later in life, including the following[23]:

- Alcoholism and alcohol abuse
- Chronic obstructive pulmonary disease (COPD)
- Depression
- Fetal death
- Ischemic heart disease (IHD)
- Liver disease
- Risk for intimate partner violence
- Multiple sexual partners
- Sexually transmitted diseases (STDs)
- Smoking
- Suicide attempts

A key point, then, is that conditions—whether favorable or adverse—during early childhood have a significant and enduring impact on population health, not simply across one individual's lifespan, but intergenerationally as well. Thus, there is little doubt that early childhood development is a significant social determinant of health, one in which physicians and health care professionals can play an important role.

3. Housing

While it is not widely taught, across a given population, knowing the zip code where an individual resides is more likely to predict his or her health outcomes than knowing his or her genetic code. There are many reasons why zip code is such an excellent predictor of health. Indeed, factors already considered (class, educational attainment, and early childhood experiences) substantially explain why zip code predicts health, insofar as populations in the United States are generally segregated along strata of class, education, and race.

The Robert Wood Johnson Foundation has characterized the impact of neighborhood and zip code on health under the heading "Place Matters."[24] The types of homes in which people reside can have an enormous impact on both individual and population health. Braveman and colleagues offer a three-level analysis emphasizing

1) physical conditions within homes, 2) conditions in the neighborhoods surrounding the homes, and 3) housing affordability.[25]

Taking these in order, one can understand how physical conditions within homes can shape overall health. For example, a home that features high levels of mold can be dangerous to its occupants, especially where one or more of the dwellers experiences some form of respiratory illness. Given the high prevalence of asthma or reactive airway disease and its disproportionate impact among children, the identification of a mold-contaminated home is extremely important. An estimated two-thirds of the time American families spend indoors is spent at home, with children being home an even larger proportion of that time.[25] This reinforces the significance of early childhood as a social determinant of health and also shows how different social determinants converge to create conditions that advance or hinder human health. Another example of a dangerous condition in the home that can disproportionately impact child health and development is the presence of lead paint. According to the US Department of Housing and Urban Development's 2011 Healthy Homes Survey, almost 35 percent of American homes (37.1 million homes total) have lead-based paint located somewhere in the relevant structure, with children younger than 6 years of age being exposed to this hazard in 3.6 million homes.[26] As with early descriptions of contributors to social determinants of health, the hazards of lead exposure are distributed along a wealth gradient, with low-income households experiencing a higher prevalence of lead-based-paint hazards.

It is not simply the conditions within homes that render housing an important determinant of population health. The notion that "place matters" considers "place" expansively, to encompass the ways in which our experiences in the vicinity of our homes (i.e., our neighborhoods) impact health. Neighborhood conditions obviously relate to housing, since homes clearly connected to the neighborhoods in which they are located. Braveman and colleagues point out the following:

> [A] neighborhood's physical characteristics may promote health by providing safe places for children to play and for adults to exercise that are free from crime, violence and pollution. . . Social and economic conditions in neighborhoods may improve health by affording access to employment opportunities and public resources including efficient transportation, an effective police force and good schools.[25]

To expand on the first point noted here, there is evidence that lighting is strongly correlated with a willingness to exercise outdoors. Because lighting is strongly correlated with perceived safety, it is understandable why poorly lit parks and recreation areas are much less likely to be used for exercise, especially in northern climates, where the days are shorter for much of the year. Additionally, neighborhoods experiencing higher crime rates and violence directly impact decisions about exercise safety as well as general mental and physical health and well-being.

Housing affordability also has significant health impact: "the shortage of affordable housing limits families' and individuals' choices about where they live, often relegating lower-income families to substandard housing in unsafe, overcrowded neighborhoods with higher rates of poverty and fewer resources for health promotion."[25] The fact that housing affordability is a determinant of health shows again how multiple social determinants of health converge to shape overall population health. The ability to afford a given level of housing is obviously connected to wealth, income, and class, which means that SEP and housing are strongly correlated. Importantly, however, SEP and housing are independent determinants of health; that is, the evidence suggests they exert significant health impact, even when controlling for one or the other. Yet, at the same time, neither exists in a social vacuum; most social determinants converge and interact in a complex matrix to impact population health.

4. Racism and Discrimination

As suggested, understanding the impact of socioeconomic conditions on population health requires knowledge of differential patterns of disease. Health inequalities cannot be understood without analysis of the social determinants of health. Although such inequalities can be tracked over a variety of demographic lines (i.e., wealth, income, gender), one of the most disturbing such lines is that of race. Across a variety of indicators, health outcomes in the United States are distributed along racial lines. Racial health inequalities have been found nearly everywhere investigators have looked, in both important measures of morbidity and mortality, and in access to health care services as well. For example, in 2013 the CDC released its Health Disparities and Inequalities Report.[27] Principal findings include the following:

- Rates of premature death (<75 years) from stroke and coronary heart disease were higher for blacks than for whites.
- Between 2006 and 2010, the preterm birth rate for black infants declined over 8 percent to 17.1 percent, which was still 60 percent higher than the rate for white infants.
- In both 2005 and 2008, the infant mortality rate for black women was almost double that for white women.
- In 2009, homicide rates for blacks were 665 percent higher than for whites.
- Members of racial/ethnic minority groups experienced higher rates of HIV diagnosis, while blacks were less likely to be prescribed antiretroviral therapy than whites.
- Members of racial/ethnic minority groups were more likely to report fair or poor self-rated health, more physically unhealthy days, and more mentally unhealthy days than white counterparts.
- Mexican-Americans with hypertension experienced poorer blood pressure control than members of all other racial/ethnic groups.
- The likelihood of working in a high-risk occupation was greatest for those who are Hispanic.
- The highest percentage of adults living below the federal poverty level were black or Hispanic.

Some of the most troubling indices are those related to the proper diagnosis and treatment of pain, which is a common illness experience in the United States and can result in significant suffering and burden. A number of studies have examined how pain is assessed and treated in a variety of clinical settings, with a consistent finding that patients of color, both children and adults, wait much longer for a diagnosis and receive appropriate treatment far less frequently than comparable white patients.[28]

Researchers have suggested that genetic predispositions can explain some of the noted racial health inequalities, but the evidence generally does not support such a claim. Similar racial health inequalities exist all over the world among divergent genetic ancestry groups.[13,29] Instead, most social epidemiologists argue that the primary explanation is "structural racism—a self-perpetuating form of bias built into structures and institutions, even when conscious intent to discriminate is no longer present."[30] Braveman elaborates as follows:

For example, a legacy of racial residential segregation continues to track many blacks and Latinos into neighborhoods not only with directly unhealthy influences on nutrition and physical activity, but also with poor employment opportunities and poorly performing schools. Because educational attainment shapes employment opportunities, racial segregation propagates the inter-generational transmission of poverty and the ill health that accompanies it.[30]

Gee and Ford offer the useful metaphor of the iceberg in describing the differences between structural and individual or person-centered racism.[31] Obvious acts of racism, such as cross-burnings, are the visible tip, while inequitable and discriminatory policies and procedures form the hidden base of the iceberg below the waterline. Interventions directed at the former may do little to address the latter. Widespread social segregation in the United States may be one of the most pernicious and health-adverse dimensions of structural racism. Such segregation "may influence health by concentrating poverty, environmental pollutants, infectious agents, and other adverse conditions."[30,31] The practice of "redlining" is a primary factor responsible for racial residential segregation, and refers to the practice of refusing a loan or the underwriting of an insurance policy to someone due to a belief that the individual lives in an area of high financial risk. Even the Federal Housing Administration (FHA) itself redlined between 1930 and 1950, typically assigning black homeowners to the highest-risk category.

Mortgage funds were channeled away from fourth category African-American neighborhoods and were typically redirected from communities that were located near a black settlement or an area expected to contain black residences in the future. As a result of these policies, the vast majority of FHA mortgage loans went to borrowers in white middle-class neighborhoods and very few were awarded to black neighborhoods in central cities.[32]

Private lenders tracked FHA practices, rendering redlining widespread in American society for the middle decades of the twentieth century. Such a standard fueled the racial residential segregation that exists to the present with significant inequitable consequences for population health.

Unconscious or implicit bias plays an important role in structural racism. Unconscious bias refers to "effortless, automatic, evaluative processes" by which humans respond to a particular stimulus.[33] A large body of evidence demonstrates that people in the United States harbor significant negative implicit biases against a variety of marginalized groups (including blacks and Latinos). "Cultural racism can trigger unconscious bias that can lead to unequal access to health enhancing economic opportunities and resources."[33] Physicians and other health care professionals are not immune to implicit bias, as numerous studies show the existence of such biases and their impact on metrics of quality care, such as perceived quality of communication and overall patient evaluations of the quality of the medical encounter.[33]

Moreover, there is increasing evidence suggesting that the experience of racism itself may be a determinant of health.[33-35] That is, even after controlling for all conceivable confounders, members of social groups subjected to persistent racism and discrimination get sicker and die more quickly than their counterparts.[10,33-35] Given that these inequalities persist even after controlling for other major determinants of health, the inference is that, largely because of racism, race itself is predictive of poorer health. A causal model is still needed to explain how experiencing racism and discrimination might result in poorer health, by explaining the epidemiologic evidence linking this social condition to health outcomes.

D. Causation Versus Correlation

As noted earlier, the vast majority of the evidence regarding social determinants of health rests on correlations. Correlation is obviously not causation, and scientists and researchers have not ignored this problem. A variety of causal models have been proposed and evaluated to assess the ways in which social conditions impact health outcomes. Arguably, the most-promising and most-studied model is known as the *allostatic load hypothesis.*[36]

The allostatic load hypothesis begins with the neuroendocrine system and the fight-or-flight response. When an individual is exposed to a noxious stimulus, the fight-or-flight response kicks in; our bodies are flooded with the stress hormone cortisol, which enables us to take the action needed to neutralize or avoid the stimulus. At that point, the physiologic response shuts off, and the body gradually returns to its prior relative homeostasis (at least, more so than during the active fight-or-flight response).[36]

The relevant question is this: what happens if the fight-or-flight response does not shut off? What happens if it stays switched on, for days, weeks, or months at a time? Physician and epidemiologist Camara Phyllis Jones has answered the question by likening it to an automobile running at high RPMs continuously for days, weeks, and months.[10] Eventually, the automobile breaks down. The human body is not all that different in this way. Human stress responses are typically measured via the accumulation of cortisol, and persistently high cortisol levels have been strongly linked with multiple morbidities and mortalities,[36] including many of the most prevalent diseases in the United States today.[10,37-39] Moreover, the persistent accumulation of cortisol may be especially damaging during the sensitive and critical period of early childhood. Indeed, a number of studies from the Center on the Developing Child at Harvard University have documented the ways in which the accumulation of stress hormones is neurotoxic and can actually disrupt the architecture of the developing brain with lifelong (and perhaps even intergenerational) consequences.[40]

Although the allostatic load hypothesis is popular among scientists and enjoys significant evidentiary support, there are other causal mechanisms at play that can help explain the strong correlations between social conditions and health outcomes. Leading social epidemiologists Nancy Krieger and George Davey Smith argue that the idea of embodiment is crucial to understanding the ways in which social conditions cause health. They cite several examples, such as low birth weight, which "reflects socially patterned exposures (during and prior to the pregnancy) to such factors as maternal malnutrition, toxic substances. . . smoking, infections, domestic violence, racial discrimination, economic adversity in neighborhoods, and inadequate medical and dental care."[41] In turn, they point out that low birth weight is correlated with elevated mortality risk in middle age, as well as increased risk for cardiovascular disease and several forms of cancer.

With a better understanding of some of the evidence and the concepts behind the social determinants of health, a closer analysis of the roles health care professionals can play in acting on the social determinants of health is appropriate. The basic idea is that, to be maximally effective at helping individuals to achieve health and communities to achieve health equity, the health care system must be redesigned with patients' social needs in mind. The following section will address these opportunities and provide recommendations for physicians, practice teams, health systems, and communities to more broadly impact health through systematic attention to the social determinants of health.

IV. MOVING HEALTH UPSTREAM: THE ROLE OF THE CLINICAL PRACTICE, HEALTH SYSTEM, AND COMMUNITY IN IMPACTING SOCIAL DETERMINANTS OF HEALTH

A. The Need to Address Health Inequalities Within the Health Care System

As discussed earlier, health inequalities are caused by unequal distribution of and exposure to negative social determinants of health.[42] Many health care professionals equate addressing social determinants of health with acting on the upstream causes of disease that lie outside the health care system.[43] But upstream efforts, while important, largely ignore the potential for medical professionals, health systems, and communities to address social determinants within the health care delivery system.[44] However, while health care professionals recognize that unmet social needs lead to poorer health outcomes, most feel ill-prepared or unable to address them.[45] This fear prohibits some health care professionals from even asking questions of their patients about social needs. Training and gaining buy-in from all front-line staff members is critical, as they might be the ones first to identify social needs and can assist with referring patients and families to community resources. It is important to note that the impact of social determinants is not limited to vulnerable groups, but rather the upstream social determinants shape differential exposure to health risk for all.[46]

B. Opportunities for Clinical Practice and Health Systems

Health care professionals and health systems can adopt equitable practice designs that routinely assess each patient's social and economic circumstances, link patients with supportive community programs and services, include social and economic conditions in treatment planning, and advocate on behalf of individual patients and community-level improvements in the social and economic circumstances impacting health.

Though previously not a priority in a volume-driven health care system, clinical practices and health care systems are becoming more incentivized to address social determinants of health and improve health equity. The Affordable Care Act's new reimbursement policies reward population health management (ensuring equal outcomes for all patients enrolled in the system), care coordination (facilitating communication and care between office or hospital visits), and value-based purchasing (addressing the cost of interventions relative to their benefits)—all domains that require attention to social determinants of health to be successful.[47]

The following are examples of how health care organizations and health care professionals are addressing the social determinants of health.

1. Tools to Assess Social and Economic Circumstances

Detailed symptom, medical, and family histories form the foundation of accurate diagnosis and treatment plans. Similarly, a careful patient-level social needs assessment is critical to inform treatment planning, as well as referral to appropriate community resources to address the patient's needs. Awareness of social data can influence decisions about care. For example, is a patient able to afford the medication prescribed to treat his or her diabetes? Does having a better understanding of a patient's SEP help physicians and health care professionals better predict a patient's risk for heart disease, given that poverty has been linked as an independent risk factor for the disease?[48] Many decisions about preventive care, as well as acute and chronic disease care, can be influenced in a manner that improves patient engagement and outcomes.

Although there is not currently a single validated tool that comprehensively screens for social needs, several approaches have been developed for clinical settings. Simply asking the question "Do you have difficulty making ends meet at the end of the month?" has been found to be a sensitive and specific predictor for detecting individuals living below the poverty line.[49] Tools assessing social needs should be integrated into the electronic health record (EHR) so that it becomes a routine part of the clinic workflow and makes this information available for discussion as the care team prepares for their daily appointments. Questions about basic needs, such as food, shelter, and safety, can be asked by clinical staff, or paper-based or electronic questionnaires can be directly answered by patients and imported into the EHR. The Institute of Medicine's Committee on Recommended Social and Behavioral Domains and Measures for Electronic Health Records suggests a set of social determinants of health data domains recommended for inclusion in all EHRs (Table 11.1).[50] These include socio-demographic, psychological, and behavioral factors that address individual-level social determinants of health, such as race and ethnicity; education; employment; financial resources; country of origin; sexual orientation; psychological assets and stressors; health literacy; mental health issues; physical activity; nutritional patterns; tobacco, alcohol, and drug use and exposure; exposure to violence; and social connections and isolation. This information would be collected directly from each patient then entered into the EHR where it can be referenced in an ongoing fashion to help in prevention

Table 11.1 Social and Behavioral Domains for Inclusion in Electronic Health Records

Sociodemographic Domains

- Sexual orientation
- Race and ethnicity
- Country of origin/US born or non-US born
- Education
- Employment
- Financial resource strain: Food and housing insecurity

Psychological Domains

- Health literacy
- Stress
- Negative mood and affect: Depression and anxiety
- Psychological assets: Conscientiousness, patient engagement/activation,[1] optimism, and self-efficacy

Behavioral Domains

- Dietary patterns
- Physical activity
- Tobacco use and exposure
- Alcohol use

Individual-Level Social Relationships and Living Conditions Domains

- Social connections and social isolation
- Exposure to violence

From Institute of Medicine. Capturing Social and Behavioral Domains and Measures in Electronic Health Records: Phase 2. Washington, DC: National Academies Press; 2014. http://www.nap.edu/read/18951/chapter/ 6 - chapter03_ch03-en2. Accessed November 7, 2016.

and health management discussions and shared decision making.

Clinical practices should remember that social needs are not limited to underserved patients. It is important to ask these questions with all patients, in all practice settings, at every visit, not just with patients from disadvantaged areas.[51] Additionally, ongoing tracking of social data supports communication between clinical practice teams and other service providers in the health care system or community, thus expanding the capacity to better address population health needs. Finally, this information can inform health equity research, helping us to better understand the impact of social determinants on health.

The following sections include examples of screening tools that have been utilized for collection of social data on patients:

POVERTY INTERVENTION TOOL

Developed by the Ontario College of Family Physicians' Poverty Committee, this intervention tool begins with the single screening question *"Do you have difficulty making ends meet at the end of the month?"* and follows with interventions that the practice team may need to take into consideration in managing that patient (Fig. 11.1).

IHELLP

Mnemonics may serve as helpful reminders to assist practices in soliciting information about common social conditions that impact a patient's or family's ability to address their health care needs. One tool that has been studied with families who have young children is IHELLP,

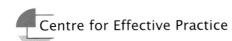 Centre for Effective Practice

Poverty: A Clinical Tool for Primary Care Providers

Poverty is not always apparent: In Ontario 20% of families live in poverty. [1]

① Screen Everyone

"Do you ever have difficulty making ends meet at the end of the month?"

(Sensitivity 98%, specificity 40% for living below the poverty line)[2]

② Poverty is a Risk Factor

Consider:

New immigrants, Women, Aboriginals, and LGBTQ are among the highest risk groups.

Example 1:

If an otherwise healthy 35 year old comes to your office, without risk factors for diabetes other than living in poverty, you consider ordering a screening test for diabetes.

Example 2:

If an otherwise low risk patient who lives in poverty presents with chest pain, this elevates the pre-test probability of a cardiac source and helps determine how aggressive you are in ordering investigations.

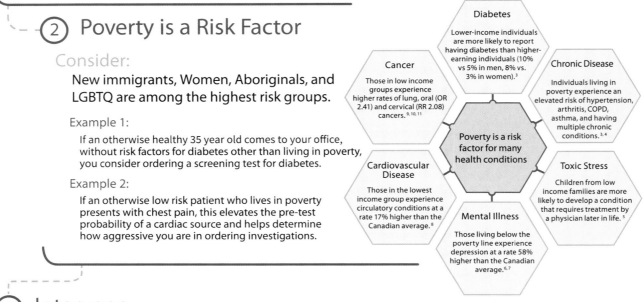

Diabetes
Lower-income individuals are more likely to report having diabetes than higher-earning individuals (10% vs 5% in men, 8% vs. 3% in women).[3]

Cancer
Those in low income groups experience higher rates of lung, oral (OR 2.41) and cervical (RR 2.08) cancers. [9, 10, 11]

Chronic Disease
Individuals living in poverty experience an elevated risk of hypertension, arthritis, COPD, asthma, and having multiple chronic conditions. [3, 4]

Poverty is a risk factor for many health conditions

Cardiovascular Disease
Those in the lowest income group experience circulatory conditions at a rate 17% higher than the Canadian average. [8]

Toxic Stress
Children from low income families are more likely to develop a condition that requires treatment by a physician later in life. [5]

Mental Illness
Those living below the poverty line experience depression at a rate 58% higher than the Canadian average. [6, 7]

③ Intervene

Ask Everyone: "Have you filled out and sent in your tax forms?"

- Ask questions to find out more about your patient, their employment, living situation, social supports and the benefits they receive. Tax returns are required to access many income security benefits: e.g. GST / HST credits, Child Benefits, working income tax benefits, and property tax credits. Connect your patients to Free Community Tax Clinics.
- Even people without official residency status can file returns.
- Drug Coverage: up to date tax filing required to access Trillium plan for those without Ontario Drug Benefits. Visit drugcoverage.ca for more options.

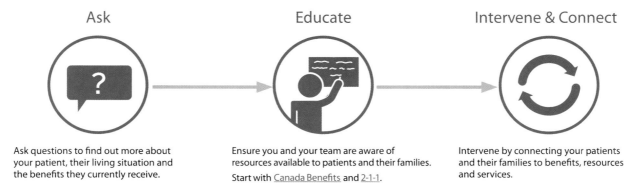

Ask

Ask questions to find out more about your patient, their living situation and the benefits they currently receive.

Educate

Ensure you and your team are aware of resources available to patients and their families.
Start with Canada Benefits and 2-1-1.

Intervene & Connect

Intervene by connecting your patients and their families to benefits, resources and services.

Fig. 11.1 **Poverty Intervention Tool.**

Table 11.2 Examples of Potential Social History Questions (Using the "IHELLP" Mnemonic) to Address Basic Needs

Domain/Area	Examples of Questions
Income	
General	Do you ever have trouble making ends meet?
Food income	Do you ever have a time when you don't have enough food?
	Do you have WIC?*
	Do you have food stamps?
Housing	
Housing	Is your housing ever a problem for you?
Utilities	Do you ever have trouble paying your electric/heat/telephone bill?
Education	
Appropriate education placement	How is your child doing in school?
	Is he/she getting the help to learn what he/she needs?
Early childhood program	Is your child in Head Start, preschool, or other early childhood enrichment?
Legal Status	
Immigration	Do you have questions about your immigration status? Do you need help accessing benefits or services for your family?
Literacy	
Child literacy	Do you read to your child every night?
Parent literacy	How happy are you with how you read?
Personal Safety	
Domestic violence	Have you ever taken out a restraining order?
	Do you feel safe in your relationship?
General safety	Do you feel safe in your home?
	Is your neighborhood safe?

*WIC includes Supplemental Nutrition Assistance Program (SNAP) for Women, Infants, and Children.

Reproduced with permission from Kenyon C, Sandel M, Silverstein M, Shakir A, Zuckerman B. Revisiting the social history for child health. *Pediatrics*. 2007; 120(3): e734–e738. http://pediatrics.aappublications.org/content/120/3/e734. Accessed November 7, 2016.

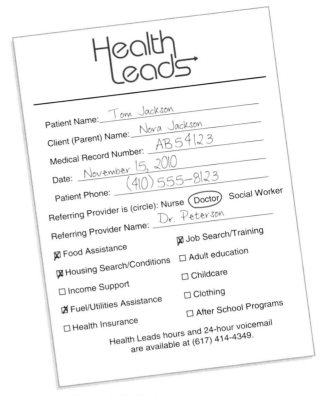

Fig. 11.2 **Health Leads sample form.**

which stands for Income, Housing, Education, Legal status/immigration, Literacy, and Personal safety.[52] Sample questions in each of these categories are shown in Table 11.2 and could be incorporated into practice workflows and EHR templates.

HEADSS

HEADSS is a mnemonic that comprises a psychosocial review of symptoms that has been used in adolescent health visits and assesses Home and environment: Education and employment; Activities; Drugs; Sexuality; and Suicide/depression.[53] This instrument, which has a series of potential questions to ask in each category, is additionally sorted by essential; use as time permits; and optional for use when the situation requires. An expanded version of this instrument includes questions regarding eating behaviors and personal safety.[54]

HELPSTEPS

Having patients or family members complete a screening tool before the visit can help streamline workflow and provide value-added time during waiting periods. Developed at Boston Children's Hospital, HelpSteps can be administered in the office via internet-based technology (e.g., a kiosk in the waiting room, an iPad in the examination room). Perhaps even more importantly, information disclosure regarding psychosocial and socioeconomic questions is enhanced using computer technology, identifying more social needs than face-to-face interviewing, especially for highly sensitive issues such as household violence and substance abuse.[55]

HEALTH LEADS

Some online instruments have been developed to lead patients to community and health system resources related to the specific needs that they express. One notable example of this is **Health Leads** (Fig. 11.2). Developed at Boston Medical Center with support from the Robert Wood Johnson Foundation, this program expands practice capacity by using trained college students as referral specialists to address basic resource needs at the root causes of poor health. Sample screening questions include: "Are you running out of food at the end of the month? Do you have heat in your home this winter?" The program then enables health care providers to prescribe basic resources like food and heat just as they do medication and refer patients to needed community resources just as they do any other specialty.

2. Beyond Screening: Additional Practice and Health System Support Recommendations

Just as a clinician might refer a patient to a specialist or to receive additional services such as physical therapy, he or she should be able to similarly refer patients to specialists in economic, environmental, and psychosocial needs.[56,57] Care managers or other trained staff can access the resources of primary care, public health, social services, and other sectors to meet a range of patient needs. Many clinical practices and health care systems have developed resource guides with referral information based on specific needs. Additionally, having pre-populated letter templates or referral pathways within the EHR improves the ease of referral and results in more appropriate transfer of information to a community specialist. In one medical-legal partnership example, EHR integration of a letter to help low-income patients with chronic conditions retain heat and electricity services resulted in a 300 percent increase in the number of completed utility protection letters.[58]

Readily available access to referral resource information increases both screening and referrals, as clinicians and staff are more likely to ask social questions when there are clear opportunities to intervene to assist patients and families in getting the resources they need.[59] Web-based programs with an updated database of service agencies loaded on laptops or tablets in the waiting room can maximize referral without disrupting the actual visit. For example, a database of nutrition resources might include not only information on healthy eating, but also links to local food pantries and farmers' markets, and referral to a nutritionist.

In the Health Leads program discussed earlier, college students are trained as advocates to work side by side with patients to connect them with the basic resources they need to be healthy (e.g., applying for nutrition-assistance program benefits, locating shelters, aiding in housing searches, or locating child care services). Use of a resource database and case management system enables these advocates to search for community resources and benefits that best match the needs of the patients they serve. With this approach, the Health Leads program has seen a 17 percent increase in patients served, a 60 percent reduction in the time required for patient intake (from 20 minutes to 8 minutes), and a 55 percent stronger agreement from partner physicians that they have adequate support to address their patients' resource needs.[60]

For practices caring for children and adolescents, the Children's Advocacy Project provides information on community resources for children, adolescents, and parents through their CAP4Kids site.[61] Developed at Drexel University, this site provides reliable, up-to-date information on community resources such as childcare, after-school programs, employment, job training, legal services, literacy, shelters, and mental health programs, as well as sample advocacy letters for special education and other services and information about local laws. Like Health Leads, CAP4Kids is available nationally with content specific to many urban centers.

3. Using Practice Data to Support Larger-Scale Change

Including data on social determinants of health as part of the overall health of a practice population will help address systemic issues that might otherwise go undetected. For example, identifying patients with uncontrolled asthma in a concentrated geography may signal substandard housing and a need for legal services to help address this underlying issue. These data can be derived from practice-entered or health care system–entered screening tools or can come from measures of social determinants of health derived from community-level geocoded data from publicly available sources (e.g., the US Census Bureau). Referred to as Community Vital Signs, this latter version of EHR-housed data avoids reliance on clinical practice or health system personnel to do all of the social data screening, thus improving efficiency and enhancing the objectivity of the data that are available for use.[62] Data from the importing of community vital signs can inform clinical recommendations for individual patients, facilitate referrals to community services, and expand understanding of factors impacting treatment adherence and health outcomes by providing an aggregated overview of the social and environmental factors impacting patient health. For example, using this approach, the EHR could identify all patients on a provider's panel who live in an area with a high proportion of fast food restaurants and then send them information about where they can purchase fresh produce along with recipes for quick, healthy meals. This information could also help care teams target disease prevention initiatives and other health improvement efforts for practices, health care systems, and public health agencies. Active data tracking of key process measures can also help a practice or health system ensure that their interventions are effectively reaching those they are intended to reach.

The health care system needs to more effectively utilize measures to understand the impact of income, education, and related issues on health. Data-driven economic arguments can help insurance companies recognize the important role that nonmedical services play in sustaining health and ensure financial support for organizations that provide vital social services.

4. Creating Equitable Practice Design

Emerging models of care, such as patient-centered medical homes (PCMHs), use multidisciplinary team members to expand the reach of the physician, enhance the comprehensiveness of care, and reduce health inequities. In addition to the additive impact that a team of health care professionals can have over that of a single physician, PCMH models also facilitate greater access to care by providing flexible office hours outside of the traditional 9 AM to 5 PM hours, using advanced-access scheduling protocols, and being located in areas where patients already are, such as in or near schools or churches. Locating within a community and being more available to those who reside there increases the likelihood that a clinical practice or other health care facility will provide culturally appropriate care that reflects understanding of the social determinants that impact health.

Waiting rooms and other patient spaces within a practice or health care facility can be intentionally designed in a way that enhances collaboration between the staff and the patients they serve. Innovative approaches provide enhanced access to community resource information, including opportunities for co-location of health and social services (e.g., behavioral health, Medicaid, and the Special Supplemental Nutrition Program for Women, Infants, and Children [WIC]), while maintaining patient privacy. Practices may also consider including services not often considered part of traditional medical care, such as emergency food boxes and on-site medical-legal partnerships.

Providing culturally informed and humble care is critical. To make the health care setting more inclusive, health systems are devoting greater attention to cultural sensitivity and to expanding the diversity of the health care workforce (see later). It is important to explicitly consider how the practice environment presents itself to all populations (e.g., refugees; low-income patients; lesbian, gay, bisexual and transgender [LGBT] individuals; individuals with disabilities) and to identify ways to be more welcoming through language, office-based literature, and even less-formal dress that can sometimes be perceived as a barrier to shared understanding.

Providing in-home care for those who cannot travel to a clinic allows health care professionals to observe patients in their own living conditions and better appreciate the social and community contexts in which they live. This principle also applies to homeless individuals, who are among those who face the biggest barriers to health care access. For example, "street medicine" provides medical care directly to those living and sleeping on the streets.[63]

C. Barriers and Facilitators to Clinical Practice Efforts to Improve Social Determinants of Health

Redesigning practice and health system approaches to better address social determinants of health requires careful thought and planning, as well as an investment in time and energy, to accomplish. Limited time is the most commonly cited barrier to screening for social considerations during an office visit and making referrals to community services. The current volume-based fee-for-service payment mechanisms provide a disincentive to take additional time with patients to improve their social determinants of health. This is anticipated to improve with a move to value-based reimbursement, but those models have not yet fully matured to answer this question.

Lack of knowledge regarding accessible and effective programs and services is another major barrier to enhancing health equity through mitigating social determinants. Even when information is available, most practices lack integration with community-based services to facilitate ease of referral. Insufficient staffing to allow time to link patients with needed resources or referrals during the regular flow of patients within a busy clinical practice setting make it less likely that this aspect of care can be provided while the patient or family is still within the visit. Finally, in more rural or remote communities, the necessary services to which to refer patients are likely not available.

Provider attitudes may interfere with the ability to help patients with social conditions that negatively impact health. These attitudes, ranging from fear of stigmatizing people living in poverty to unconscious bias, can inhibit discussions of patients' living conditions and income. Often health care professionals feel powerless to intervene in a way that improves a patient's condition, and health systems struggle to believe that their investment to improve community health will result in meaningful change over time.

To address these barriers, common facilitators can be employed to improve social determinants that impact health. These include training for health care professionals about how to screen for and address relevant social conditions and adoption of more interprofessional, team-based practice environments in which all providers are working at the top of their license in order to promote a comprehensive practice ecosystem to address these issues. Establishing relationships with community programs and service agencies for ease of facilitating referrals, and engaging the larger community to help address macro-level issues that impede health are important to improving health equity. Finally, supportive compensation models, integration of medical services and data within and across sites, and expanded potential for piloting collaborations under the Affordable Care Act are all hopeful signs of the recognition of the need to address social determinants of health in a more comprehensive fashion.

D. Community and Policy Support for Health Advocacy and Improving Health Equity

Health care systems could see greater improvements in patient outcomes if they become involved in addressing the social determinants of health in the communities in which their patients reside. By failing to address the social determinants of health at the most fundamental level, the opportunity to effect widespread, sustainable change in population health is lost.[12]

Social determinants of health can be addressed by developing a community-based health coalition of partners that defines key components of a health-promoting system.[64] Coalition members can include community-based organizations, government agencies, and private sector partners who collaborate to advance social accountability and participate in collective action to create systems that protect health.[65] Coalition partners share a vision for healthy families and offer complementary health-related missions. Bidirectional understanding of perspectives and accomplishment of a shared vision among stakeholders form the foundation of a high-functioning coalition. Communication is key, especially with the public sector, and requires using language that will allow for effective communication about the implications of social determinants of health and how these might be addressed. For example, the term *social determinants of health* itself does not register with everyone. Pointing out health disparities does not generally resonate with all audiences. Talking about equal opportunity to improve health may be more effective.[66]

A variety of health care professional and other community partners may be considered in developing coalitions to address social determinants of health:

- *Practice- or health system–based health care professionals* can contribute their expertise and influence as health advocates within communities to determine and understand strengths and needs, speak on behalf of others when needed, and support the mobilization of resources to effect change. Such activities could range from providing volunteer clinical services (e.g., sports physicals at Boys and Girls Clubs) to serving on the advisory boards of advocacy or social service organizations.
- *Social workers* and *case managers* can be front-line experts in assessing the family needs and finding appropriate community resources.
- *Community health workers* (CHWs) are becoming more prominent partners in addressing social determinants of health. These are members of the communities they serve who possess intimate knowledge of community needs and resources and are considered leaders among

their peers. They can be trained on how to initiate discussions about underlying social conditions and environment-related factors that impact health, increase access to services, identify solutions to improve neighborhood conditions, and create community opportunities. An example of this is Acción Para La Salud (Action for Health), an intervention in three Arizona border communities that utilizes an 18-month training course consisting of four workshops with the Acción CHWs and their supervisors.[67]

■ Members of the *public health* sector are natural partners, as they have large datasets that can place disease in a social context. They often engage in an ongoing basis with partners outside of the health system and can assist in relationship building with these entities for addressing underlying social determinants of health.

■ *Medical-legal partnerships* are promising clinical-community collaborations that address problems with housing, public benefits, and education.[68,69] There are situations in which lawyers can help improve health by holding schools, agencies, and landlords accountable for addressing patient and family needs. The National Center for Medical-Legal Partnership has a mission to improve the health and well-being of people and communities by leading health, public health, and legal sectors in an integrated, upstream approach to combating health-harming social conditions.[70] They provide a toolkit to guide practices and health care systems and legal institutions through the process of coordinating care and developing a medical-legal partnership.

■ *Street outreach workers* are also potential members of a community-based health care team. They have been used to provide services to disengage youth from gangs and street activity, and to connect them with resources for housing, job training, health care, and education.[71]

Coalition building requires a phased approach, beginning with joining or creating an organization to advocate both within and on behalf of communities. Examples might include enhancing support for building new public facilities for physical activity or partnering with low-resource schools to keep the gym open for classes. Starting with a small group of health care and social service organization partners to jointly define a problem and articulate a shared vision helps begin to engage the larger community.[72] After establishing these goals, the coalition can develop an action plan and secure resources. Finally, identifying how to sustain and grow the coalition requires ongoing reassessment by all partners. The more sectors that are involved in a partnership, the greater the challenges around development of shared goals, aligned leadership, communication, and data sharing. It is better to start with a small group of partners and expand as capacity is developed. Ensuring action as well as follow-through can be enhanced by having the medical provider introduce the patient to behavioral health or other supporting resource personnel in real time, sharing monthly data, and developing connections from the EHR directly to community partners.

Adaptation and utilization of available tools can save time and limited resources when working with community partners:

■ The WHO developed a Health Impact Assessment, which can be used to provide a better understanding of the potential impacts of a proposed policy, regulation, or project while it is being developed.[73]

■ The Prevention Institute developed the Toolkit for Health and Resilience In Vulnerable Environments (THRIVE) as a method to help community members shift from focusing on a discrete health problem to focusing on the factors that underlie the problem. THRIVE provides a structured flow and process that is easily accessed by all partners involved and is organized so that community members with little experience can understand the role that physical, social, and economic environments play in shaping the health and safety of their community and to identify potential solutions.[74] The tool is divided into three domains, subdivided into factors associated with health:

1. Equitable opportunity
   ■ Racial justice
   ■ Jobs and local ownership
   ■ Education
2. People
   ■ Social networks and trust
   ■ Participation and willingness to act for the common good
   ■ Norms/customs
3. Place
   ■ What is sold and how it is promoted
   ■ Look, feel, and safety
   ■ Parks and open space
   ■ Getting around
   ■ Housing
   ■ Air, water, and soil
   ■ Arts, culture, and entertainment

Community stakeholders are asked to rate the importance of each factor in an assessment and then to respond to a number of probing questions. The final stage of THRIVE is to engage stakeholders in developing action plans that incorporate policies and social conditions contributing to health inequities. In one example of the use of THRIVE, community members from a frontier county in New Mexico rated safety, jobs, housing, and education among the top health issues. Community leaders integrated these health priorities in a countywide strategic planning process.[75]

E. Health Literacy

Health literacy is the ability to read, comprehend, and analyze information, instructions, symbols, charts, and diagrams to make appropriate health decisions.[76] Limited health literacy affects people of all ages, races, incomes, and education levels, but its impact disproportionately affects lower socioeconomic, immigrant, and minority groups.[77–80] Patients with low health literacy may experience difficulty understanding prescription labels and navigating the complex health forms and systems, resulting in poorer health outcomes and higher costs. Addressing health literacy for all patients is a necessity that includes the need to provide verbal and written information that is appropriate for all patients.

F. Health Professions Education

Health professions education programs foster acquisition of the foundational knowledge, skills, and attitudes that define the practice norms for future health providers and systems. Although most traditional curricula do not address screening, identification, or provision of resources for social and financial risks, several schools have recently developed new curricula that address the social determinants of health and community partnerships. For example, the Human Rights and Social Justice Scholars Program at the Icahn School of Medicine at Mount Sinai uses longitudinal policy and advocacy service projects in collaboration with community partners to train preclinical medical students in social medicine.[81] The University of California, Los Angeles, School of Dentistry teaches a holistic approach to dental care that considers social and environmental determinants.[82] Such academic-community partnerships, with meaningful input from health consumers, create positive and lasting impact on learner knowledge, skills, and attitudes.[83] As discussed earlier, busy health care professionals are influential allies when speaking alongside and for communities to campaign for better social conditions. Some educators feel that skill-based curriculum in advocacy should be mandatory for all medical trainees.[84]

Training in social determinants must continue beyond professional school. Resident physicians report discomfort in identifying families that face social, economic, or environmental difficulties and feel inadequately prepared to counsel and refer them to community resources.[85–87] Curricula focused on social determinants increases resident self-reported competence in screening for housing, benefits, and educational concerns.[88] Service-learning experiences that include mindful attention to preparation, service, and reflection can illuminate the social determinants of health.[89] Such training and reflection may be especially impactful with these learners, who are also competent providers in direct health care, to further appreciate the impact of community allies on health. Fair and Mallery's article[89] summarizes additional exemplars on how academic medical centers and teaching hospitals are addressing the social determinants of health (Fig. 11.3).

The attitudes of physicians and other health care professionals may be the most important driver toward actualizing actions related to the social determinants of health. While knowledge and skills are clearly required, an open attitude is critical, especially as current health professions students will be working with an increasingly diverse patient population. Self-awareness, self-reflection, and remaining humble and sensitive to differences are key characteristics of culturally competent providers.[90] All health professions trainees need cultural competency training. The recently published American Association of Colleges of Nursing Cultural Competencies for Graduate Nursing Education sets national standards for graduate-level nurses to promote health equity through education, clinical practice, research, scholarship, and policy.[91] The other health professions have similar expectations, and some are defined by the community of interest. For example, the American College of Physicians developed a new set of recommendations to achieve health equity for LGBT individuals including enhanced physician understanding of how to provide culturally and clinically competent care for LGBT individuals and addressing environmental and social factors that can affect their mental and physical well-being.[92] There are similar published recommendations for topical areas, such as health literacy competencies for trainees before graduation, and tools for starting medical-legal partnerships.[70]

Students sometimes call upon their personal experiences to address these needs, but the health workforce does not match the patient population in terms of social or economic background.[93,94] For example, most medical students are children of parents with high levels of education.[95] Roughly one-half of medical students' fathers have a graduate degree compared with 12 percent of men in the US population. Similarly, roughly one-third of medical students' mothers have a graduate degree compared with approximately 10 percent of US women. The same holds true for parental income.[96] The fraction of medical students from the lowest quintile of parental income in the United States has never been greater than 5.5 percent. Again, the same is true when the difference between race and ethnicity of physicians is compared to the US population. As an example, in California, less that 5 percent of physicians self-identify as Latino, whereas nearly 40 percent of Californians report Latino ethnicity.[97] According to the American Association of Colleges of Nursing, nursing students from minority backgrounds represented 28 percent of students in entry-level baccalaureate programs, 29 percent of master's students, and 28 percent of research-focused doctoral students.[98] Men composed 11 percent of students in baccalaureate programs, 10 percent of master's students, 8 percent of research-focused doctoral students, and 10 percent of practice-focused doctoral students.[98] These differences simply point to the need to educate learners on cultural humility. Cultural humility incorporates a "lifelong commitment to self-evaluation and self-critique, to redressing the power imbalances in the patient-physician dynamic, and to developing mutually beneficial and nonpaternalistic clinical and advocacy partnerships with communities on behalf of individuals and defined populations."[99] Cultural humility is applied to all interactions, regardless of professional degree or year in training. It encourages providers to approach each patient as a teacher so physicians and other health care professionals are less dependent on their own knowledge and experiences.

V. CASE STUDY 1 CONCLUSION

In listening to Mrs. H's story, you begin to wonder if there are other unmet needs in the family. You take a humble approach and recognize that there may be sensitive issues underlying the children's behavior and Mrs. H's illness. You use the IHELLP mnemonic to ask her about concerns related to income, housing, education, legal status/immigration, literacy, and personal safety. She shares with you that she has had trouble paying her bills and has not refilled her medications since she lost her job 2 months ago. She admits to having trouble using the new glucometer that was provided when her insurance changed this year. She worries that the children's asthma has worsened because of the poor heating in her apartment. As you develop a treatment plan for Mrs. H, you refer her to the Legal Aid attorney and Health Leads advocate in the office and ask that she meet with the pharmacist to review the glucometer and asthma action plans.

VI. CHAPTER SUMMARY

This chapter addresses the role that the social determinants of health play in health systems science. The chapter begins by examining the historical and epidemiologic evidence

How Can Academic Medical Centers and Teaching Hospitals Address the Social Determinants of Health?

Malika Fair, MD, MPH, director, Public Health Initiatives, Diversity Policy and Programs, Association of American Medical Colleges, and Taniecea Arceneaux Mallery, PhD, director, Equity, Diversity and Community Engagement, University of Louisiana at Lafayette

Social determinants of health are the conditions in which people are born, grow up, live, work, age, and receive health care.[1] Academic medical centers and teaching hospitals are uniquely positioned to address these factors and have a powerful impact on the health of communities.

Basic Necessities

- The availability of basic necessities such as healthy food and clean water is vital for the health of communities.
- Decreased rates of obesity and increased life expectancy can be partly attributed to better nutrition.[2]

- **Gundersen Lutheran Health System** has been committed to the health of its communities by working with local restaurants, convenience stores, and other retailers to offer healthy food choices to its community.[3]

Built Environment

- Health is influenced by the safety and physical surroundings of homes, neighborhoods, and workplaces.
- Inadequate housing, dangerous streets, and blighted neighborhoods all have a negative impact on health.[2]

- As a prominent institution within a city challenged with crime, extreme poverty, and poor living conditions, **Henry Ford Health System** has partnered with several institutions to improve local neighborhoods and develop safe and affordable housing for the residents of Detroit.[3]

Education

- Educational opportunity can lead to positive health outcomes.
- People with more educational opportunities have better jobs, more affluence, greater health, and improved quality of life.[2]

- **Johns Hopkins University**, in collaboration with Morgan State University, has developed a new public school in one of the poorest neighborhoods in east Baltimore. The school, named Henderson-Hopkins, is part of a major redevelopment project that includes new science and technology buildings, a park, retail development, and mixed-income housing.[4]

Community

- Social connectedness and a sense of community is important to achieving good health.
- Social cohesion, defined as the ability to obtain social support from family, friends, and community members, is associated with lower mortality rates.[2]

- **Florida International University** has developed the Green Family Foundation NeighborhoodHELP (Health Education Learning Program), which exposes students to the delivery of health care from a family and community perspective that will shape the way they interact with patients for the rest of their careers.[5]

Economic Stability

- Economic factors play a key role in the health of communities.
- The unemployment rate has an impact on rates of domestic violence, substance abuse, depression, and physical illness.[2]

- **University Hospitals** launched *The UH Difference: Vision 2010*, which aimed to direct as much spending as possible toward local minority- and female-owned businesses to produce lasting change in northeast Ohio.[6]

References

1. Office of Disease Prevention and Health Promotion. Healthy People 2020. http://www.healthypeople.gov/2020/topicsobjectives2020/overview.aspx?topicid=39. Accessed September 15, 2015.
2. Community Tool Box. Section 5: Addressing social determinants of health and development. http://ctb.ku.edu/en/table-of-contents/analyze/analyze-community-problems-and-solutions/social-determinants-of-health/main. Accessed September 15, 2015.
3. Zuckerman D. Hospitals building healthier communities: Embracing the anchor mission. March 1, 2013. http://community-wealth.org/content/hospitals-building-healthier-communities-embracing-anchor-mission. Accessed September 15, 2015.
4. Kimmelman M. Reading, writing and renewal (the Urban Kind). N Y Times. March 18, 2014. http://www.nytimes.com/2014/03/18/arts/design/reading-writing-and-renewal-the-urban-kind.html. Accessed September 15, 2015.
5. Florida International University, Herbert Wertheim College of Medicine. Green Family Foundation NeighborhoodHELP. http://medicine.fiu.edu/about-us/departments/clinical/humanities-health-society/overview/index.html. Accessed September 15, 2015.
6. Serang F, Thompson JP, Howard T. The anchor mission: Leveraging the power of anchor institutions to build community wealth. February 2, 2013. http://community-wealth.org/content/anchor-mission-leveraging-power-anchor-institutions-build-community-wealth. Accessed September 15, 2015.

Author contact: mfair@aamc.org

Fig. 11.3 How academic medical centers and teaching hospitals are addressing the social determinants of health. (From *Academic Medicine*. 2016;91[3]. http://www.aahci.org/Portals/1/AIM_Best_Practices/Social_Determinants_Health/How_Can_Academic_Medical_Centers_Teaching_Hospitals_Address_Social_Determinants_Health.pdf. First published online January 5, 2016. © by the Association of American Medical Colleges.)

demonstrating that the social and economic conditions in which people live, work, and play are the prime determinants of health and its distribution in populations. Although most people in the United States, including most health care professionals, tend to think of population health largely as a function of access to health care services, strong evidence shows that such access is only a relatively minor determinant of health. While health care is crucial for the sick and injured, the root causes of ill health are powerfully correlated with conditions such as socioeconomic position, educational attainment, housing, and exposures to racism and discrimination. Moreover, promising, evidence-based causal models give compelling rationales for believing that the connections between social determinants and health outcomes are causally related. And, of course, where social and economic conditions are primary drivers of population health, it is not surprising that inequalities in those conditions beget inequalities in health outcomes.

Given this evidence, the logical question is how attention to the social determinants of health may be integrated into a clinical practice focused on improving population health. The chapter details exemplar programs that facilitate health care professionals' ability to screen for the myriad ways in which social and economic conditions contribute to health outcomes for their patients. Beyond screening, the chapter also details how additional practice support resources and professionals outside the traditional boundaries of health systems can help address the social determinants of health. Crafting more equitable practice designs and using practice data to drive broader structural changes may also assist in alleviating the inequitable toll that adverse social conditions take on health. All of these approaches should incorporate community organization, participation, and advocacy, and the chapter details a variety of programs that do so effectively.

Finally, the chapter addresses pathways to integrating attention to the social determinants of health into health professions education. Special emphasis must be placed on the significance of health literacy and on the cultivation of cultural humility within health care professional practice. Especially where professional attitudes toward disadvantaged groups have a great impact on quality of care, lifelong learning is essential to action on the social determinants of health.

QUESTIONS FOR FURTHER THOUGHT

1. What is meant by the sentence "Health is not equivalent to health care"?
2. What is the difference between a critical period and a sensitive period in relation to epidemiologic risk?
3. What are some examples of the impact of race on inequalities in morbidity and mortality rates?
4. Why are differences in educational attainment correlated with health inequalities?
5. How can different health care professionals and community partners contribute to a coalition designed to create a community-based, health-promoting system?

Annotated Bibliography

Gottlieg I, Sandel M, Adler NE. Collecting and applying data on social determinants of health in health care settings. *JAMA Intern Med.* 2013;173(11):1017–1020.

This article proposes a framework for how interventions related to social determinants of health can be considered in the health care system and describes ways to collect data and target interventions at the level of the patient, the institution, and the broader population. Collection of patient data can be used to adjust individual disease risk and inform interventions to improve vulnerable patients' social circumstances. Some of the interventions reviewed include colocation of health and social services and improvement of referral capacity. Opportunities and barriers to accomplishing this are presented.

Klein MD, Kahn RS, Baker RC, Fink EE, Parrish DS, White DC. Training in social determinants of health in primary care: does it change resident behavior? *Acad Pediatr.* 2011;11(5):387–393.

This paper evaluates whether a 1-year-long education intervention for primary care residents on the social determinants of health changed attitudes and knowledge. The study divided 38 pediatric residents in a large urban academic outpatient clinic into an experimental arm (n=20) and a control arm (n=18). Using a presurvey and postsurvey design, the authors found that participants in the experimental arm (i.e., those receiving the educational intervention) reported more comfort with and greater knowledge of the social issues their patients and families experienced. Participants in the experimental arm also documented use of more social history questions, suggesting changes in social screening that may be a pathway to integrating attention to the social determinants of health in primary care residency training.

Link BG, Phelan J. Social conditions as fundamental causes of disease. *J Health Soc Behav.* 1995;(Spec No):80–94.

This paper introduces a new theory for linking social conditions with health outcomes: the idea of fundamental causes. For a variable to qualify as a fundamental cause, it must 1) be linked with multiple diseases, 2) be linked with multiple risk factors, and 3) persist over time. Link and Phelan give a number of examples of fundamental causes and show how social conditions such as income and social status qualify as such causes. Finally, Link and Phelan consider the implications of fundamental cause theory for health policy and suggest directions for future research.

Swain GR, Grande KM, Hood CM, Inzeo PT. Health care professionals: opportunities to address social determinants of health. *WMJ.* 2014;113(6):218–222.

This article discusses the "upstream" causes of health and illness, focused on employment, income, and education, as well as social cohesion, social support, community safety, affordable housing, and food security. Policy case examples are presented for these as examples of how advocacy can help address these negative factors on health outcomes. Implications for practice are discussed, and a helpful mnemonic "IHELLP" is presented to assist with screening of individual patients.

Taylor R, Rieger A. Medicine as social science: Rudolf Virchow on the typhus epidemic in Upper Silesia. *Int J Health Serv.* 1985;15(4):547–559.

This paper provides one of the first English-language translations of Virchow's 1848 report On a Typhus Epidemic in Upper Silesia, *which is regarded as one of the most historically significant texts in the modern history of public health. Taylor and Rieger both situate the tract in its larger social context and analyze the implications of Virchow's argument for contemporary medicine and public health. This paper is crucial in explicating Virchow's concept of social medicine—a practice of medicine that integrates awareness of and attention to the social and political realities that patients experience.*

References

1. Stonington S, Holmes SM. Social medicine in the twenty-first century. *PLoS Med.* 2006;3(10):e445.
2. World Health Organization. Health impact assessment: glossary of terms used. http://www.who.int/hia/about/glos/en/index1.html. Accessed November 29, 2015.
3. Taylor R, Rieger A. Medicine as social science: Rudolf Virchow on the typhus epidemic in Upper Silesia. *Int J Health Serv.* 1985;15(4):547–559.
4. Anderson MR, Smith L, Sidel VW. What is social medicine? *Monthly Rev.* 2005;56(8). http://monthlyreview.org/2005/01/01/what-is-social-medicine/. Accessed January 24, 2016.

5. The Commonwealth Fund. Mirror, mirror on the wall, 2014 update: how the US health care system compares internationally. http://www.commonwealthfund.org/publications/fund-reports/2014/jun/mirror-mirror. Accessed November 29, 2015.

6. MacDorman MF, Mathews TJ, Mohangoo AD, Zeitlin J. International comparisons of infant mortality and related factors: United States and Europe, 2010. *Nat Vit Stats Rep.* 2014;63(5):1–7.

7. Ingraham C. Our infant mortality rate is a national embarrassment. *The Washington Post.* https://www.washingtonpost.com/news/wonk/wp/2014/09/29/our-infant-mortality-rate-is-a-national-embarrassment/. Accessed November 29, 2015.

8. Kindig D, Stoddart G. What is population health? *Am J Public Health.* 2003;93(3):380–383.

9. Kindig D. What are we talking about when we talk about population health? Health Affairs Blog. http://healthaffairs.org/blog/2015/04/06/what-are-we-talking-about-when-we-talk-about-population-health/. Accessed November 29, 2015.

10. *Unnatural Causes.* [DVD]. California Newsreel: United States; 2008.

11. Marmot M. Social determinants of health inequalities. *Lancet.* 2005;365(9464):1099–1104.

12. *Closing the Gap in a Generation: Health Equity Through Action on the Social Determinants of Health.* Final Report of World Health Organization's Commission on Social Determinants of Health. http://www.who.int/social_determinants/final_report/csdh_finalreport_2008.pdf. Accessed November 29, 2015.

13. Braveman P, Gottlieb L. The social determinants of health: it's time to consider the causes of the causes. *Public Health Rep.* 2014;129(suppl 2): 19–31.

14. Marmot M, Wilkinson R. *Social Determinants of Health.* 2nd ed. New York: Oxford; 2006.

15. Low MD, Low BJ, Baumler ER, Huynh PT. Can education policy be health policy? Implications of research on the social determinants of health. *J Health Polit Policy Law.* 2005;30(6):1131–1162.

16. Low BJ, Low MD. Education and education policy as social determinants of health. *Virtual Mentor.* 2006;8(11):756–761.

17. Ben-Shlomo Y, Kuh D. A life course approach to chronic disease epidemiology: conceptual models, empirical challenges and interdisciplinary perspectives. *Int J Epidemiol.* 2002;31(2):285–293.

18. Hayward MD, Gorman BK. The long arm of childhood: the influence of early-life social conditions on men's mortality. *Demography.* 2004;41(1):87–107.

19. Osler M, Andersen AM, Lund R, Holstein B. Effect of grandparent's and parent's socioeconomic position on mortality among Danish men born in 1953. *Eur J Public Health.* 2005;15(6):647–651.

20. Pungello EP, Campbell FA. Poverty and early childhood intervention. http://www.law.unc.edu/documents/poverty/publications/pungelloandcampbellpolicybrief.pdf. Accessed November 29, 2015.

21. Campbell F, Conti G, Heckman JJ, et al. Abecedarian & health: improve adult health outcomes with quality early childhood programs that include health and nutrition. http://heckmanequation.org/sites/default/files/F_Heckman_AbecedarianHealth_062615.pdf. Accessed November 29, 2015.

22. The Heckman Equation. http://heckmanequation.org/heckman-equation. Accessed November 29, 2015.

23. The Centers for Disease Control Division of Violence Prevention. ACE study: major findings. http://www.cdc.gov/violenceprevention/acestudy/. Accessed September 6, 2016.

24. Exploring the intersection of health, place and economic justice. The Robert Wood Johnson Foundation Culture of Health Blog. http://www.rwjf.org/en/culture-of-health/2013/10/exploring_the_inters.html. Accessed November 29, 2015.

25. Braveman P, Dekker M, Egerter S, Sadegh-Nobari T, Pollack C. Robert Wood Johnson Foundation issue brief #7: housing and health. http://www.rwjf.org/content/dam/farm/reports/issue_briefs/2011/rwjf70451. Accessed November 29, 2015.

26. US Department of Housing and Urban Development, Office of Healthy Homes and lead Hazard Control. *American Healthy Homes Survey: lead and Arsenic Findings.* http://portal.hud.gov/hudportal/documents/huddoc?id=AHHS_REPORT.pdf. Accessed November 29, 2015.

27. The Centers for Disease Control Health Disparities and Inequalities Report (2013). http://www.cdc.gov/minorityhealth/CHDIReport.html. Accessed November 29, 2015.

28. Institute of Medicine. *Relieving Pain in America: A Blueprint for Transforming Prevention, Care, Education, and Research.* Washington, DC: National Academies Press; 2011.

29. Chaufan C. How much can a large population study on genes, environments, their interactions and common diseases contribute to the health of the American people? *Soc Sci Med.* 2007;65(8):1730–1741.

30. Braveman P. Health inequalities by class and race in the US: what can we learn from the patterns? *Soc Sci Med.* 2012;74(5):665–667.

31. Gee GC, Ford CL. Structural racism and health inequities: old issues, new directions. *Du Bois Rev.* 2011;8(1):115–132.

32. Seitles M. The perpetuation of residential racial segregation in America: historical discrimination, modern forms of exclusion, and inclusionary remedies. *J Land Use & Envtl L.* archive.law.fsu.edu/journals/landuse/Vol141/seit.htm. Accessed November 29, 2015.

33. Williams DR, Mohammed SA. Racism and health I: pathways and scientific evidence. *The American Behavioral Scientist.* 2013;57(8):10.

34. Krieger N. Does racism harm health? Did child abuse exist before 1962? On explicit questions, critical science, and current controversies: an ecosocial perspective. *Am J Public Health.* 2003;93(2):194–199.

35. Krieger N, Sidney S. Racial discrimination and blood pressure: the CARDIA Study of young black and white adults. *Am J Public Health.* 1996;86(10):1370–1378.

36. McEwen BS. Stress, adaptation, and disease: allostasis and allostatic load. *Ann N Y Acad Sci.* 1998, May 1;840:33–44.

37. Seeman TE, McEwen BS, Rowe JW, Singer BH. Allostatic load as a marker of cumulative biological risk: MacArthur studies of successful aging. *Proc Natl Acad Sci U S A.* 2001;98(8):4770–4775.

38. Seeman T, Epel E, Gruenewald T, Karlamangla A, McEwen BS. Socioeconomic differentials in peripheral biology: cumulative allostatic load. *Ann N Y Acad Sci.* 2010;1186:223–239.

39. Seeman T, Gruenewald T, Karlamangla A, et al. Modeling multisystem biological risk in young adults: the Coronary Artery Risk Development in Young Adults Study. *Am J Hum Biol.* 2010;22(4):463–472.

40. Harvard Center on the Developing Child. http://developingchild.harvard.edu/science/. Accessed November 29, 2015.

41. Krieger N, Davey Smith G. "Bodies count," and body counts: social epidemiology and embodying inequality. *Epidemiol Rev.* 2004;26(1):92–103.

42. Farrer L, Marinetti C, Cavaco YK, Costongs C. Advocacy for health equity: a synthesis review. *Milbank Q.* 2015;93(2):392–437.

43. Link BG, Phelan J. Social conditions as fundamental causes of disease. *J Health Soc Behav.* 1995;(Spec No):80–94.

44. Gottlieg I, Sandel M, Adler NE. Collecting and applying data on social determinants of health in health care settings. *JAMA Intern Med.* 2013;173(11):1017–1020.

45. Goldstein D. 2011 Physicians Daily Life Report. Harris Interactive. Prepared for the Robert Wood Johnson Foundation. http://www.rwjf.org/content/dam/web-assets/2011/11/2011-physicians-daily-life-report. Published 2001. Accessed November 23, 2015.

46. Sadana R, Blas E. What can public health programs do to improve health equity? *Public Health Rep.* 2013;128(suppl 3):12–20.

47. Swain GR, Grande KM, Hood CM, Inzeo PT. Health care professionals: opportunities to address social determinants of health. *Wisconsin Medical J.* 2014;113(6):218–222.

48. Fiscella K, Tancredi D, Franks P. Adding socioeconomic status to Framingham scoring to reduce disparities in coronary risk assessment. *Am Heart J.* 2009;157(6):988–994.

49. Brcic V, Eberdt C, Kaczorowski J. Development of a tool to identify poverty in a family practice setting: a pilot study. *Int J Fam Med.* 2011;2011:812182.

50. Institute of Medicine. *Capturing Social and Behavioral Domains and Measures in Electronic Health Records: Phase 2.* Washington, DC: National Academies Press; 2014.

51. Canadian Medical Association. Physicians and health equity: opportunities for practice. http://healthcaretransformation.ca/wp-content/uploads/2013/03/Health-Equity-Opportunities-in-Practice-Final-E.pdf. Published 2012. Accessed November 23, 2015.

52. Kenyon C, Sandel M, Silverstein M, Shakir A, Zuckerman B. Revisiting the social history for child health. *Pediatrics*. 2007;120:e734–e738.

53. Cohen E, MacKenzie RG, Yates GL. HEADSS, a psychosocial risk assessment instrument: implications for designing effective intervention programs for runaway youth. *J Adolescent Health*. 1991;12(7):539–544.

54. Goldenring JM, Rosen D. Getting into adolescent heads: an essential update. *Contemp Pediatr*. 2004;21:64.

55. Gottlieb L, Hessler D, Long D, Amaya A, Adler N. A randomized trial on screening for social determinants of health: the iScreen Study. *Pediatrics*. 2014;134:e1611–e1618.

56. Margolis PA, Stevens R, Bordley WC, et al. From concept to application: the impact of a community-wide intervention to improve the delivery of preventive services to children. *Pediatrics*. 2001;108(3):E42. http://pediatrics.aappublications.org/content/pediatrics/108/3/e42.full.pdf. Accessed on November 23, 2015.

57. Henize AW, Beck AF, Klein MD, Adams M, Kahn RS. A road map to address the social determinants of health through community collaboration. *Pediatrics*. 2015;136(4):e993–e1001.

58. Pelletier SG. Addressing social determinants of health: merging social determinants data into EHRs to improve patient outcomes. *AAMC Reporter*. May 2015.

59. Klein MD, Kahn RS, Baker RC, Fink EE, Parrish DS, White DC. Training in social determinants of health in primary care: does it change resident behavior? *Acad Pediatr*. 2011;11(5):387–393.

60. Health Leads Blog. Making connections. https://healthleadsusa.org/2013/11/clientconnect-strengthens-health-leads-program/. Accessed November 29, 2015.

61. Cap4Kids: The Children's Advocacy Project of America. What is Cap4Kids? http://cap4kids.org/whatiscap4kids.html. Accessed November 15, 2015.

62. Bazemore AW, Cottrell EK, Gold R, et al. "Community vital signs": incorporating geocoded social determinants into electronic records to promote patient and population health. *J Am Med Inform Assoc*. 2016;23(2):407–412.

63. Street Medicine Institute. http://streetmedicine.org/wordpress/. Accessed November 29, 2015.

64. Garg A, Sandel M, Dworkin PH, Kahn RS, Zuckerman B. From medical home to health neighborhood: transforming the medical home into a community-based health neighborhood. *J Pediatr*. 2012;160(4):535–536.

65. Ingram M, Schacter KA, Sabo SJ, et al. A community health worker intervention to address the social determinants of health through policy change. *J Prim Prev*. 2014;35(2):119–123.

66. Silberberg M, Castrucci BC. Addressing social determinants of health. In *Practical Playbook: Public Health and Primary Care Together*. New York: Oxford; 2015.

67. Acción Para La Salud. Curricula. http://azprc.arizona.edu/sites/default/files/Background%20%20&%20references.pdf. Accessed September 6, 2016.

68. Klein MD, Beck AF, Henize AW, Parrish DS, Fink EE, Kahn RS. Doctors and lawyers collaborating to HeLP children—outcomes from a successful partnership between professions. *J Health Care Poor Underserved*. 2013;24(3):1063–1073.

69. Weintraub D, Rodgers MA, Botcheva L, et al. Pilot study of medical-legal partnership to address social and legal needs of patients. *J Health Care Poor Underserved*. 2010;21(2 suppl):157–168.

70. National Center for Medical-Legal Partnership. http://medical-legalpartnership.org. Accessed November 30, 2015.

71. Cleek EN, Wofsy M, Boyd-Franklin N, Mundy B, Howell TJ. The family empowerment program: an interdisciplinary approach to working with multistressed urban families. *Fam Process*. 2012;51(2):207–217.

72. Toolbox overview for building needle-moving community collaborations. www.serve.gov/sites/default/files/ctools/CommunityCollaborativeToolkit_all%20_materials.pdf. Published 2014. Accessed November 23, 2015.

73. World Health Organization. Health impact assessment. http://www.who.int/hia/en/. Accessed November 14, 2015.

74. The Prevention Institute. THRIVE: Toolkit for Health & Resilience in Vulnerable Environments. Final Project Report September 2004. http://minorityhealth.hhs.gov/assets/pdf/checked/thrive_finalprojectreport_093004.pdf. Accessed November 23, 2015.

75. Davis R, Cook D, Cohen L. A community resilience approach to reducing ethnic and racial disparities in health. *Am J Public Health*. 2005;95(12):2168–2173.

76. US Department of Health and Human Services. *Healthy People* [with Understanding and Improving Health (vol. 1) and Objectives for Improving Health (vol. 2)]. 2nd ed. Washington, DC: US Government Printing Office; 2010.

77. Berkman ND, DeWalt DA, Pignone MP, et al. *Literacy and Health Outcomes* (AHRQ Publication No. 04-E007-2). Rockville, MD: Agency for Healthcare Research and Quality; 2004.

78. Chamberlain LJ, Wang NE, Ho ET, Banchoff AW, Braddock 3rd CH, Gesundheit N. Integrating collaborative population health projects into a medical student curriculum at Stanford. *Acad Med*. 2008;83(4):338–344.

79. Geppert CM, Arndell CL, Clithero A, et al. Reuniting public health and medicine at The University of New Mexico School of Medicine Public Health Certificate. *Am J Prev Med*. 2011;41(4 suppl 3):S214–S219.

80. Meurer LN, Young SA, Meurer JR, Johnson SL, Gilbert IA, Diehr S. The urban and community health pathway: preparing socially responsive physicians through community-engaged learning. *Am J Prev Med*. 2011;41(4 suppl 3):S228–S236.

81. US Department of Health and Human Services, Office of Disease Prevention and Health Promotion. *National Action Plan to Improve Health Literacy*. Washington, DC: Author; 2010.

82. Bakshi S, James A, Hennelly MO, et al. The Human Rights and Social Justice Scholars Program: a collaborative model for preclinical training in social medicine. *Ann Glob Health*. 2015;81(2):290–297.

83. Ramos-Gomez FJ, Silva DR, Law CS, Pizzitola RL, John B, Crall JJ. Creating a new generation of pediatric dentists: a paradigm shift in training. *J Dent Educ*. 2014;78(12):1593–1603.

84. Happell B, Bennetts W, Platania-Phung C, Tohotoa J. Exploring the scope of consumer participation in mental health nursing education: perspectives from nurses and consumers. *Perspect Psychiatr Care*. 2016;52(3):169–177.

85. Bhate TD, Loh LC. Building a generation of physician advocates: the case for including mandatory training in advocacy in Canadian medical school curricula. *Acad Med*. 2015;90(12):1602–1606.

86. Weitzman CC, Freudigman K, Schonfeld DJ, Leventhal JM. Care to underserved children: residents' attitudes and experiences. *Pediatrics*. 2000;106(5):1022–1027.

87. Weissman JS, Campbell EG, Gokhale M, Blumenthal D. Residents' preferences and preparation for caring for underserved populations. *J Urban Health*. 2001;78(3):535–549.

88. O'Toole JK, Burkhardt MC, Solan LG, et al. Resident confidence addressing social history: is it influenced by availability of social and legal resources? *Clin Pediatr (Phila)*. 2012;51(7):625–631.

89. Fair M, Mallery TA. How can academic medical centers and teaching hospitals address the social determinants of health? *Acad Med*. 2016;91(3):443.

90. Wells AL, Martinez IL, Gillis M. Community service learning in Florida undergraduate medical education. *Florida Fam Physician*. 2014;63(1):12–14.

91. Martinez IL, Artze-Vega I, Wells AL, Mora JC, Gillis M. Twelve tips for teaching social determinants of health in medicine. *Med Teach*. 2014, Nov 6:1–6.

92. Clark L, Calvillo E, Dela Cruz F, et al. Cultural competencies for graduate nursing education. *J Prof Nurs*. 2011;27(3):133–139.

93. Daniel H, Butkus R. Health and Public Policy Committee of American College of Physicians. Lesbian, gay, bisexual, and transgender health disparities: executive summary of a policy position paper from the American College of Physicians. *Ann Intern Med*. 2015;163(2):135–137.

94. Serwint JR, Thoma KA, Dabrow SM, et al. Comparing patients seen in pediatric resident continuity clinics and national ambulatory medical care survey practices: a study from the Continuity Research Network. *Pediatrics*. 2006;118:e849–e858.

95. O'Toole JK, Solan LG, Burkhardt MC, Klein MD. Watch and learn: an innovative video trigger curriculum to increase resident screening for social determinants of health. *Clin Pediatr*. 2013;52:344–350.

96. Grbic D, Garrison G, Jolly P. Analysis in brief: diversity of US medical students by parental education. Volume 9, Number 10. Association of American Medical Colleges. https://www.aamc.org/download/142770/data/aibvol9_no10.pdf. Published August 2010. Accessed November 30, 2015.

97. Jolly P. Analysis in brief: diversity of US medical students by parental income. Volume 8, Number 1. Association of American Medical Colleges; January 2008.

98. Paxton C. California Health Care Almanac. http://www.chcf.org/almanac. Published July 2010. Accessed November 30, 2015.

99. American Association of Colleges of Nursing. Enhancing diversity in the workforce. http://www.aacn.nche.edu/media-relations/fact-sheets/enhancing-diversity. Accessed November 30, 2015.

12

Health Care Policy and Economics

Matthew M. Davis, MD, MAPP, Elizabeth Tobin-Tyler, JD, MA, and Mark D. Schwartz, MD

LEARNING OBJECTIVES

1. Understand the core principles of the formation and implementation of health care policy in the United States.
2. Understand how the economic aspects of the US health care system dominate reform efforts and how health care professionals, health plans, and patients can affect health care spending.
3. Understand central themes of health care reform in the United States over the last century and how they relate to the main components of the Affordable Care Act.

Health policies reflect and shape historical and contemporary political philosophies and priorities and also drive governmental actions. The overarching objective of this chapter is to demystify the health policy process—to help readers understand the interplay among multiple stakeholders, why these individuals and organizations behave the way they do, and how their decisions interact to become the form and function of the US health care system. A major emphasis of this chapter is health care economics because concerns about the affordability and high costs of health care continue to motivate policymaking at the federal and state levels. The chapter includes an examination of major health care reform efforts in the United States over the past century with a focus on major provisions of the Affordable Care Act to provide readers with a helpful rubric for understanding the core elements of this complex, recent major reform effort. This chapter enables a level of awareness and understanding of the principles of policy and economics that will permit readers to make sense of the differential impacts of health care policies on multiple different stakeholders.

CHAPTER OUTLINE

I. INTRODUCTION

For many observers and participants in the US health care system, health care policy appears to be a bewildering array of overlapping programs, puzzling acronyms, chronically acrimonious political debate, and conflicting special interests. The often arcane nature of health care policy is further complicated by the fact that policy can occur at many different levels. Examples include requirements to use electronic health records to document encounters between patients and physicians; immunization requirements affecting nursing staff within hospitals; decisions about which medications will be included in a formulary in a state Medicaid program; and how much tax will be levied on American workers in order to finance the federal Medicare program. The aggregate effect of these characteristics of health care policy lead many patients, health care professionals, and other stakeholders to feel that policy is something done *to* them, rather than *with* them or *by* them.

The overarching objective of this chapter is to demystify the policy process—to help current and future health care professionals understand the interplay of multiple stakeholders, why these individuals and organizations behave the way they do, and how their decisions interact to shape the form and function of the US health care system. The key starting point is to understand that policy, from the Greek word *polis,* meaning "city," can be made any time there is a decision that affects more than one individual. Policies are a necessary part of any system, in order to create efficiencies, establish and deliver on expectations, and specify consequences for failure to behave in acceptable ways. Policies also provide mechanisms through which failings and inequities in a system can be addressed.

These positive aspects of policies are counterbalanced, however, by two key caveats. The first is the so-called *law of unintended consequences:* that health care policies, no matter how well-intentioned, have unforeseen effects on stakeholders. While some unintended consequences are minor, others may lead to circumstances that are worse than the situations they were intended to address. For example, a childhood vaccine against a disease called pertussis (whooping cough) was found to cause too many serious side effects, so a new vaccine against pertussis was developed and substituted for the older version. While the new vaccine caused fewer side effects, it failed to sustain immunity as long—leading to the unintended consequence of increasing outbreaks (i.e., less effective prevention) of pertussis in children and adults. When unintended policy consequences occur, recognizing them and addressing them promptly and comprehensively can help achieve the original goals of a new policy with minimal long-term impact to the stakeholders whose interests who were adversely affected.

The second caveat, particularly relevant in the US health care system, is that policies run contrary to the paradigmatic American focus on the individual. A policy that advantages one individual may well inconvenience or disadvantage another. Effects on the latter individual tend to be emphasized more in the media and popular narrative than the perspective that a policy may have accomplished the utilitarian goal of "the greatest good for the greatest number." The tension between benefits for individuals versus benefits for the population is a frequent, highly visible challenge in health care policymaking in the United States. For example, legislators in Congress often lament how many taxpayer dollars are spent on the federal Medicare program, while individual Medicare-covered patients' pleas for expensive therapies with questionable benefit and value often appear on the home page of media outlets.

These caveats notwithstanding, health care policy is a dominant force for change in the US health care system. This chapter presents the fundamental principles that undergird health care policymaking and also presents central stakeholders and themes that strongly influence the direction of policies related to health and health care. In this chapter, the reader will also find many examples of health care policies that have shaped the health care system in the United States as it functions today and will inform what reforms are attempted in the future. To examine every major health care policy would require many books; instead, this chapter highlights instructive, influential policies across many aspects of the system.

Another major emphasis of this chapter is health care economics, because common questions such as "Who pays for health care?" and "What can an individual do if he or she cannot afford health care?" continue to motivate health care policymaking at federal and state levels in the United States. While it is possible to understand US health care policy at a basic level without fully grasping economics, this chapter enables a level of awareness and understanding of economic principles and phenomena in the US health care system that will permit readers to make sense of the differential impacts of policies on multiple different stakeholders.

II. BASIC PRINCIPLES OF HEALTH POLICY

Health policy is a dynamic blend of social strategies, laws, regulations, and funding decisions, most often embodied in constitutions, legislative actions, rules, and judicial decisions. Health policies reflect and shape historical and prevalent philosophies and priorities and drive governmental actions.[1] While public policy aims to distribute finite resources to the public as appropriate, health policy is a nexus of policy, politics, procedure, and science, but not always in that order. It has been said that if health policy is chess, then it is chess while playing rugby on a speeding train.[2]

A. Political Will

Health policy is generated or changed most often when three forces align: the scientific evidence base, social strategy, and political will (Fig. 12.1).[3] Scientific evidence refers to sound data regarding the nature of the problem to be addressed by policy. Social strategy is the actual detailed policy plan or approach to address a problem along with the social infrastructure (systems) in place to support the strategy. Political will is public understanding and support for the resources needed to implement the strategy and achieve the solution. *Public* in this context refers to both government leadership and the broader community of constituents that the policy will affect.[4] In health policy, evidence and strategies abound, but unified political will is increasingly precious. Yet, no policy change happens without it.

In the example of the Affordable Care Act (ACA), there had been broad agreement for a long time on the nature of the problem: unsustainable growth in the cost of health care with diminishing returns in health outcomes. As a proportion of the US gross domestic product (GDP; national economic activity, expressed as the sum of all goods and services produced annually), national health care expenditures in the United States more than tripled from 5 percent ($27.4 billion) in 1960 to 17.4 percent ($2.6 trillion) in 2010 (Fig. 12.2).[5] While the United States spends more per capita on health care ($8508 in 2011) than all other countries in the world, it lags behind all peer industrialized nations in health outcomes,

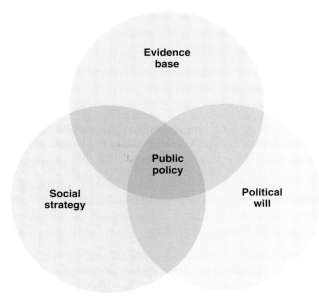

Fig. 12.1 **Model of public policy.** (Adapted from Richmond JB, Kotelchuck M. Political influences: rethinking national health policy. In: Mcquire C, Foley R, Gorr A, Richards R, eds. *Handbook of Health Professions Education.* San Francisco, CA: Jossey-Bass Publishers; 1993:386–404.)

access, efficiency, equity, and overall ranking, in an annual assessment by the Commonwealth Fund.[6] There is no shortage of evidence and agreement that something must be done to improve this value equation in the US health care system.

Over recent decades, many policy approaches to addressing this problem have been proposed from across the political spectrum. In fact, many of the core provisions in the ACA had been developed, argued, and refined over the years by both political parties, including insurance marketplaces, mandates to purchase insurance, standardized benefits, a ban on denying coverage based on a pre-existing medical condition, and so on.

One of the major reasons that the majority of US presidents over the last century tried and failed to reform the country's health care system was not for lack of evidence or good ideas, but rather for lack of political will. Political will has been called "the slipperiest concept in the policy lexicon," "the sine qua non of policy success which is never defined except by its absence."[7] A reasonable definition is that political will is "the extent of committed support among key decision makers for a particular policy solution to a particular problem."[8] Political will has both binary and continuous properties and is a complex, multifaceted construct that must be understood in its particular context.

In more pragmatic terms, there are four principal stakeholders in health policy that can influence political will: Patients, Providers, Payers, and Public entities ("four *Ps*"). Patients are, of course, the ultimate beneficiaries and consumers of health policy and health care. However, individual citizens usually lack the political clout of larger constituencies to influence health policy decision makers. Providers are often divided between two key players: physicians (and other health care professionals) and hospitals. Although aligned in their core mission to provide health care services to patients to reduce suffering and prolong healthy lives, physicians and hospitals are often in conflict in their respective business models and self-interests.[9] Payers of health care include insurance companies, employers, federal and state government, and consumers themselves. Health care is ultimately financed by consumers through premiums, taxes, and salary offsets via insurance companies (private and public) and employers that offer health coverage. Public entities (government and public

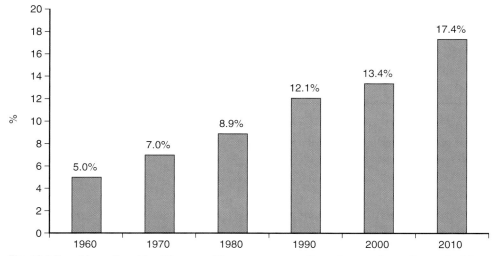

Fig. 12.2 **Trend in national health expenditures as a proportion of gross domestic product in the United States, 1960 to 2010.** (From National Health Expenditure Data, Centers for Medicare and Medicaid Services, US Government. https://www.cms.gov/research-statistics-data-and-systems/statistics-trends-and-reports/nationalhealthexpenddata/nationalhealthaccountshistorical.html. Accessed November 21, 2015.)

health agencies) are increasingly important players that regulate and provide health insurance and direct health care services through Medicare, Medicaid, and public clinics and hospitals. Public health officials at local, state, and national levels also contribute their expertise and efforts regarding surveillance for acute and chronic diseases, as well as outreach to promote preventive health practices.

B. The Iron Triangle

While the four *P*s discussed earlier are key stakeholders in health policy, the so-called *Iron Triangle* of US health care drives the federal policymaking apparatus (Fig. 12.3). The Iron Triangle describes the tightly interdependent relationships among three major forces in shaping political decision making: the administration (executive), the Congress (legislative), and interest groups (constituencies). Small groups dominate the three sides of the Iron Triangle: government bureaucrats in executive positions, a legislative committee with jurisdiction and authority on the issue, and a corporate or professional interest group or coalition of groups. This "sub-government" is quite stable and often impenetrable. The actors organize into mutually reinforcing relationships between regulated interests and regulators. In the United States, power is exercised in Congress and particularly in its committees and subcommittees. By aligning itself with selected constituencies, an administrative agency may be able to affect policy outcomes directly in legislative committees.

The classic example is the triangle formed by the US House and Senate Committees on Armed Services, the federal Department of Defense, and the defense contractors, often called the *military-industrial complex*.[10] An example in health care is the triangle formed by the House Ways and Means Subcommittees on Health, the Office of the National Coordinator on Health Information Technology (ONCHIT) (representing the administration) in the federal Department of Health and Human Services (HHS), and the electronic health record vendors—represented by their trade association, the Electronic Health Record Association (EHRA). These relationships are echoed at state and local levels as well. For many years, the sophisticated tobacco lobby successfully worked with state legislatures and health agencies to limit restrictions on tobacco sales, often by shifting the debate from public health to economics and freedom of choice concerns.[11]

In the daily work of health policy decision making, interest group constituencies are valued and powerfully influential partners of the congressional committees that authorize and fund policy and the federal agencies that operationalize and regulate the law. As political bodies, congressional committees and federal agencies seek to develop their power base to maximize their influence and impact. They typically work with constituencies that will provide the most political clout in a policy arena. As a result, committees and agencies tend to ally themselves with the powerful interest groups more often than with the citizens that are the target of a particular policy or service.

"Constituents" are politically active members who share a common interest or goal. They are not necessarily aligned with the citizens who are the expected recipients of goods or services provided by a governmental agency through the policy being considered. Interest groups are the stakeholders and core constituencies of the committees and agencies. They are the major health industries, and their lobbying groups including trade associations, voluntary health associations,

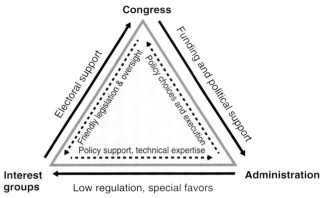

Fig. 12.3 **The Iron Triangle of health policy.**

professional societies, academia and think tanks, unions, and other stakeholders. These groups are wealthy, well-organized, and well-connected. They can move money and votes, exerting their influence through direct lobbying, making campaign contributions, and providing valued technical expertise in the applicable policy.

These alliances provide efficient and manageable access by Congress and the administration to expertise and political clout. In contrast, consumer-citizens are usually loosely organized, have divergent views, and lack political and financial muscle. Thus, most consumers, even those organized into small groups, have limited influence on policymakers. This tends to produce policies that often do not adequately reflect the priorities of the ultimate beneficiaries.

C. Health Policy Trifecta

There is broad agreement that the three core aims of health reform are to improve health care access, improve health care quality, and constrain costs. This health policy "trifecta" is embodied in the pursuit of the Triple Aim as initially described by the Institute for Healthcare Improvement: improving the experience of care, improving the health of populations, and reducing per capita costs of health care (Fig. 12.4).[12] A high-value health care system requires attention to all three of these interdependent and sometimes conflicting aims. Most health policy initiatives seek to address one or more of these aims. Policy to fund recommended vaccinations for children is a rare example of the trifecta, improving access and quality outcomes while reducing the cost of preventable illnesses. More commonly, improving access or quality of care requires more resources and increases costs, depending on how the time horizon and economic perspective is defined. Investment in prevention may reduce health care costs, but often only after years or decades of efforts.

As an example of the complexity of the Triple Aim, the ACA's Hospital Readmissions Reduction Program penalizes hospitals up to 3 percent of Medicare reimbursement when a substantial proportion of their patients return to the same or another acute hospital setting within 30 days of discharge.[13,14] In 2015, 80 percent of US hospitals were penalized under this law, averaging less than 1 percent penalty per hospital.[15] Initiated in 2013, within 2 years the policy focused on patients admitted with five common conditions (heart attack, heart failure, pneumonia, chronic obstructive pulmonary disease, and hip or knee replacement) and anticipates adding more conditions. The program incentivizes

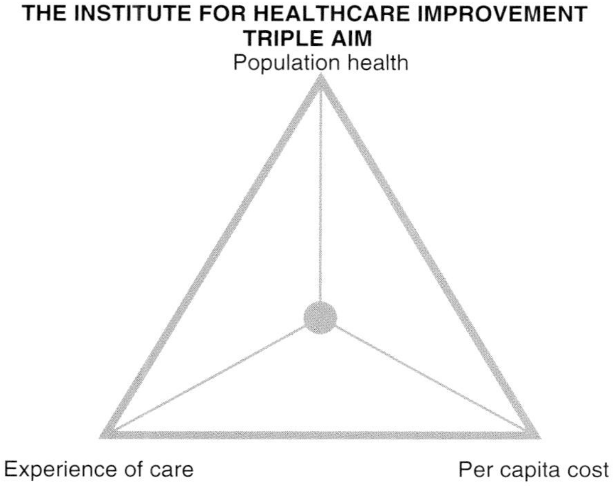

THE INSTITUTE FOR HEALTHCARE IMPROVEMENT
TRIPLE AIM

Fig. 12.4 The Triple Aim of health care reform.

hospitals to invest in improved discharge planning and coordinated services among hospitals, physicians, patients, and community services. These additional costs may in time be offset by reduced penalties to hospitals and reduced societal costs as re-admission rates have declined by as much as 17.5 percent for Medicare patients with these conditions, translating to an estimated 150,000 fewer hospital re-admissions across the country annually.[16] However, hospitals that care for chronically ill and low-income patients are far more likely to be penalized than other institutions, with safety net hospitals twice as likely to be penalized than other hospitals.[17]

Therefore, while the Triple Aim is a worthy pursuit in health care reform, policies aiming for the trifecta require comprehensive and detailed scrutiny to anticipate and monitor downstream consequences.

III. BASIC PRINCIPLES OF HEALTH CARE ECONOMICS

When it comes to paying for health care, the bottom line is that the patient (often called the *consumer*) pays. While there may be health insurance plans that help pay for health care, consumers pay premiums that finance the plans; insurance plans pay for health care principally from the premium dollars already paid to them. While there may be government-sponsored health programs such as Medicare and Medicaid, consumers pay the taxes that finance those programs. Increasingly, patients who seek health care are asked to "cost-share" with their insurance plans and government programs, thereby emphasizing consumers' central role in paying for care. With so many moving parts in the US health care system regarding paying for health care, it is easy to forget that consumers ultimately pay—if not always individually, then certainly collectively as a nation.

A. Why Health Insurance?

A common question is "What is the need for so many different ways to pay for health care in the United States, if consumers are the ultimate payers?" The answer is that health care in the United States is more expensive than the average consumer can afford, especially when it comes to a sudden need for complex health care in the highest-cost settings (e.g., hospitals).

Insurance as a financial mechanism is designed to help dampen the economic shock of an unexpected, costly event for an individual and his or her family—whether that event is a house fire, a car wreck, or a fractured hip. The central premise of insurance is that a company, by pooling the risks of various unexpected events over a large enough group of consumers (policyholders) and asking those consumers to pay regularly (premiums) into a central account, will have enough money to help the consumers pay the large bills that come due for unexpected, expensive events that actually occur (claims).

Given that US consumers depend on health insurance plans for financial help at some of their most vulnerable times, the financial well-being of health insurance companies (also called *carriers*) is a key issue in the functioning of the US health care system. Carriers' financial status depends greatly on their abilities to anticipate the types of health problems that consumers will experience and the corresponding amount of health care that consumers seek. If the insurance company charges an amount for its premiums that is acceptable to consumers and has fewer claims to pay than it expected, then the company will do well. If the insurance company faces more claims than it anticipated for the premiums that it charged, then the company will struggle. Furthermore, if the insurance company charges too much for its premiums in an effort to do well, it will likely lose customers to another company with similar benefits in its plan that is charging lower premiums.

In this basic example, the financial pressures on insurance carriers are clearly evident. The challenge for patients is that health insurance carriers, as businesses, often find ways to share those financial pressures with their policyholders. We discuss these strategies in the following section.

B. Key Concepts in Health Insurance

Health insurance is often described as a "benefit" that is accessible to employees of companies in the United States that make health plans available as part of benefit packages (i.e., as part of a compensation package, other than wages). In another sense, each health insurance plan is itself a package of benefits—the types of health care which, if sought by the policyholder, will be recognized by the insurance carrier as part of the plan and for which the carrier is prepared to pay some share of the costs.

Benefits in health plans have many facets, often described as what a plan "covers." One aspect of benefits is the type of setting in which health care is received. For example, a plan may cover visits to the hospital, emergency department, or primary care office, but may not cover visits to a mental health or dental health professional. Another facet of benefits may be quantity-based, such as a limit on the number of visits to a mental health professional that will be covered in a given year. A third facet of benefits is network-based, in which the plan contracts with a limited set of health care professionals with whom it has a preferred relationship. These professionals are within the "network" of the plan, and care sought from other health care professionals (whether intentionally or accidentally) is "out-of-network" and not covered in the same way by the insurance carrier. A fourth aspect of benefits is based on preferred lists related to specific prescription drugs, diagnostic tests, and durable medical equipment that a plan will cover.

Without a benefit specified as part of a health insurance plan policy, a consumer will find it exceedingly difficult to receive help from an insurance carrier in paying for care. Yet even when a benefit is specified as being covered by a plan, the interaction of a policyholder with a health plan revolves around the interaction of benefits with the cost-sharing structure. The cost-sharing structure involves a small set of components:

■ *Premium:* The price paid by the consumer to hold the insurance plan, usually for 1 year at a time, and commonly paid in monthly installments. The premium must be paid regardless of whether the policyholder uses any health care.
■ *Deductible:* The amount of a health care bill from a health care professional or institution (e.g., hospital) that a patient must pay *before* the health insurance plan begins to help. In other words, this is the amount deducted from what the carrier pays.
■ *Co-insurance:* The share of a health care bill remaining to be paid after the deductible has been applied for which the policyholder is responsible. A typical co-insurance amount is 20 percent.
■ *Co-pay:* The flat fee for health care use that is applied at the location where care is received (e.g., primary care office, pharmacy).

To ensure their financial well-being, insurance carriers apply these components of cost-sharing as an interwoven set to attract potential policyholders and influence the health care–seeking behavior of consumers. For instance, lower premiums are paired with higher deductibles in order to attract consumers with more modest incomes who find the premiums more affordable and who may be willing to tolerate higher deductibles for the relatively infrequent health care that they seek. On the other hand, patients who anticipate frequent health care use often opt for the most affordable higher-premium plan they can find, which typically has lower "user fees"; for example, the deductible, co-insurance, and/or co-pays are more modest than in the lower-premium plans.

By packaging benefits and cost-sharing in ways that attract groups of consumers with particular shared concerns and circumstances, health insurance carriers try to optimize their financial outcomes in ways that may also benefit consumers. The better that an insurance carrier can anticipate the costs of costly, unexpected events in a group of insured individuals (also called *covered lives*) who have access to a plan with certain benefits, the better that the carrier can set a premium and cost-sharing for that plan that will be closer to the real cost of the health care sought by the policyholders. Theory holds that a financial model that is closer to the real cost will be advantageous to consumers in terms of yielding a fairer price. In contrast, when a carrier has a plan with a more heterogeneous group of policyholders, it is typically more difficult for the carrier to anticipate the costs it will face. As a consequence, the carrier will likely build in a cost-structure cushion in the plan to account for uncertainty; the consumers typically experience the cushion as greater cost-sharing and a consequently less affordable plan.

Importantly, one of the most common forms of health insurance in the United States today is private health insurance that is sponsored by employers. Employees are able to pay premiums for such plans with their pre-tax workplace earnings, thereby reducing their taxable income. Moreover, employers commonly pay for a portion of the annual premiums as part of employees' compensation. So-called *group health insurance* of this type has the advantage of making insurance plans more widely available to consumers who may have had difficulty finding a similar plan that was affordable to them in the individual insurance plan market. On the other hand, such plans attract more heterogeneous groups of policyholders, thereby driving up premiums and cost-sharing for the policyholders and their employers.

C. Rising Health Care Costs—Everyone's Concern?

An additional concern for health insurance carriers, over which they have less control, is the cost of health care incurred by policyholders. The following is a fundamental equation in microeconomics:

$$\text{Cost} = \text{Price} \times \text{Quantity}$$

In other words, health care costs rise when prices are higher and/or when the quantity of health care sought by consumers increases. Cost-sharing arrangements involving higher deductibles and co-insurance are known to discourage consumers' use of health care services (although consumers may avoid using necessary as well as unnecessary services), and thereby mitigate increases in quantity. However, the aging population in the United States and the ability of modern medical therapies to help patients live with a reasonable quality of life, despite one or more chronic health conditions, has meant that the frequency of health care encounters has been increasing over time. As costs of health care increase, carriers pass on their higher spending to their consumers.

Another core principle of microeconomics is that prices are driven by the costs of goods and the costs of labor. In the health care context, the costs of goods include the prices of widely used pharmaceuticals and diagnostic tests, which continue to advance in their sophistication and their prices. Some experts have estimated that advances in medical technology such as diagnostic tests and pharmaceuticals have been responsible for as much as 50 percent of the increase in medical spending in the United States over the last several decades. While some of this increased spending is related to broader use (e.g., more patients are undergoing magnetic resonance imaging than in the past), a large component of higher spending is related to the higher price per unit good as well.

In the health care environment, the costs of labor are another major concern. Physicians in the United States are the best paid physicians in the world, but they also face major educational debt liabilities that may limit their incomes. The United States does not have a public system of medical education like peer nations in Europe. The ratio of subspecialty-trained physicians to primary care physicians in the United States is essentially the mirror image of other industrialized nations, which also increases the costs of labor as a per-encounter average. Advanced practice nurses and physician assistants are increasingly involved in primary and subspecialty care settings in the United States and are able to provide high-quality care at lower per-employee costs than physicians. Some physician groups have challenged the scope of practice of advanced practice nurses and physician assistants, which may limit their participation in patient care and thereby limit competition for physicians. While there are evolving interprofessional models of practice involving teams of physicians and other health care professionals that illustrate many efficiencies, especially in pediatric care and some surgical subspecialties, these models have not yet been widely adopted.

As a result, health insurance carriers have turned to various approaches to limit their exposure to higher prices related to the costs of labor. One such approach—network-based benefits design—was discussed earlier. Another approach is related to how health insurance carriers pay health care professionals for services that they provide. In the United States, the original form of payment by insurers is called *fee-for-service*, in which insurance carriers pay health care professionals for services as charged (e.g., by the visit and by the procedure). Fee-for-service arrangements are simple, but they may encourage health care professionals to provide unnecessary care because they will be paid more for doing more.

In contrast, in managed care arrangements, a health insurance carrier contracts with health care professionals on a per-patient (also called *capitated*) basis, in order to set a fee that will be paid from the carrier to the professional regardless of the amount of health care sought by the patient. From the patient perspective, managed care plans are advantageous because they encourage health care professionals to anticipate health care needs and adopt a preventive approach to care (e.g., by administering influenza vaccination) in order to minimize the need for future unexpected visits (e.g., hospitalization for influenza) to manage acute health needs or exacerbations of chronic conditions. From the insurance carrier perspective, managed care arrangements can work well because they provide more certainty for the carrier about how much it will pay health care professionals in a given month.

From the health care professionals' perspective, however, managed care arrangements are sometimes criticized as restricting autonomy and clinical decision making. Health care professionals who provide care that is more expensive than the capitated payment they received from the carrier are left at a financial disadvantage. Anticipating unfavorable financial outcomes can sometimes lead to adversarial, rather than collaborative, relationships between health care professionals and their patients. Frustration with capitation-related limits on care, such as tests that can be performed and medications that can be prescribed, may lead patients and health care professionals alike to place blame on health insurance carriers, while insurance carriers are often working to keep costs within reach of average patients.

In summary, in health insurance plans, consumers and health care professionals are increasingly aware that, while health plans make it possible for patients to get access to expensive health care, the increasing costs of health care related to increasing prices for goods and labor are threatening the very fabric of health care today. That is why measures of health care quality are so important, to help assure that patients and their health care professionals are working toward the same goals of improving care and outcomes. (See Chapters 5 and 6 for more on health care quality and safety.)

D. Government-Sponsored Coverage for Health Care

When the market for private insurance does not provide an affordable option for an individual, that consumer may seek coverage through a government-sponsored program. Government-sponsored programs such as Medicare, Medicaid,

the Veterans Affairs Health System, the TriCare system for active duty military personnel and their dependents, and the Indian Health Service are not health insurance, although they are often referred to that way in the media and general conversation. Rather, these are programs that provide direct benefits for health care to the program enrollees, called *beneficiaries*. Just as a privately insured individual has coverage for health care expenses through a private health insurance plan, an individual enrolled in Medicare also has coverage, but through a different mechanism. Stated another way: All health insurance is a form of health care coverage, but not all health care coverage is health insurance.

As discussed in detail later in this chapter, government-sponsored programs grew out of a need for health care coverage for special populations (e.g., seniors, poor children, veterans, native populations) who were perceived to have particular medical needs that were not being served through the private health insurance market. Such programs are funded by taxpayers and therefore have a fundamentally different responsibility to the public in their financial management than do private insurance plans.

As a result, programs like the Veterans Health Administration (VHA) and Medicare have led the way in implementing cost-control efforts. For example, the VHA contracts with pharmaceutical companies for a limited formulary of prescription drugs for its entire beneficiary population (over 8 million veterans), thereby keeping its acquisition costs low and passing those savings on to the veterans. While the veterans' health care professionals must prescribe within a narrower formulary than many other health care professionals, the superior health outcomes of veterans versus same-age Medicare beneficiaries with regard to heart disease and diabetes suggest that such formulary limits are not limiting appropriate care.

Medicare has pioneered the concept of the accountable care organization (ACO) across the United States in an effort to encourage health care professionals to work together across multiple different settings (emergency department, hospital, primary care, rehabilitation care) to optimize patient outcomes while controlling growth in costs. Under an ACO, Medicare provides a capitated benefit for a broad group of health care professionals and institutions, including hospitals—a substantially broader approach than for managed care contracts of the past. Although the goals of improved quality and controlled cost growth were somewhat challenging for many institutions in the early years of ACOs, there is increasing evidence of the promise of this model. (ACOs are discussed further later in the chapter in remarks about the ACA.)

While these are positive examples of innovations in care financing by government-sponsored programs in the United States, there are also negative examples. For instance, in 2015 the VHA was widely criticized for long wait times for its patients that had been exacerbated by tight budgets for staff. In Medicare, efforts to control hospital-related spending by declaring brief hospital admissions as "observation" stays had the consequence of shifting the majority of costs of hospital care to the beneficiaries, whose Medicare benefits would have otherwise covered the bulk of costs if the brief admissions were designated as routine hospitalizations.

The proportion of the US population with government-sponsored coverage continues to grow steadily, as a result of three phenomena. First, there are demographic shifts. The share of the US population 65 years of age and older has grown, and the proportion of the US population covered by Medicare has increased. The same is true for the number of military veterans in the United States. Second, there are changes in government program eligibility related to persistent poverty and near-poverty in the population. As the income eligibility requirements for Medicaid have become more generous, because of reforms such as the ACA, more poor and low-income individuals have qualified for Medicaid. Third, fewer employers are offering group health insurance plans to their employees over time. As a result, proportions of adults and children covered under private health plans are decreasing, and these individuals have had to seek coverage through government sources (as eligibility permits) or become uninsured.

IV. THEORIES OF HEALTH CARE REFORM

Much of American economic and political ideology is grounded in the market theory first espoused by Adam Smith in the late 1700s: Markets unfettered by government interference are most efficient, producing the appropriate amount of goods or services demanded by consumers through a price mechanism.[18] In the context of the delivery of health care services, however, the producer-to-consumer relationship is not so neatly defined. Is health care a commodity that is sold to consumers like other market commodities? If so, do the usual economic theories that govern the market apply to health care?

Another core component of Smith's theory is that producers and consumers must have symmetric information for a market to function well. In other words, consumers can act in their best interests when they know the true costs of goods and labor that producers face in making a product or delivering a service. Consumers in the US health care system have imperfect information; because they do not know the actual costs of the medical services they receive, they cannot bargain for a better price.[18] Furthermore, consumers with health insurance do not have as much incentive as an uninsured patient to know the costs of health care because most insurance plans shield them from experiencing the full costs of a typical encounter. Another major challenge is that consumers also have imperfect information in choosing their health insurance plans; consumers who are insufficiently informed about the costs of health care cannot make optimal decisions in the choice of insurance plans with different payment structures and benefits. The asymmetry in information among the provider, insurer, and patient leads to what economists call *market failure*. So far, attempts to develop health care cost transparency tools have shown little efficacy in providing consumers with meaningful information in order to inform their decision making.[20]

A. How Much Government Regulation Is Best for US Health Care?

Some government regulation of health insurance, therefore, is needed to maintain a competitive insurance market, protect against monopolies, and provide consumers with information so that they can make informed decisions.[21] The question for health policymakers and reformers interested in improving the health care market is: How much and what types of government regulation can ensure an efficient

market? As discussed later, many of the provisions of the ACA are focused on regulation of the health insurance market to improve competition and create more transparency for consumers.

However, government regulation of the health insurance market is clearly not the only consideration in the debate about the role of government in health care. What about individuals who are outside of the health care market because they have difficulty accessing health insurance and health care in the first place? What is the role of government in ensuring that its citizens have access to health care? These pivotal questions are at the heart of major efforts to reform the US health care system over the last half-century. There are many competing values and principles involved in health system reform efforts. While discussion of all of these considerations is beyond the scope of this chapter, Table 12.1 provides a list of important considerations.

Some of those who argue that the government should play a strong role in health care take issue with the idea that health care services should even be considered a market commodity. Instead, they argue that health care should be considered a right that must be distributed equitably across the population. Some theorists argue that health care is special and different from other social goods because of its impact on equality of opportunity; the government, therefore, has an obligation to ensure fair access to health care in order to enable its people to participate in political, social, and economic systems.[22] Under this theory, health care reform efforts should include considerations of equitable distribution of health care resources.

B. The Politics of Health Care Reform

A lack of shared values and goals has made health care reform difficult in the United States. A majority of Americans do not believe that it is the responsibility of the government to ensure that all citizens have health insurance.[23] Slightly more than one half (54 percent) of Americans rate the quality of health care in the United States as excellent or good, although 79 percent rate their own health care as excellent or good. Yet, the majority believe the health care system has major problems, with one in five believing that it is in a state of crisis.[24]

Table 12.1 Objectives and Corresponding Benchmarks of Fairness in Health Care

Equity	Efficiency	Accountability
Intersectoral public health	Efficacy, efficiency, and quality improvement	Democratic accountability
Financial barriers to equitable access	Administrative efficiency	Patient and provider autonomy
Nonfinancial barriers to access		
Comprehensiveness of benefits and tiering		
Equitable financing		

Adapted from: Daniels N. *Just Health: Meeting Health Needs Fairly*. Cambridge University Press; 2007:246.

In addition to the lack of consensus among policymakers and the American public about the values and goals for health care reform, or even the need for it, the current "system" is a "patchwork of public and private insurance plans; federal, state and local governments; and institutions and individual providers who are often unconnected to one another."[25] In structuring reform efforts, policymakers have had to determine which aspects of the system may be influenced by government regulation, what level of government (federal, state, local) should be charged with administering policy changes, and how much to intervene in the core relationships among health care institutions, providers, and patients in order to improve the system. Furthermore, while there is a great deal of fragmentation in the delivery of health care across multiple settings such as hospitals and primary care, reforms addressing one aspect of the system (e.g., cost containment) inevitably affect other aspects in another (e.g., access to and quality of care).

C. A Brief History of Health Care Reform in the United States

Perhaps the best way to trace the ways in which reform theories, public opinion, and politics have influenced health care policy in the United States is to trace the history of reform successes and failures. Understanding this history is fundamental to providing appropriate historical context for the passage of the most significant recent change to health policy, the ACA in 2010.

1. Proposals for Universal Coverage

For more than 100 years, health care reformers have called for some form of national health insurance. As a Progressive Party candidate in 1912, Theodore Roosevelt proposed a social insurance plan, which included health insurance.[26] His cousin, President Franklin Delano Roosevelt, tried multiple times to enact national health insurance, including attempting to tie it to the Social Security Act of 1935. Yet he was unsuccessful, in part due to the strong opposition from powerful interest groups, particularly physician groups and state medical societies who linked national health insurance to socialism.[26]

President Harry Truman ran on a platform that included national health insurance, winning re-election in 1948. However, he failed to convince Congress, and opposition remained strong from employers and physician groups.[25]

It was not until the 1970s that universal coverage once again reached the national policy debate. Building on the enactment of the Medicare and Medicaid programs in 1965 (discussed in more detail later), Democratic Senator Edward (Ted) Kennedy introduced the Health Security Act in 1970, which would create a single federally operated health insurance program.[29] In response, Republican President Richard Nixon proposed his own comprehensive plan mandating that employers provide private insurance coverage for employees and providing that a government-sponsored program cover everyone else. The Watergate scandal in 1974 derailed these efforts, and it was not until the 1990s that serious attempts were made to provide universal coverage.[26] It is also notable that the Nixon administration was the first to focus policy initiatives on addressing rising health care costs, such as supporting managed care models like health maintenance

organizations (HMOs) to promote "restraint, efficiency and the health of the patient."[25]

In the late 1980s, Physicians for a National Health Program proposed a government-financed health insurance plan, a "single-payer" program, which would replace the multipayer private insurance system. While versions of the single-payer plan were introduced in Congress, none succeeded.[25]

Upon taking office in 1992, President Bill Clinton made health care reform a centerpiece of his administration. His wife, Hillary Clinton, led a White House Task Force leading to a proposed plan called the Health Security Act.[26] In an attempt to achieve universal coverage while emphasizing cost containment, the proposal did not shift coverage from private to public like many prior proposals. Instead, it proposed to create regional "health alliances" that would include various plans competing for business among employers and individuals. To provide for cost containment, it established regional spending limits and caps on premium increases.[25] These proposals, however, were formulated largely behind closed doors, out of sight of an increasingly skeptical Congress. Moreover, the health care insurance industry perceived a strong threat to its market control and organized a successful public marketing campaign to convince mainstream Americans that their private health insurance plans were under attack.

As with many of his predecessors' proposals for reform, President Clinton's plan met with failure in Congress. As health policy expert John McDonough notes, "This failure taught Democrats lessons galore, among them: the president should not micromanage the congressional process and the effort should not threaten coverage of Americans who want to keep what they have." These lessons "weighed on the minds of political veterans who reengaged in 2008"[26] as they once again attempted reform through the ACA.

D. Major Milestones in US Health Care Reform

While many US health care reform efforts met with failure, others have profoundly shaped the system as it exists today. The most momentous change occurred with the passage of the Medicaid and Medicare programs in 1965, but smaller more incremental reforms also set the stage for passage of the ACA in 2010. A few of these are highlighted in the following sections.

1. Medicare and Medicaid

The most significant health care legislative achievement of the twentieth century in the United States came in 1965, when President Lyndon Johnson collaborated with strong Democratic majorities in the US House of Representatives and Senate to win approval for Medicaid and Medicare. Discussed in greater detail later in the chapter, Medicaid and Medicare were structured as safety net programs designed to provide government-funded coverage to those unlikely to access the private insurance market—older adults, disabled individuals, and poor children.

Medicare was financed exclusively by the federal government. In contrast, Medicaid was financed through a combination of federal and state funds, building on a shared financing model for health care for the indigent established over prior years in the federal Kerr-Mills Act. Many believed at the time that Medicaid and Medicare were the precursors to publicly funded universal coverage.[26]

2. Health Insurance Portability and Accountability Act of 1996

Despite the failure of President Clinton's Health Security Act in 1994, he signed the Health Insurance Portability and Accountability Act (HIPAA) into law in 1996. Accomplished through the bipartisan leadership of Democratic Senator Ted Kennedy and Republican Senator Nancy Kassebaum, Title I of the HIPAA addresses concerns about the continuity of coverage for workers and their families upon losing or leaving a job with private employer-based insurance coverage. The law creates a guarantee for eligible workers, so they can obtain health insurance in the group market.

Title II of the law includes provisions for administrative simplification geared toward reducing bureaucratic burdens on health care providers and institutions. One important result of the HIPAA is the rapid expansion of health information technologies (HIT).[26] The HIPAA is perhaps most well-known for its "privacy rule," regulating restricted use and disclosure of protected health information.

3. The State Children's Health Insurance Program

Another bipartisan achievement was the creation of the Children's Health Insurance Program (CHIP) through the Balanced Budget Act of 1997. Republican Senator Orrin Hatch and Democratic Senator Ted Kennedy worked together to establish a 10-year block grant to states to expand health insurance coverage for low-income children, whose family income is too high to meet eligibility requirements for Medicaid.[26] President George W. Bush vetoed re-authorization legislation for the CHIP in 2007 when the initial grant expired, instead signing a temporary expansion. President Barack Obama passed re-authorization legislation in 2009, extending funding until 2013. The ACA extended the program until 2019 with appropriation of funding through 2015.[25] Subsequent legislation enacted in 2015 appropriated CHIP funding through 2017.

E. State Health Care Reform

While the history and milestones in health care reform at the federal level are important for understanding the context for passage of the ACA in 2010, so are examples of state-level health care reforms. A few examples of state reforms that influenced the structure and approach of the ACA are discussed in the following sections.

1. Hawaii

An early state law aimed at expanding health insurance coverage was Hawaii's *Prepaid Health Care Act,* passed in 1974. The law expanded health insurance coverage by mandating that employers provide health insurance to employees working at least 20 hours per week. It also required that employers pay a minimum of 50 percent of the cost of the premium. The employees' share of the premium cannot exceed 1.5 percent of wages.[39] The employer mandate was a precursor to a similar mandate in the ACA.

2. Vermont

In 2011, Vermont enacted *An Act Relating to a Single Payer and Unified Health System,* intending to create the first state single-payer health system in the United States. The law created Green Mountain Care, "a state-funded-and-managed insurance pool that would provide near-universal coverage to residents with the expectation that it would reduce health care spending."[40] The legislation required the legislature to draft a plan for Green Mountain Care by 2013, but the plan was not completed until late 2014. In December 2014, the governor announced that the universal plan would be too costly for the state, requiring a significant tax increase, and the effort was abandoned.[41] The Vermont experience demonstrated the difficulty of achieving major health care system transformation, such as the creation of a single-payer system, without a clear pathway to affordable financing for such a system.

3. Massachusetts

The state health care reform law that most influenced the approach taken in the ACA was the 2006 Massachusetts law signed by Republican Governor Mitt Romney, entitled *An Act Providing Access to Affordable, Quality, Accountable Health Care.* The law contains the following provisions: a mandate that nearly all state residents obtain a minimum level of insurance coverage; sliding-scale subsidized health coverage for individuals with incomes below 300 percent of the federal poverty level (FPL), with fully subsidized coverage for those below 150 percent of the FPL; establishment of the Massachusetts Health Connector, an insurance exchange where consumers can select from private, subsidized, and free health insurance plans depending on their income and eligibility; and a requirement that employers with more than 10 full-time employees provide health insurance.[42]

As apparent later in the chapter, the Massachusetts law strongly influenced the approach taken to expansion of coverage in the ACA. A study of the law's implementation after 6 years concluded that Massachusetts successfully achieved near-universal coverage and improved access to care for its residents, but struggled with rising health care costs that have led to increasing prices for premiums and cost-sharing experienced by Massachusetts consumers.

V. THE PATH TO THE AFFORDABLE CARE ACT

While many of the reforms and milestones at the federal and state levels focused on expansion of coverage, other aspects of the health care system—rising health care costs, research demonstrating poor quality of care, and evidence that US population health outcomes were far worse than peer nations—began to drive the discourse around health care reform. In other words, health services research increasingly pointed to the deficiencies in the health care system itself, not just problems with access to it.

Perhaps most significantly, evidence that the percentage of health care expenditures in the United States had almost doubled between 1980 and 2010 and now far surpassed peer nations led to calls for comprehensive reform. As health policy expert John McDonough notes: "Though the United States spent far more than any other advanced society on medical services, its health system's quality, effectiveness, efficiency, equity, and public health indicators were mediocre at best by international standards."[43]

Reformers began to frame the need for systemic change as multifaceted, recognizing that expanding access without reducing costs or that attempting to reduce costs without attention to quality measurement would be ineffective. The Institute for Healthcare Improvement's Triple Aim provided a framework for addressing the interconnected problems with the system. But despite the calls for reform from health policy advocates, no serious reform would be possible without political leadership, the support of key interest groups, bipartisan compromise, and some indication that health care reform was a priority for the American public.

A. Leadership

During the 2007 primary election, polls indicated that Democratic voters still viewed health care reform as a priority, ranking it second after the economy. Democratic candidates Barack Obama and Hillary Clinton both put forth comprehensive health care proposals, as did Republican candidate John McCain. With the financial crisis of 2008, many thought the newly elected President Obama might not pursue a major piece of legislation focused on health care reform.

However, against the advice of some of his advisors, Obama made health care reform a priority at the beginning of his administration. Aided by the leadership of Senate Majority Leader Harry Reid and House Speaker Nancy Pelosi, Obama held steadfast in pushing comprehensive legislation, despite many setbacks including the loss of former Senator Tom Daschle, his choice to lead the White House Office on Health Reform, to individual tax problems; the death of longtime Democratic champion of health care reform in the Senate, Ted Kennedy, who was replaced by a Republican, Scott Brown; and the challenges of managing multiple competing interests within the Democratic party—liberals pushing for a "public option" health plan to compete with private plans in a newly created marketplace for subsidized health plans versus more conservative Democrats skeptical of too much government involvement.[25]

B. Interest Groups

One of the lessons from President Bill Clinton's failure to pass comprehensive health reform was that without the support of key interest groups, legislation would likely fail. For the first time, interest groups that historically opposed health care reform added their voices to support it. Most notably, the American Medical Association (AMA), which had historically rejected reform efforts focused on expanding coverage and regulating costs, listed health care reform as one of its top priorities. In addition to the AMA, somewhat surprisingly, other key interest groups came to the table: the Pharmaceutical Research and Manufacturers of America, the Federation of American Hospitals, and health insurance industry representatives.[25]

C. Opposition and the Rise of the Tea Party

A new political movement known as the *Tea Party,* consisting of libertarian, conservative, and Republican activists, made defeating Obama's health care initiative the focus of their platform. The Tea Party and other opponents of the law successfully used the media to attack it as a "government takeover" of health care. For example, a provision in the law

creating funding for consultation with Medicare recipients for advanced care planning once every 5 years or more frequently if they became seriously ill was characterized as the creation of "death panels," in which bureaucrats would determine whether or not to provide medical care to older adults and disabled individuals. Although the claim was discredited, it resonated with some Americans, who were already skeptical about a larger role for government in health care.[44]

D. Compromise

While Obama favored the public option strongly supported by liberal Democrats, ultimately political pragmatism won out over principle to achieve successful passage of reform legislation. The Obama administration also made concessions to the insurance and pharmaceutical industries to achieve their support.[45] As Jonathan Oberlander explains, the final bill was the result of multiple compromises to ensure passage: "Political pragmatism carried the day as reformers made compromises on a range of additional issues—abortion, cost control, the scope of benefits, the narrowing of universal into 'near' universal coverage—in order to pass legislation. The all-or-nothing mind-set that more than once has sunk health care reform was history."[45]

E. Passage of the Affordable Care Act

President Obama signed the ACA into law after a year-long national debate. The law was passed by a Democratic-controlled House and Senate, without any Republican support. Despite the lack of support from Republicans, the final law is more reflective of prior proposals by Republicans for employer mandates for private insurance than by Democrats for single-payer or expanded publicly funded options. In fact, as discussed earlier, the ACA is modeled on the Massachusetts law supported by Republican Governor Mitt Romney.[29] Polls continue to show that public opinion is deeply divided about the law, with the majority of Democratic voters in favor of the law and the majority of Republican voters against it. As of January 2016, 65 percent of Democrats supported the law, while less than 15 percent of Republicans did.[46]

F. The Major Components of the Affordable Care Act

Although the ACA has 10 titles, or major sections (Table 12.2), it is easier to break the key components of the law into four categories: 1) expanded access to health insurance, 2) consumer benefits and protections, 3) cost-saving mechanisms, and 4) quality improvement measures. Each of these is discussed briefly in the following sections.

G. Expanded Access to Health Insurance

The ACA strives for near-universal access to coverage for all Americans through several important mechanisms. All of these provisions went into effect by 2014.

1. The Individual Mandate

First, the law creates an "individual mandate" requiring that all individuals maintain "minimum essential health

Table 12.2 Ten Central Components of the Affordable Care Act

Title	Name	Purpose
I	Quality Affordable Coverage	To expand private health insurance coverage and to strengthen federal regulation of health insurance industry
II	Role of Public Programs	To expand and improve Medicaid for lower-income adults and families
III	Improving Quality and Efficiency in Health Care	To improve the quality, efficiency, and effectiveness of medical care, especially in the Medicare program
IV	Preventing Chronic Disease and Improving Public Health	To advance health promotion and disease prevention, and to strengthen public health
V	Healthcare Workforce	To increase the numbers and improve the quality of the US healthcare workforce
VI	Transparency and Program Integrity	To combat fraud and abuse, to promote transparency in healthcare, to advance comparative effectiveness research
VII	Innovative Medical Therapies	To permit the manufacture, marketing, and sale of biopharmaceutical similar to drugs (biosimilars)
VIII	Community Living Assistance Services and Supports	To create an insurance program to provide cash assistance to disabled persons (repealed on 1/1/2013)
IX	Revenue Provisions	To establish new taxes and fees to pay for the programs and benefits created in the law
X	Strengthening Healthcare for All Americans	Composed of amendments and new additions to title I-IX

From McDonough JE. The United States health system in transition. *Health Systems & Reform.* 2015;1:1, 39–51.

coverage" or pay a fine implemented as part of paying federal taxes. The individual mandate is necessary in order to create a large risk pool of premium-paying individuals to support the other insurance reforms required in the Act. Specifically, for insurers to provide coverage to previously uninsured individuals, particularly less healthy ones, the pool must include younger and healthier individuals whose premiums help to support these individuals.

2. The Employer Mandate

In addition to the individual mandate, the law requires employers with 50 or more employees to offer affordable health insurance or pay a penalty.

3. Premium Subsidies

The law makes it possible for low-income individuals (between 100 percent and 400 percent of the FPL), who do not qualify for Medicaid or may not have access to employer-sponsored plans, to purchase insurance by subsidizing (providing a tax credit toward) the cost of the premium.

4. Health Insurance Exchanges

To create a stronger and more regulated insurance market in order to offer consumers more transparency and lower-cost insurance options, the law creates health insurance exchanges. These exchanges serve as a competitive marketplace through which individuals can select and purchase insurance.

5. Medicaid Expansion

The ACA provides federal support to states to expand their Medicaid programs to cover all eligible US citizens and legal immigrants with incomes below 133 percent of the FPL. As

discussed in the following sections, the original intent of the law was that all states would expand their Medicaid programs, but a Supreme Court decision made this provision optional for states.

H. Consumer Benefits and Protections

One of the fundamental changes made by the law to the insurance industry was to restrict certain insurance company practices such as pre-existing conditions exclusions and discriminatory enrollment practices based on health status. The law also maintains coverage for young adults, who may have difficulty finding coverage through employment or affording it on their own by guaranteeing dependent coverage (through their parents' plan) until 26 years of age.

Insurers must also provide under the plan a set of "essential health benefits" through one of four categories of plans, known as *bronze, silver, gold,* and *platinum* within defined cost-sharing limits. To promote preventive care, the law requires that new health insurance plans must cover certain preventive services for free, without cost sharing. These include: services with an "A" or "B" rating from the US Preventive Services Task Force; immunizations recommended by the Centers for Disease Control and Prevention (CDC); and screening and preventive care for women based on guidelines from the Health Resources and Services Administration.

I. Cost-Saving Mechanisms

The ACA is financed primarily through savings that are expected to be realized from changes to Medicaid and Medicare, as well as tax provisions and fees. Some of the Medicare cost savings will be achieved by reducing payments for preventable hospital re-admissions and hospital-acquired infections; reducing reimbursement rates and imposing cost-sharing limits for Medicare-managed care plans; and increasing the Medicare Part A (hospitalization) tax rate and reducing Medicare Part D (prescription drug) subsidies for high-income beneficiaries.

Reduction in Medicaid spending comes from reduced payments to Disproportionate Share Hospitals (DSH), which have traditionally received federal funds to provide uncompensated care in low-income communities. This provision was based on the expectation that the expansion of Medicaid would lead to fewer uninsured patients using hospital services. Savings are also expected to be realized through rebates to Medicaid programs from drug manufacturers.

The law also includes several taxes and fees. For example, the ACA imposes a tax on indoor tanning services and medical devices and imposes annual fees on the pharmaceutical manufacturing industry.[25]

CASE STUDY 1

Jacinta and Evelyn are cousins in their mid-fifties. They both have diabetes and take oral medications, but with progressively worse blood sugar control over the past few years. Jacinta lives in Michigan, which expanded income eligibility for low-income adults through its Medicaid program in 2014 with support from the ACA. Evelyn lives in Georgia, which chose not to expand its Medicaid eligibility. Both Jacinta and Evelyn hold a combination of part-time jobs that do not offer health insurance benefits. Both have incomes that place them just below the poverty line.

Although they were both uninsured as recently as 2013, their respective state programs now present quite different options for the cousins. In Michigan, Jacinta has signed up for the expanded Medicaid program and now has health insurance that covers hospitalizations, doctor visits, emergency care, prescription medications, mental health visits, and dental care. In Georgia, Evelyn is not eligible for the Medicaid program, which only provides coverage for individuals at lower incomes than hers. She cannot find a health plan that is affordable for her.
- What policy decisions led to the differing circumstances for these women regarding availability of government-sponsored health insurance?
- How does having health insurance alter Jacinta's behavior regarding seeking health care?
- How does not having health insurance alter Evelyn's behavior regarding seeking health care?
- What are some policy options that might make health care more affordable for both cousins, while also constraining growth in health care spending?

J. Quality Improvement Measures

The architects of the ACA sought to not only address access and cost savings, but support for quality improvement measures as well. The law establishes the National Quality Strategy, led by the Agency for Healthcare Research and Quality (AHRQ), to set priorities for quality improvement and to develop quality measures. Also established was the Patient-Centered Outcomes Research Institute (PCORI), to "identify critical research questions, fund patient-centered comparative clinical effectiveness research, and disseminate the results."[47]

K. Linking Quality Improvement and Payment Reform

In addition to establishing these initiatives, the law supports a range of demonstration and pilot programs designed to improve the quality and safety of care while also reducing unnecessary costs. These include models of care that shift to a managed care approach that emphasizes quality of care with a focus on reducing costs by improving the coordination of care. These include ACOs and patient-centered medical homes, discussed later in the chapter.

L. Prevention and Public Health

As noted earlier, in addition to addressing increasing health care costs, reformers were also guided by the increasing body of research pointing to poor US population health outcomes. The ACA contains a range of provisions aimed at prevention and public health, including the establishment of the National Prevention, Health Promotion and Public Health Council, whose primary task is to create and implement the National Prevention Strategy (NPS), and a Prevention and Public Health Fund to support initiatives aimed at improving public health and reducing medical costs. The Prevention and Public Health Fund, for example, provides grants to local communities to implement proven practices to improve nutrition and physical activity, reduce tobacco use, and control blood pressure and cholesterol.

Perhaps most importantly, the ACA fosters collaboration between health care, public health departments, and community organizations to address population health needs. The law requires that, in order for nonprofit hospitals to maintain their tax-exempt status, every 3 years they must conduct a community health needs assessment and develop an implementation plan to address identified needs. In creating its plan, the hospital must include "input from people who represent the broad interests of the community served by the hospital facility, including those with special knowledge of, or expertise in, public health."[48] The IRS regulations governing community health needs assessments take an expansive view of community health: hospitals should identify "not only the need to address financial and other barriers to care but also the need to prevent illness, to ensure adequate nutrition, or to address social, behavioral, and environmental factors that influence health in the community."[49]

M. Health Equity

Parts of the ACA also explicitly focus on reducing health disparities and promoting health equity. These include requirements regarding the collection and reporting of data by race, ethnicity, and language; expansion of workforce diversity; support for cultural competence education and model curricula; promotion of health disparities research; prevention initiatives targeted at underserved communities; and expanding access to insurance coverage.[50] Some of these provisions are highlighted briefly here.

1. Equity in Insurance Rates

There are significant racial/ethnic disparities in insurance coverage. Latinos are more than three times as likely to be uninsured as non-Hispanic whites, while African-Americans are nearly twice as likely to be uninsured.[50] Since passage of the ACA, uninsured rates have declined for both African-Americans and Latinos. Between 2010 and 2014, uninsured rates for African-Americans declined from 24 percent to 18 percent. The uninsured rate for Latinos declined from 39 percent to 34 percent.[51]

These rates were expected to decline even more with the insurance expansions of the ACA, but because roughly one-half of the states decided not to expand their Medicaid programs, declines in the uninsured rates have not been as robust as expected. One-quarter of Latino adults who live in states that expanded their Medicaid programs were uninsured by the end of 2014, while nearly one-half remain uninsured in states that had not.[51]

2. Access to Care

The ACA significantly expanded funding for community health centers, which provide primary care to predominantly low-income and diverse patient populations. In addition to expansion of access through community health centers, the ACA contains other provisions aimed at improving access to care for underserved populations, such as support for nurse-managed health centers, community health workers, and school-based health centers.[50]

3. Expanded Civil Rights Protections

Prior to the ACA, civil rights laws enforced by the US Department of Health and Human Services Office for Civil Rights (OCR) barred discrimination in health care based on race, color, national origin, disability, or age. Section 1557 of the ACA extends civil rights protections to ban sex discrimination in health programs, and applies those protections to "Health Insurance Marketplaces, any health program that HHS itself administers, and any health program or activity, any part of which receives funding from HHS, such as hospitals that accept Medicare patients or doctors who treat Medicaid patients."[52]

Some of the key civil rights provisions under the ACA and proposed HHS rules are as follows:

- Prohibits women from being charged more than men for health insurance coverage or discrimination in health services.
- Prohibits categorical exclusions on coverage of all care related to gender transition and ensuring that individuals must also be treated consistent with their gender identity, including in access to facilities.
- Provides requirements regarding provision of language services, such as oral interpreters and written translations for patients with limited English proficiency, including in health insurance exchanges.
- Provides requirements for the provision of auxiliary aids and services and accessibility of programs offered through electronic and information technology for individuals with disabilities.[52]

CASE STUDY 2

Joe is a car mechanic, and his wife Susan works for the local grocery store in their rural community. Together they earn about $2400 a month. What are their options for health insurance?

Option 1: Joe and Susan are covered by an insurance plan administered by the federal government. The insurance plan is funded by taxes paid by Joe and Susan's employers, a relatively small tax paid by Joe and Susan on their wages, with the rest financed by federal income taxes.

Option 2: Joe and Susan pay a percentage of their income into a regional health insurance fund. Their employers are mandated to pay into the fund as well, based on a state formula, and the state government pays the remaining amount to cover Joe and Susan under a state-administered health insurance plan.

Option 3: While some employers (those with 50 or more employees) are mandated to offer health insurance to their employees, neither Joe nor Susan's employers fall under this requirement. Instead, Joe and Susan are required to purchase health insurance through a state-run health insurance exchange. They can purchase a plan based on their needs and desires with regard to what services will be covered, how large a deductible they will pay, and the monthly premium.

Consider the pros and cons of each of these options. Which one would you prefer?

- If you were Joe or Susan?
- If you were a government official?
- If you were a health insurer?
- If you were a health care provider?

N. The Affordable Care Act: Implementation Successes and Challenges

The law has been subject to legal challenges, technology disasters, delays, and repeated criticism, including over 50 votes in the House of Representatives to repeal it. The Senate joined the House in late 2015 in voting to repeal the ACA but did not have enough votes to override a veto from President Obama. On the other hand, the ACA has also had some important successes, highlights of which are outlined in the following sections.

1. Legal Challenges

Immediately after the ACA was passed, legal challenges were brought by opponents of the law, claiming that some of its provisions violated the US Constitution. Other lawsuits followed, alleging that the ACA violated federal law protecting religious rights and asking the court to interpret the law's provisions as not allowing for insurance subsidies to individuals living in states that used the federal health insurance exchange instead of a state exchange. Three of these cases made it to the Supreme Court.

2. National Federation of Independent Business v. Sebelius (2012)

Brought by 26 states, several individuals, and the National Federation of Independent Business, this lawsuit challenged the constitutionality of the individual mandate and Medicaid expansion under the ACA. First, the suit alleged that Congress did not have the authority to require individuals to carry health insurance. The Supreme Court upheld the law's individual mandate. Second, the suit alleged that the mandatory expansion of Medicaid under the ACA was overly coercive of the states because it threatened that if a state did not participate, it would lose all of its federal Medicaid funding. On this point, the court agreed that the law was unconstitutional.[52]

Essentially, the court said that states may decide whether to participate in Medicaid expansion, making this portion of the ACA optional. Approximately one-half of the states have chosen to participate, thereby undermining a major component of coverage expansion on which ACA proponents had founded estimates of impact of the law.

3. Burwell v. Hobby Lobby (2014)

This case challenged the contraception requirements adopted by the HHS under the ACA provisions for the types of preventive care for women that should be covered in certain employer-based health plans. HHS exempted certain employers, including religious organizations.

Hobby Lobby, a closely held for-profit corporation, filed suit under the federal Religious Freedom Restoration Act (RFRA), arguing that it should not be required to provide coverage for four specific types of contraception (morning after pills and intrauterine devices) to which it objected based on religious beliefs. Citing the importance of protections for religious beliefs, the Court held that the government's contraceptive requirement was not the "least restrictive" means of ensuring access to contraceptive care. It is the first time that the Court has allowed a corporation to claim a religious exemption.[53]

4. King v. Burwell (2015)

This suit challenged the authority of the federal HHS to issue regulations regarding both state-run and the federal health insurance exchanges, arguing that the language in the ACA only allowed for subsidies for individuals who obtained their insurance through state exchanges, not federal exchanges. The challenge was particularly important because nearly 5 million people had obtained their insurance through federal exchanges at the time of the lawsuit, and because, if the challenge to the ACA was successful, people in the thirty-four states that had not set up state insurance exchanges for federally subsidized plans would lose their insurance subsidies.

The Supreme Court rejected the argument that the language in the ACA only refers to exchanges set up by the states. Many saw the case as critical to survival of the ACA since, had the court found that the subsidies only applied to insurance obtained through the small number of state exchanges and not the federal exchange, it would have substantially undermined the insurance expansion goals that were fundamental to the Act.[54]

5. Delays and Problems with Launch of the Federal Exchange

Implementing a law as complex as the ACA and that substantially reorders the health insurance industry has faced major logistic challenges. While the Obama administration engaged in a substantial effort to issue regulations in order to implement the law on schedule (reportedly more than 20,000 pages of regulations), parts of the law were delayed. The employer mandate was delayed by 1 year for larger employers and 2 years for smaller employers. Deadlines for consumers to purchase insurance have been delayed more than once.

The most notable implementation problem was with the launch of the federal exchange website: www.healthcare.gov. While some states implemented their own exchanges, most did not and consumers from these states were reliant on the federal exchange to purchase insurance. The federal exchange website was scheduled to launch on October 1, 2013, with a deadline for consumers to purchase insurance by January 1, 2014, or face a penalty. However, major technology problems with the federal website meant that the deadline was extended to April 15, 2014, and the information technology gaffes initially undermined public confidence in the program.

6. Enrollment

After the 2014 deadline, the Obama administration reported that 8 million individuals enrolled in private insurance plans through either a state exchange or the federal exchange.[55] An additional 4.8 million individuals enrolled in Medicaid in the states that expanded their programs.[43] Another 7.8 million adults between 19 and 25 years of age were enrolled in parents' plans under the provisions of the ACA enacted in late 2010, 6 months after the law was enacted.[56] The Congressional Budget Office estimates that by 2017, 25 million formerly uninsured individuals will have enrolled in ACA-sponsored coverage initiatives.

While substantial strides in health insurance coverage have been made since 2014, it is estimated that 13 percent of nonelderly adults are still uninsured. Fig. 12.5 illustrates the reasons given for being uninsured among adults. Many still view insurance as simply too expensive. Another notable factor for remaining uninsured is whether or not a low-income individual lives in a state that did not expand its Medicaid program. States that expanded Medicaid were twice as likely to see drops in uninsured rates as states that did not.[57]

7. Systems and Payment Reforms

As discussed earlier, the ACA contains multiple provisions for reforming the health care delivery system. The following is a progress report on some of those provisions as of late 2015. These reforms are all intended to achieve the Triple Aim, but the long-term effects of these innovations on the health care system remain to be determined:

- Four hundred Shared Savings ACOs serving nearly 7.2 million beneficiaries, roughly 14 percent of the Medicare population: A study in 2013 found that less than one-half of the ACOs met quality and spending benchmarks and generated roughly $315 million in shared savings. The remaining ACOs failed to fulfill requirements to measure the quality of care delivered to patients or did not reduce spending enough to meet the minimum criteria to share in savings.[58]
- Nearly 7000 practices have achieved patient-centered medical home status.[43]
- As of October 1, 2015, 1618 participants including acute-care hospitals, physician group practices, home health agencies, inpatient rehabilitation facilities, long-term care hospitals, and skilled nursing facilities were

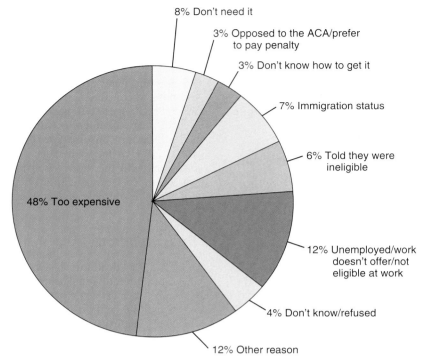

Fig. 12.5 **Reasons for being uninsured as provided by uninsured adults* during the Affordable Care Act era.** *Note: Includes uninsured adults 19 to 64 years of age. (From Kaiser Family Foundation. *Key Facts about the Uninsured Population.* October 5, 2015. http://kff.org/uninsured/fact-sheet/key-facts-about-the-uninsured-population/.)

participating in the Centers for Medicare and Medicaid Services' (CMS) Bundled Payments for Care Improvement Initiative.[59]

Case Study 3

Michael Weatherstone is a 60-year-old family physician who has practiced in a small town since he finished residency. He has been in practice for so long in the same community that he has treated two and sometimes three generations of families. He knows his patients by name, often runs into them in the supermarket, and even sometimes makes house calls in the middle of the night, if necessary.

Dr. Weatherstone's daughter, Sarah, is finishing her family medicine residency at a primary care clinic in an urban hospital. She has two small children and does not want to have the kind of perpetually on-call lifestyle that her father has had in his career. She prefers a salaried job that allows her more work-life balance; yet she also hopes to develop strong relationships with her patients and to be engaged in the larger community where she will practice.

- With the changing health care system, what type of practice might Sarah find or develop that will allow her to fulfill her professional objectives?
- How might Sarah team up with other health care professionals to achieve her practice goals?
- What role might technology play in Sarah's practice?
- How will Sarah's practice likely be different from that of her father?
- How will provisions of the ACA affect her patients' coverage?

O. The Effect of the Affordable Care Act on Health Care Delivery

1. Patients

The most significant impact of passage of the ACA on patients is expanded access to affordable health insurance and the creation of exchanges that should make obtaining insurance easier and more transparent. Support for consumers through patient navigation and community-based outreach efforts continue to be important in ensuring that individuals, particularly those from vulnerable populations, are able to access care.

The newly insured, in particular, need support and education about how to be "informed and empowered" health care consumers.[60] Additionally, as discussed earlier, there remain substantial gaps in coverage for some groups of Americans. Even with full implementation of the ACA, there will continue to be a substantial number of Americans who do not have health insurance and who lack a regular source of primary care, making them vulnerable to both poor health and potentially unaffordable out-of-pocket costs.

On the other hand, many patients who were previously uninsured or who were underinsured will see improved coverage under the ACA's essential health benefits provisions. Preventive services for which they may have previously had to pay for out of pocket, or that included large co-pays, are now fully covered.

Beyond expansion of coverage, the ACA places a focus on patient-centered care and shared decision making. Regulations under the ACA emphasize the use of patient satisfaction surveys, and many of the quality measures described in the ACA are linked to patient experience of care. Additionally, provisions encouraging patient voices in research (such as PCORI) offer patients an opportunity to advocate for better health care.

Finally, the ACA's emphasis on care integration, accountability for population health, and community-based health improvement initiatives also have the potential to both strengthen the patient experience of care as well as to improve overall health.[61]

2. Health Care Professionals

Recognizing the need for expanded access to primary care as more individuals become insured, the ACA included a 10 percent bonus for primary care professionals working in underserved areas between 2011 and 2015. It also increased Medicaid reimbursement for certain services to create parity with Medicare to encourage more doctors to accept newly enrolled Medicaid patients in 2013 and 2014.[62] The extent to which the increased need for primary care will lead to physician shortages is debated, with some suggesting that the system will experience serious shortages[63] and others asserting that the system will be able to absorb new patients.[64]

As the ACA shifts payment for medical services away from fee-for-service toward other methodologies such as bundled payments, patient-centered medical homes, and ACOs, physicians will need to adapt not only to the new payment structure, but also to the cultural changes to the practice of medicine brought about by these payment reforms.

Through incentives under the ACA for reform, clinical decision making is shifting toward a team-oriented approach in which the physician works with other health care professionals to provide patient care. In addition, efforts to reduce costs and better coordinate care rely on technology, particularly the electronic health record. Finally, consolidation of the health care market will mean that physicians are more likely to work for larger entities than they have in the past.

3. Health Care Institutions

The ACA contains many provisions aimed at improving quality and decreasing costs in hospital care. One particular focus is on reducing rates of hospital re-admissions. Many of these provisions tie quality measures to payment to incentivize institutional reforms and encourage a movement away from fee-for-service payment. The ACA holds hospitals accountable for their 30-day re-admission rates for several conditions (e.g., heart attacks) and for hospital-acquired infections with financial penalties.

An additional challenge for hospitals located in states that chose not to expand Medicaid is the ACA's cut to Disproportionate Share Hospital (DSH) payments. These payments are made to hospitals that serve a large number of Medicaid and uninsured patients to help cover the costs of uncompensated care. The architects of the ACA anticipated that hospitals' provision of uncompensated care would decline substantially as more low-income individuals enrolled in Medicaid. However, even with full implementation of ACA provisions, over 10 percent of nonelderly adults are expected to be uninsured and will likely continue to need hospital care. These include poor adults living in states that did not expand Medicaid, immigrants who are not eligible for coverage, and those individuals who choose not to or cannot afford insurance even with the subsidies provided under the ACA. Moreover, hospitals in states that chose not to expand Medicaid face serious budgetary crises when these cuts go into effect in 2018 as they remain on the hook for uncompensated care.[65]

VI. POLICY CONTROVERSIES AND UNFINISHED BUSINESS

A. Legislation Versus Rule Making

Establishing and implementing public health policy is a two-part process requiring legislative law and administrative law, respectively. Legislative law, or *statute* (how a bill becomes a law), is the underlying legal language, written in precise form, like the computer programming code for a smart phone app. Administrative law, or *rule* (how a law becomes a rule), is the translation of the statute into the more operational language of a rule to authorize and guide how public agencies establish or modify programs that provide goods or services. This more prosaic process is like the graphic user interface and operating manual for your smartphone app.

A law is enacted when a bill is introduced by a member (sponsor) of Congress, passed by a majority of the relevant subcommittee and then full committee with jurisdiction over the issue, then by the House (at least 218 votes) and Senate (at least 51 votes) in identical form, and finally signed by the president. Most bills never see the light of day in the subcommittee, let alone be considered or voted on by the House or Senate or make it to the president's desk.

While that is challenging enough, it is only half the battle with regard to implementing a health policy change. In the federal rulemaking process, the Executive Branch agency authorized in the law must prepare a Notification of Proposed Rulemaking (NPRM)—the draft language for the administrative law. For health care policy, this is usually one of the agencies in the HHS, such as the CMS, the Food and Drug Administration (FDA), the National Institutes of Health (NIH), the CDC, the AHRQ, and so on. The proposed rule is open for public comment for 1 to 3 months. The agency then compiles and considers the comments and revises the NPRM into a final rule in the context of the authorizing statute.

In practice, law and rule making is often an iterative process, with congressional and agency staff consulting with each other as they draft language. Key stakeholders and constituencies (interest groups and citizens) have multiple opportunities to advocate and to shape a particular policy through both the legislative and administrative lawmaking process (Fig. 12.6). Each provides several decision points and opportunities for leverage by advocates.

B. Health Care Workforce Policy

Health care in the United States is delivered by a multitude of health care professionals, including physicians, nurses, nurse practitioners, physician assistants, pharmacists, dentists, and many others.[66] The size and distribution of this health care workforce (by profession, specialty, geography, gender, race/ethnicity, and so on) is shaped more by local practice models, marketplaces, reimbursement, and educational pipelines than by public policies to align the workforce with society's health care needs.[67] Unlike many peer nations, the United States does

Opportunities for Health Policy Advocacy

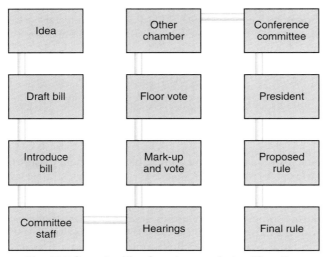

Fig. 12.6 **Opportunities for advocacy in health policy.**

not have a centralized body to shape the size or distribution of the health care workforce in response to needs for equitable access, geographic distribution, or workforce efficiency.

Members of Congress and their staff regularly meet with representatives of the various professional and specialty groups of health care providers. Groups of providers frequently project a shortage in their ranks and advocate for policies to remedy this gap. Without an unbiased source of information regarding workforce demand and supply, Congress has been reluctant to weigh in on this issue. Policies to shape workforce generally create winners and losers and, thus, happy and unhappy political constituents.

To address this shortcoming in federal health care workforce policy, the ACA included a provision (Sec. 5101) to authorize the establishment of a new National Health Care Workforce Commission, tasked with reviewing health care workforce and projected workforce needs. The Commission would provide comprehensive, unbiased information to Congress and the Administration about how to align health care workforce resources with national needs. Congress would use this information when providing appropriations to discretionary programs or in restructuring other federal funding sources.

However, as with many new authorizing statutes, no activity is permitted until Congress also appropriates funds for that purpose. To date, Congress has not passed the appropriation of $3 million required to establish the Workforce Commission and initiate its work. This level of funding is small, and thus the lack of appropriation is an expression of political opposition to the ACA.

C. Authorization Versus Appropriation Legislation (and Three Kinds of Money)

Action by authorizing and appropriation committees of the Congress is required for many policies to be fully implemented. Authorizing Committees establish or modify programs. In health policy, these committees in the House of Representatives are Ways and Means (W&M), Energy and Commerce (E&C), and Education and Labor (E&L). Their counterparts in the Senate are the Senate Finance Committee (SFC) and the Health, Education, Labor, and Pensions (HELP) Committee.

Appropriations committees (12, each paired in the House and Senate) determine how much federal funding is allocated to discretionary programs for each fiscal year through the federal budgeting process, across all federal agencies. About one-third of all federal spending goes to these discretionary programs (e.g., funding for NIH research, CDC, transportation, housing, education), and their funding levels must be appropriated annually. For health-related programs, the appropriation committees in the House and Senate determine these funding levels. This is a highly contentious, political process because increasing funds to one program generally requires reducing funds to another in this zero-sum game in each year's budget negotiations.

In contrast to discretionary funding, about two-thirds of all federal spending is direct or mandatory (e.g., Medicare, Social Security), which guarantees funds for these services for as many Americans as are eligible; such services are referred to as *entitlement programs.* Mandatory funding does not require annual appropriations and can only be changed by modifying the underlying authorizing statute.

Besides mandatory and discretionary spending, there is a third kind of money in federal policy: tax spending. Operating with much less public attention than the first two kinds, tax spending is also a powerful and stealthy lever in shaping policy. Tax spending is "revenue foregone," money that would normally have come in as taxes but is, instead, kept by the taxpayer for other uses. This is usually implemented via a tax deduction or tax credit. Since the money never actually comes into the US Treasury, tax spending is an indirect form of spending. It may seem odd to refer to tax policy as a form of federal spending, but for budgeting purposes, money that is not collected as taxes is equivalent to money that comes in and then goes out. Tax spending is rarely noted as part of the federal budget; few realize that in addition to the $3.5 billion in mandatory and discretionary spending in 2011, the United States spent $1.1 billion in such tax spending. The two largest sources of tax spending are the home mortgage interest deduction and the pretax deduction of health insurance premiums.

D. Graduate Medical Education Policy

Graduate medical education (GME) is the pathway through which resident physicians in all specialties develop the competence to practice independently. As another example of the decentralized processes shaping the US physician workforce, GME policy is mostly controlled by medical professional regulatory bodies—the Accreditation Council for Graduate Medical Education (ACGME) and the American Board of Medical Specialties (ABMS)—and influenced by powerful hospital and physician interest groups. Examples include the Association of American Medical Colleges (AAMC) and the AMA. These groups generally advocate for expanded GME funding and for lifting the caps for the number of Medicare-funded residency positions that have been frozen at 1996 levels, but also promote innovation in medical education.[66,67]

However, many professional organizations agree that the guaranteed federal funding policy of GME (more than $15 billion annually, mainly via Medicare and Medicaid) is not well-aligned with the health care needs of the nation.[68,69] In a critical report in 2014, the Institute of Medicine (IOM) described a number of concerns about the US system of GME, including a mismatch between the health needs of the population and the specialty makeup of the physician workforce; persistent geographic maldistribution of physicians; insufficient diversity in the physician population; a gap between new physicians' knowledge and skills and the competencies required for current medical practice; and a lack of fiscal transparency. The IOM recommended significant reforms to GME financing and regulatory policy to address these concerns, rationalizing and aligning GME policy with US physician workforce needs, and promoting innovation, and increase accountability and transparency of GME programs.

With growing pressure toward fiscal austerity and responsible stewardship of taxpayer dollars, GME funding is perceived as vulnerable. This could provide an opportunity to reform the GME financing system and to use such policy change to reshape the physician workforce.

VII. CHAPTER SUMMARY

Health policy in the United States is inherently complex—just as clinical medicine is complex. Today's evolving health care system in the United States, with the highest per capita spending of any country in the world, is the result of a century of progressively increasing public demand for technologically advanced medical care delivered by a subspecialty-dominated workforce, paid for through a uniquely American combination of private insurance plans and government-sponsored programs. Political debates about health care have been some of the most acrimonious political struggles of the last 50 years, yet have also led to programmatic lynchpins of the current system (Medicare, Medicaid) that currently provide coverage for almost 120 million Americans.

Moreover, there are disparities in health and health care for patients in the United States based on socio-demographic characteristics and geography—such as whether or not an individual lives in a state that decided to expand Medicaid eligibility under the ACA. While health care professionals can address some of these disparities through the care they provide, health policy presents an indispensable avenue for standardizing approaches across the US health care system and ensuring that high-quality, affordable care is accessible to as many patients as possible.

The long-term sustainability of the US health care system, especially as paid for through government programs, rests on successful containment of perpetually rising health care costs that are progressively consuming greater shares of the GDP. State-level health care reforms that set the stage for the ACA, and the ACA itself, principally focused on expanding coverage rather than controlling costs. While cost control is not a broadly popular focus for policy reform because the public perceives that such reforms will limit their access to care, financial realities for government programs and private health insurance plans are likely to lead to increasing pressures on health care professionals and patients to adjust to a system with more constraints than they have experienced previously.

By understanding core principles and aspects of health policy in the United States today, physicians and other health care professionals can appreciate essential contextual details at the federal, state, and local levels that will help them provide high-quality care that is affordable for their patients. Individuals who are inclined toward advocacy may also decide to support future reforms in the US health care system. After all, despite multiple reform initiatives and clinical care that is popularly perceived as second to none in the world, the US population has poorer population health outcomes than in peer nations, despite spending substantially more per person on health care.

QUESTIONS FOR FURTHER THOUGHT

1. Describe core components of the Affordable Care Act that attempt to address the Triple Aim.
2. Why does the US health care system include such a patchwork quilt of private health insurance plans and government-sponsored coverage?
3. What is the difference between health coverage and health insurance? Why are some forms of health coverage not health insurance?
4. For a health policy question that concerns you, consider which stakeholders influence how that policy has been formed and how it affects the US health care system today. Which stakeholders currently seem most influential? Which stakeholders seem least influential? What would have to change to shift the balance of influence among stakeholders?

Annotated Bibliography

Askin E, Moore N, Shankar V, Peck W. *The Health Care Handbook: A Clear and Concise Guide to the United States Health Care System*. 2nd ed. St. Louis, MO: Academic Publishing Services, Washington University School of Medicine; 2014.
This is a very clear user's manual that explains the US health care system and the policies that will change it. It is an excellent guide to the people, organizations, and industries that make up the US health care system and major issues the system faces today. It is rigorously researched and scrupulously unbiased yet written in a conversational and humorous tone.
Blumenthal D, Morone J. *The Heart of Power: Health and Politics in the Oval Office*. Los Angeles, CA: University of California Press; 2010.
This engaging text offers a detailed examination of how several US presidents (from Franklin D. Roosevelt to George W. Bush) have wrestled with health policy challenges of the nation while also frequently facing health problems for themselves and their families.
McDonough JE. *Inside National Health Reform*. New York: Milbank Memorial Fund; 2011.
This book offers a fascinating look at the inside politics of health reform, with a detailed account of the passage and provisions of the Affordable Care Act.
Teitelbaum JB, Wilensky SE. *Essentials of Health Policy and Law*. 3rd ed. Burlington, MA: Jones & Bartlett; 2016.
This book covers the essentials of health policy and law, with topics ranging from health care economics to health care reform to the public health system. It is very accessible for readers who are not well-versed in health policy and includes discussion questions and case studies. It is regularly updated to keep up with the changing policy landscape.

References

1. Coggon J. *What Makes Health Public? A Critical Evaluation of Moral, Legal, and Political Claims in Public Health*. Vol. 15. Cambridge University Press; 2012.
2. Schwartz MD. Rules of the game. In: Sessums S, Moran B, Rich E, Dennis L, Liebow M, eds. *Clinicians and Health Care Advocacy*. New York: Springer; 2011.
3. Richmond JB, Kotelchuck M. Political influences: rethinking national health policy. In: Mcquire C, Foley R, Gorr A, Richards R, eds. *Handbook of Health Professions Education*. San Francisco, CA: Jossey-Bass Publishers; 1993:386–404.
4. Atwood K, Colditz GA, Kawachi I. From public health science to prevention policy: placing science in its social and political contexts. *Am J Public Health*. 1997;87(10):1603–1606.

5. Centers for Medicare and Medicaid Services, US Government. National health expenditure data. https://www.cms.gov/research-statistics-data-and-systems/statistics-trends-and-reports/nationalhealthexpenddata/nationalhealthaccountshistorical.html. Accessed November 21, 2015.

6. Davis K, Stremikis K, Schoen C, Squires D. Mirror, mirror on the wall, 2014 update: how the U.S. health care system compares internationally. The Commonwealth Fund. http://www.commonwealthfund.org/publications/fund-reports/2014/jun/mirror-mirror. Published June 2014. Accessed November 21, 2015.

7. Hammergren L. *Political Will, Constituency Building, and Public Support in Rule of Law Programs.* Center for Democracy and Governance; Bureau for Global Programs, Field Support, and Research; U.S. Agency for International Development. http://pdf.usaid.gov/pdf_docs/PNACD023.pdf. Published August 1998. Accessed November 8, 2016.

8. Post LA, Raile AN, Raile ED. Defining political will. *Politics & Policy.* 2010;38(4):653–676.

9. Moses 3rd H, Matheson DM, Dorsey E, George BP, Sadoff D, Yoshimura S. The anatomy of health care in the United States. *JAMA.* 2013;310(18):1947–1964.

10. Adams G. *The Iron Triangle: The Politics of Defense Contracting.* New York: Council on Economic Priorities; 1981.

11. Givel MS, Glantz SA. Tobacco lobby political influence on US state legislatures in the 1990s. *Tob Control.* 2001;10(2):124–134.

12. Berwick DM, Nolan TW, Whittington J. The Triple Aim: care, health, and cost. *Health Aff.* 2008;27(3):759–769.

13. Kocher RP, Adashi EY. Hospital readmissions and the Affordable Care Act: paying for coordinated quality care. *JAMA.* 2011;306(16):1794–1795.

14. Boozary AS, Manchin III J, Wicker RF. The Medicare Hospital Readmissions Reduction Program: time for reform. *JAMA.* 2015;314(4):347–348.

15. Boccuti C, Casillas G. Aiming for fewer hospital U-turns: the Medicare Hospital Readmission Reduction Program. Kaiser Family Foundation Issue Brief. http://files.kff.org/attachment/issue-brief-aiming-for-fewer-hospital-u-turns-the-medicare-hospital-readmission-reduction-program. Published January 2015. Accessed November 21, 2015.

16. U.S. Department of Health & Human Services. New HHS data shows major strides made in patient safety, leading to improved care and savings. https://innovation.cms.gov/Files/reports/patient-safety-results.pdf. Published May 7, 2014. Accessed November 21, 2015.

17. Jha AK. Readmissions penalty at year 3: how are we doing? Ounce of Evidence: Health Policy Blog. https://blogs.sph.harvard.edu/ashish-jha/readmissions-penalty-at-year-3-how-are-we-doing/. Accessed November 21, 2015.

18. Patel K, Rushefsky M. *Health Care Politics and Policy in America.* 3rd ed. Armonk, NY: M.E. Sharpe; 2006.

19. Deleted in review.

20. Government Accounting Office. *Health Care Transparency: Actions Needed to Improve Cost and Quality Information for Consumers.* http://www.gao.gov/products/GAO-15-11. Published October 2014. Accessed November 8, 2016.

21. Nichols LM. Government intervention in health care markets is practical, necessary, and morally sound. *J Law Med Ethics.* 2012;40(3):547–557.

22. Daniels N. Justice, health, and healthcare. *Am J Bioeth.* 2001;1(2):2–16.

23. Gallup Poll. November 20, 2014. http://www.gallup.com/poll/179501/majority-say-not-gov-duty-provide-healthcare.aspx.

24. Gallup Poll. November 25, 2013. http://www.gallup.com/poll/165998/americans-views-healthcare-quality-cost-coverage.aspx.

25. Teitelbaum JB, Wilensky SE. *Essentials of Health Policy and Law.* 2nd ed. Burlington, MA: Jones & Bartlett; 2013:45.

26. McDonough JE. *Inside National Health Reform.* New York: Milbank Memorial Fund; 2011:20.

27. Deleted in review.

28. Deleted in review.

29. Bodenheimer T, Grumbach K. *Understanding Health Policy: A Clinical Approach.* 6th ed. New York: McGraw Hill; 2012:190.

30. Deleted in review.

31. Deleted in review.

32. Deleted in review.

33. Deleted in review.

34. Deleted in review.

35. Deleted in review.

36. Deleted in review.

37. Deleted in review.

38. Deleted in review.

39. State of Hawaii, Department of Labor and Industrial Relations Disability Compensation Division. Highlights of the Hawaii Prepaid Health Care Act. http://labor.hawaii.gov/dcd/files/2013/01/PHC-highlights.pdf.

40. Marcy J. Vermont edges toward single-payer health care. *Kaiser Health News.* http://khn.org/news/vermont-single-payer-health-care/.

41. Wheaton S. Why single payer died in Vermont. *Politico.* December 20, 2014. http://www.politico.com/story/2014/12/single-payer-vermont-113711.

42. Kaiser Family Foundation. The Massachusetts health care reform law: six years later. https://kaiserfamilyfoundation.files.wordpress.com/2013/01/8311.pdf. Published May 2012.

43. McDonough JE. The United States health system in transition. *Health Systems & Reform.* 2015;1(1):39–51.

44. Nyhan B. Why the "Death Panel" myth wouldn't die: misinformation in the health care reform debate. *The Forum.* 2010;8(1):1–24.

45. Oberlander J. Long time coming: why health reform finally passed. *Health Aff.* 2010;29(6):1112–1116.

46. Kaiser Family Foundation. Kaiser Health tracking poll: the public's views on the ACA. http://kff.org/interactive/kaiser-health-tracking-poll-the-publics-views-on-the-aca/#?response=Favorable–Unfavorable&aRange=twoYear&group=Party%2520ID::Democrat.

47. Patient-Centered Outcomes Research Institute. Why PCORI was created. http://www.pcori.org/about-us/why-pcori-was-created.

48. Crossley M, Tobin-Tyler E, Herbst J. Tax-exempt hospitals and community health under the affordable care act: identifying and addressing unmet legal needs as social determinants of health. *Public Health Rep.* 2016;131(1):195–199.

49. 79 Fed. Reg. 78954 (December 31, 2014).

50. Joint Center for Political and Economic Studies. Patient Protection and Affordable Care Act of 2010: Advancing Health Equity for Racially and Ethnically Diverse Populations. http://jointcenter.org/sites/default/files/Patient%20Protection%20and%20Affordable%20Care%20Act.pdf. Published July 2010. Accessed November 8, 2016.

51. The Commonwealth Fund. Latinos have made coverage gains but millions are still uninsured. http://www.commonwealthfund.org/publications/blog/2015/apr/latinos-have-made-coverage-gains. Published April 27, 2015.

52. US Department of Health and Human Services. HHS takes next step in advancing health equity through the Affordable Care Act. http://www.hhs.gov/about/news/2015/09/03/hhs-takes-next-step-advancing-health-equity-through-affordable-care-act.html.

53. *Burwell v. Hobby Lobby,* 573 US ___; 2014.

54. *King v. Burwell,* 576 US ___; 2015.

55. U.S. Department of Health and Human Services. ASPE Report: Health Insurance Marketplace: summary enrollment report for the initial annual open enrollment. http://aspe.hhs.gov/report/health-insurance-marketplace-summary-enrollment-report-initial-annual-open-enrollment-period.

56. Blumenthal D, Collins SR. Health care coverage under the Affordable Care Act—a progress report. *N Engl J Med.* 2014;371:275–281.

57. Kaiser Family Foundation. Key facts about the uninsured population. http://kff.org/uninsured/fact-sheet/key-facts-about-the-uninsured-population/. Published October 5, 2015.

58. The Commonwealth Fund. The Affordable Care Act's payment and delivery system reforms: a progress report at five years. http://www.commonwealthfund.org/publications/issue-briefs/2015/may/aca-payment-and-delivery-system-reforms-at-5-years. Published 2015.

59. Centers for Medicare & Medicaid Services. Bundled Payments for Care Improvement (BPCI) Initiative: general information. https://innovation.cms.gov/initiatives/bundled-payments/.

60. Patel K, Parker R, Villarruel A, Wong W. *Amplifying the Voice of the Underserved in the Implementation of the Affordable Care Act (Discussion Paper)*. Washington, DC: Institute of Medicine; 2013. https://nam.edu/wp-content/uploads/2015/06/BPH-AmplifyingtheVoice.pdf. Accessed November 8, 2016.

61. Millenson ML, Macri J. Will the Affordable Care Act move patient-centeredness to center stage? *Urban Institute*. March 2012. http://www.rwjf.org/content/dam/web-assets/2012/03/will-the-affordable-care-act-move-patient-centeredness-to-center.

62. Askin E, Moore N. *The Health Care Handbook*. 2nd ed. St. Louis: Washington University; 2014:151.

63. Association of American Medical Colleges. The Complexities of Physician Supply and Demand: Projections from 2013 to 2025. https://www.aamc.org/download/426242/data/ihsreportdownload.pdf?cm_mmc=AAMC-_-ScientificAffairs-_-PDF-_-ihsreport. Published March 2015. Accessed November 8, 2016.

64. Glied S, Ma S. How will the Affordable Care Act affect the use of health care services? Commonwealth Fund Issue Brief. http://www.commonwealthfund.org/~/media/files/publications/issue-brief/2015/feb/1804_glied_how_will_aca_affect_use_hlt_care_svcs_ib_v2.pdf. Published February 2015.

65. Kaiser Family Foundation. How are hospitals faring under the Affordable Care Act? Early experiences from Ascension Health. Issue Brief. http://kff.org/report-section/how-are-hospitals-faring-under-the-affordable-care-act-early-experiences-from-ascension-health-issue-brief/. Published April 30, 2015.

66. Association of American Medical Colleges. Physician shortages to worsen without increases in residency training. https://www.aamc.org/download/150584/data/physician_shortages_factsheet.pdf. Published 2010. Accessed November 8, 2016.

67. Frieden J. AMA expands consortium of innovative medical schools. *MedPage Today*. November 4, 2015. http://www.medpagetoday.com/PublicHealthPolicy/MedicalEducation/54484. Accessed Feb 25, 2016.

68. Iglehart J. Financing graduate medical education—mounting pressure for reform. *N Engl J Med*. 2012;366:1562–1563.

69. Jackson A, Baron RB, Jaeger J, Liebow M, Plews-Ogan M, Schwartz MD, for the Society of General Internal Medicine Health Policy Committee. Addressing the nation's physician workforce needs: the Society of General Internal Medicine (SGIM) recommendations on graduate medical education reform. *J Gen Intern Med*. Published online April 15, 2014.

Application of Foundational Skills to Health Systems Science

Sara Jo Grethlein, MD, and Jose Azar, MD

LEARNING OBJECTIVES

1. Describe how an evidence-based, data-driven approach can frame and address systems-level challenges.
2. Recognize the advantages and pitfalls in using technology to enhance communication skills.
3. Summarize the importance of cultural competence in the success of systems initiatives.
4. Understand the critical role of interprofessional and hidden teams as well as unprofessional behavior on health care system function.

Learning content without applying it may lead to limited comprehension and practice. This chapter will explore and provide examples of skills in the application of evidence-based medicine, communication, cultural competence, teamwork, and professionalism that were presented in previous chapters. How can we operationalize adherence to the best evidence in care? What are the pros and cons of using patient portals to communicate with patients? Practically, how can we provide culturally competent care that accommodates less common belief systems or gender identities? How do health care providers and leaders balance competing interests such as finance and ethics? This chapter walks through examples of where institutions and individuals got it right or wrong to learn key lessons from the past.

I. INTRODUCTION: FOUNDATIONAL SKILLS FOR HEALTH CARE DELIVERY

Learning to bat and field are critical skills that baseball players need, but there are additional, more complex competencies required to succeed as a team member playing a game. Previous chapters have explored foundational information in patient safety, quality improvement, teamwork, leadership, clinical informatics, and other domains critical to health systems science (HSS).

This chapter reviews the skills needed by health care professionals to be successful across the HSS domains and explores examples of successful and ineffective approaches to demonstrate the importance of these skills. These cross-cutting skills generalize across system-related and provider-based competencies and may merge both areas through broader system awareness.

Physicians and other health care professionals are rarely presented with simple, straightforward, unidimensional issues. More commonly, they must identify interwoven threads and apply multifaceted approaches to provide patient-centered, high-value care for individual patients and populations of patients. Although we focus on one or two key domains in each example, the ability to communicate well, engage with colleagues, and inspire others through example underlies the successful execution of each of these illustrations.

II. EVIDENCE-BASED MEDICINE

Evidence-based medicine is the practice of identifying and applying the best available scientific evidence to guide practice and reduce unnecessary variation in health care delivery. This practice is required to ensure that care is effective, one of the six dimensions of quality from the Institute of Medicine reviewed in Chapter 4. Unnecessary variation is the variation in medical care when there is identified evidence for best practice. Research from Dartmouth Medical School shows that 30 percent to 40 percent of patients in the United States do not receive care consistent with current evidence, and that 20 percent to 25 percent of care provided is unnecessary or potentially harmful.

As a clinical example, the use of beta blockers for patients with congestive heart failure has been shown to reduce mortality and improve overall outcomes; however, studies have shown significant variability in their use depending on the clinical setting and variability in the dosing. Registry studies in the mid-2000s reported rates of beta blocker use in heart failure patients of 34 percent to 57 percent in primary care, 66 percent to 74 percent in heart failure specialty clinics, and exceeding 80 percent in clinics with process improvement efforts. A study conducted by the Department of Medicine at Baylor University showed that 50 percent of heart failure patients received suboptimal doses of beta blockers at discharge and up to 2 years later.[1] As discussed in previous chapters, unnecessary practice variation in care delivery is a common cause of unintended patient harm, reduced efficiency, suboptimal treatment effectiveness, and high costs of care.

Effective implementation of best evidence in daily practice remains a major challenge, with only 14 percent of published knowledge widely incorporated into daily practice.[2–4] Numerous barriers hamper successful implementation, including 1) poor generalizability of the evidence to the real world since most studies are conducted in academic medical settings, 2) lack of systems designed to support best practice, 3) complexity of the intervention or new practice, 4) lack of readiness for adoption of change, and 5) underuse of effective strategies, approaches, and tools to facilitate change such as behavioral economics, change management, Lean, and Six Sigma tools. In order to improve the adoption and implementation of best evidence into daily practice, health care delivery systems can deploy several strategies, including practice guidelines, evidence-based pathways, and drug formularies.

A. Clinical Practice Guidelines and Clinical Pathways

Since the 1990s, clinical practice guidelines have been developed and published to enhance the adoption of best evidence in clinical practice. Clinical practice guidelines, when consistently adopted, may enhance the practice of medicine by helping to reduce inappropriate practice variation and to improve the quality and safety of health care.[5] Guidelines are typically published by large national networks, professional societies, and government agencies; therefore their recommendations are based on consensus, include multiple possible evidence-based options, and are not localized to a specific practice or health care delivery system.

Clinical pathways are standardized, evidence-based clinical decision tools developed to guide practice at the local level. They are integrated management plans that provide the sequence and timing of specific clinical actions aimed to achieve specific clinical goals. Clinical pathways aim to standardize clinical processes in order to improve clinical effectiveness and efficiency. Therefore, they are tools used by physicians and other health care professionals to treat patients with specific diagnoses or conditions according to evidence-based medicine. They are also used by health care teams and practice leaders to identify, define, and implement the best process for their organization. Clinical pathways may help health care systems reduce variation in clinical performance, identify patients who are eligible for clinical trials, improve the efficiency of care delivery, improve the quality and outcomes of patient care, improve the safety of care delivery, and reduce the costs of care.

In order to optimize the successful implementation and compliance with clinical pathways, a health care system should incorporate the pathways into the routine workflow of its clinicians and, preferably, simplify the use of the pathways by integrating them into the electronic health record (EHR). Pathways cannot be followed in 100 percent of cases because a clinician needs to personalize the therapy by taking into account the patient preferences, comorbidities, and the acuity of their presentation. Therefore, pathways become a tool to balance the need to reduce variation in practice among clinicians while allowing for personalization of therapy. It is generally accepted that pathways apply to 80 percent of cases, and personalization of the pathway is needed 20 percent of the time. It is essential that the personalization is based on the individual patient rather than the personal preferences and biases of clinicians. Cost and resource savings derived from the reduction of unnecessary variation can become assets that can be applied to the provision of care for the outlying 20 percent of patients. Pathways will not capture the uniqueness of all patients, but, for example, reducing hospitalizations for average-risk patients with community-acquired pneumonia will make beds available for those patients the physician still determines need admission due to factors not accounted for by the pathways.

Adult oncology specialty practice in the United States provides a successful example of development and utilization of practice guidelines as well as standardized clinical pathways in three ways: 1) guiding clinical decision making and facilitating insurance prior authorizations and pay-for-performance programs, 2) defining quality care and facilitating external quality monitoring, and 3) improving the quality of cancer care (efficiency and effectiveness) through implementation of clinical pathways through an electronic health record.

1. Guiding Clinical Decision Making and Facilitating Insurance Prior Authorizations and Pay-for-Performance Programs

The National Comprehensive Cancer Network (NCCN) is an alliance of 26 of the world's leading cancer centers dedicated to improving the quality and effectiveness of care provided to patients with cancer.[6] The NCCN has developed guidelines for treatment of 35 major cancers as well as for supportive care and cancer screening in order to help guide decision making in oncology. Because these guidelines are a consensus at a national level, the majority of the recommendations issued in the NCCN guidelines are developed from lower levels of evidence but with uniform expert opinion. Nevertheless, NCCN guidelines are the most comprehensive and widely used oncology standard in clinical practice in the world. These guidelines are accepted by the Centers for Medicare and Medicaid Services and most private insurance companies and are used to facilitate prior authorizations for diagnostic tests and cancer therapy. These guidelines are also under consideration to be used as the reference for **pay-for-performance** programs by third-party payers.

CASE STUDY 1

Chemotherapy regimens are a complex set of orders that include orders for the chemotherapeutic agents, supportive care medications, laboratory tests, nursing orders, and parameters for modifying the dose or withholding the chemotherapy infusion. For example, a standard chemotherapy infusion order set includes the chemotherapy agents, the dosing of each chemotherapy agent, the route and rate of administration, and the parameters for dose reduction. In addition to the chemotherapy agents, the order plans include orders for laboratory tests, intravenous fluids, supportive care medications for prevention of nausea and vomiting, prophylactic antibiotics for prevention of infections, and colony-stimulating factors. The order sets also include nursing orders that provide instructions regarding the sequence and relative timing of the infusions, frequency of clinical monitoring, call orders regarding specific parameters such as vital signs and laboratory results, and discharge information. The order sets can include references for the chemotherapy regimen publication and supporting evidence.

Computerized physician order entry (CPOE), if appropriately implemented with careful consideration for workflow and coordination of care, can be an effective tool to manage the complexity of the order sets. The electronic orders allow for asynchronous workflow, where multiple team members can be working on different aspects of the regimen in parallel rather than in sequence (synchronous process in the case of paper order sets that can be used by one team member at a time), therefore allowing for a more efficient process. For example, after the physician enters the orders electronically, the precertification clerk can work on the insurance approval process while the clinic secretary schedules the infusion time, the clinical pharmacist can double-check the accuracy of the orders and review any medication adverse interactions while the infusion nurse is providing the patient chemotherapy education, and the staff pharmacist can start mixing the chemotherapy agents.

In addition, CPOE can provide the possibility of efficient and frequent communication among team members through electronic messages that allow for clarification of specific modifications to the chemotherapy regimen as well as exchange of information relevant to the planning and administration of therapy. For example, traditional paper order entry (synchronous workflow) can be bypassed, and it is possible for the pharmacist to prepare the chemotherapy agents before the insurance approves to cover the regimen. Or the nurse may start giving the prophylactic medications before the pharmacist has started preparing the chemotherapy agents.

While CPOE has a great deal of potential in this situation, disruptions to the traditional sequential workflow introduce a risk for serious errors and unintentional patient harm (financial or medical). How can this challenge be overcome? What other health systems science principles can further improve the care of cancer patients?

2. Defining Quality Care and Facilitating External Quality Monitoring

The American Society of Clinical Oncology (ASCO) developed the Quality Oncology Practice Initiative (QOPI) in 2006 as a voluntary quality reporting program. The QOPI assesses the quality of cancer care by measuring adherence to evidence- and consensus-based **process measures.**[7] QOPI measures are aimed at supporting an environment for practice improvement and chemotherapy safety. The QOPI has demonstrated mixed results regarding compliance with guidelines. For measures regarding chemotherapy where evidence is widely accepted, the QOPI has identified minimal gaps in care. For other measures that reflect adoption of more recently published high-level evidence (e.g., testing for mutations in intracellular molecular targets, such as KRAS, that can impact treatment decisions for patients with metastatic colon cancer), the QOPI identified initial gaps in care that have been reduced over the course of a few years. In other QOPI measures, a wide gap and lack of improvement has been observed. Such challenging measures include psychosocial distress assessment, smoking cessation counseling, fertility preservation, and chemotherapy treatment summary.

3. Improving the Quality of Cancer Care (Efficiency and Effectiveness) Through Implementation of Clinical Pathways Through an Electronic Health Record

In 2012, Mount Sinai Medical Center in New York implemented the chemotherapy module of their EHR.[8] In addition to the usual goals of implementing an EHR such as increased legibility, record accessibility, and a more efficient order entry system, they aimed to increase the use of evidence-based chemotherapy regimens and supportive care medications. Their primary goals were to reduce errors, improve practice efficiency, reduce the cost of care, and improve adherence with evidence-based practice. To accomplish these goals, they created an interprofessional chemotherapy council that reviewed and validated 600 evidence-based protocols that were integrated into standardized pathways. They also developed an electronic tool to track practice variation regarding the protocols, which allowed them to monitor compliance, improve their practice, and improve the protocols. The implementation of these standardized protocols allowed them to achieve 86 percent compliance with evidence-based practice, improve appropriate anti-emetic use by 20 percent, and increase their infusion volume without compromising patient wait times or patient safety.

B. Formularies

A formulary is a continually updated list of medications and related information representing the clinical judgment of physicians, pharmacists, and other experts in the diagnosis, prophylaxis, or treatment of disease and promotion of health. A formulary includes, but is not limited to, a list of medications and medication-associated products or devices, medication-use policies, important ancillary drug information, decision-support tools, and organizational guidelines.

A **formulary system** is the ongoing process through which a health care organization establishes policies regarding the use of drugs, therapies, and drug-related products and identifies those that are most medically appropriate and cost-effective to best serve the health interests of a given patient population. Formulary systems are used in many different settings, including hospitals, acute care facilities, home care settings, and long-term-care facilities, as well as by payers such as Medicare, Medicaid, insurance companies, and managed care organizations.

Formulary systems are considered an essential tool for health care organizations. Formularies have grown from simple drug lists to comprehensive systems of medication use policies intended to ensure safe, appropriate, and cost-effective use of pharmaceuticals in patient care.

The pharmacy and therapeutics (P&T) committee at each health care institution is responsible for managing the formulary system. It is composed of actively practicing physicians, other prescribers, pharmacists, nurses, administrators, quality improvement managers, and other health care professionals and staff who participate in the medication-use process. The P&T committee should be responsible for overseeing policies and procedures related to all aspects of medication use within an institution. Other responsibilities of the P&T committee include evaluation of medication use, adverse drug event monitoring and reporting, medication error prevention, and development of clinical care plans and guidelines. P&T decisions should be evidence-based through unbiased reviews of the literature and address conflict of interest in its decision-making process. In addition, the P&T committee should systematically address patient safety in its decision-making process by taking into consideration the potential for medication errors related to ordering, sound-alike or look-alike names, dosing, storage, preparation, and administration of medications. The P&T committee should consistently monitor medication errors and near-misses and make recommendations to prevent future events by ensuring that policies address the potential risks or by conducting improvement projects to reduce these risks.

Antimicrobial stewardship is one of the activities conducted and monitored by the formulary system[9] and used to improve care delivery (decreasing unnecessary variation and improving safety). Antimicrobial stewardship is a method by which health care institutions manage the appropriate selection, dosing, route, and duration of antimicrobial therapy. It is primarily aimed at improving quality of care and patient safety by optimizing clinical outcomes while minimizing the unintended consequences of antimicrobial use, including the emergence of resistance and selection of pathogenic organisms, such as *Clostridium difficile*. *C. difficile* infection rates, disease severity, and associated mortality rates are rising amid growing concern for rising treatment failure rates and emergence of more virulent strains. According to the Centers for Disease Control and Prevention, *C. difficile* was estimated to cause almost one-half million infections in 2011, and 29,000 patients with *C. difficile* infection died within 30 days of the initial diagnosis. The associated economic burden is also significant. Nosocomial *C. difficile* infections increase the cost of otherwise matched hospitalizations by fourfold, translating to a cost reported up to $4.8 billion per year in the United States.

Antibiotic use is a major risk factor for the development of *C. difficile* infection. Antimicrobial stewardship programs have been successfully used as a method to regulate antibiotic use and reduce the rate of these infections. For example, the Michael E. DeBakey Veterans Affairs Medical Center and the Department of Medicine at the Baylor College of Medicine have reduced the rate of *C. difficile*–associated disease (CDAD) by nearly 50 percent through the implementation of an antibiotic stewardship program (Fig. 13.1).[10] In their 550-bed hospital, the rate of CDAD remained constantly elevated despite multiple interventions such as hand hygiene and isolation procedures. Therefore, after 3 years of unsuccessful interventions, they decided to implement an antibiotic stewardship program. Under this program, prescriptions for most parenteral antibiotics required approval by an infectious disease physician or clinical pharmacist. The program included a list of acceptable antibiotics that did not require prior approval; daytime orders for all other antibiotics outside the list were only honored if approved. Overnight orders for formulary antibiotics were honored until the following day, when the pharmacist and infectious disease specialist reviewed them, either approving the order or making other recommendations. Implementation of the antibiotics stewardship program was associated with a reduction in the rate of all cases of CDAD from a baseline of 3.3 cases per 1000 bed-days to 1.7 cases per 1000 bed-days during the ensuing 12 months, a 47.2 percent decrease with a p value of 0.001 by t-test.

III. COMMUNICATION SKILLS VIA NEW TECHNOLOGY

The physician-patient relationship has evolved over decades from a paternalistic relationship where the physician is the primary decision maker to a partnership where the patient is an autonomous and competent partner in the decision-making process. In order to be an active partner in this relationship, the patient must be empowered and well informed. Communication during a clinic visit is the foundation of the relationship between the patient and the physician, but there is often information (such as a laboratory test result) that is not available and therefore cannot be exchanged during the clinic visit. In addition, patient-centered care and efforts to provide high-value care and advance the **Triple Aim** require a mechanism for patients to interact with care teams with concerns or questions that do not require face-to-face visits. A patient-centered communication system also ensures patient access to their medical record. Traditionally, health care systems have relied on phone communication or providing paper copies of records by mail, fax, or in person. In order to more actively and efficiently engage patients in their own care and improve patient satisfaction, health care delivery systems may leverage information technology by designing and implementing **electronic patient portals** and engaging in the use of social media. The federal government is working to ensure implementation of these communication mechanisms by auditing them as part of their assessment of adherence to the meaningful use standards of the HITECH Act, which was passed as part of the American Recovery and Reinvestment Act of 2009.

If one imagines a simple goal such as increasing a practice's footprint within a geographic area, it quickly becomes apparent that there are a myriad of elements to consider. Setting aside the business assessments that would be important

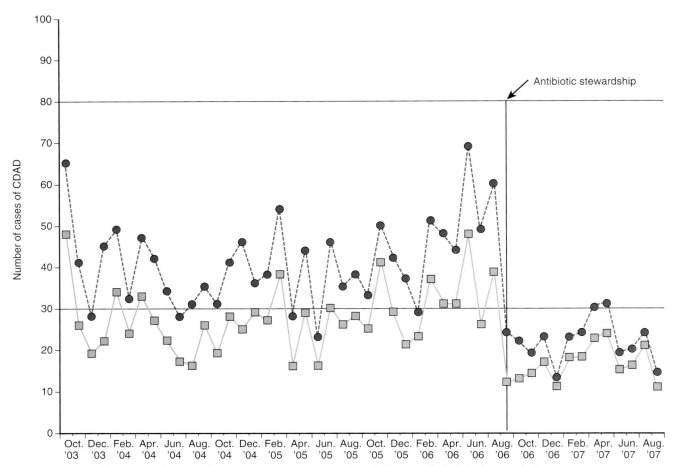

Fig. 13.1 Incidence of *Clostridium difficile*–associated disease (CDAD), before and after implementation of the antibiotic stewardship program. *Upper dashed line,* total number of cases of CDAD, as defined in the Centers for Disease Control and Prevention criteria during the years under study; *lower solid line,* number of first-time cases, as determined from the EHR. (From Nuila F, Cadle RM, Logan N, Musher DM; Members of the Infectious Disease Section of the Michael E DeBakey VA Medical Center. Antibiotic stewardship and *Clostridium difficile*–associated disease. *Infect Control Hosp.* 2008;29[11]:1096–1097.)

to any expansion, a robust understanding of the community's characteristics, medical practices, and beliefs would be an asset to help design an ideal communication system. If striving to improve services to elderly nursing home residents, a communication strategy built on social media platforms would likely be ineffective, and similarly, a preventive health program for teens that relies on traditional mail would be suboptimal.

Case Study 2

Becoming a physician is a transformative event. Society has expectations of physician behavior that may make it difficult for physicians to have full expectations of privacy, especially in the age of social media. As students transition to their professional role, they may not fully comprehend this challenge. Patients and potential employers may make judgments about their character or qualifications based on their media presence. Health care professionals do not always live up to the professionalism they use in person in their virtual lives.[62] A published survey of medical schools found that students were identified as

using profanity, appearing intoxicated, and sharing sexually suggestive material commonly in their social media presence. More concerning was the finding that 13 percent of schools reported students sharing patient information online. Three schools reported student dismissals due to their online behavior, and 67 percent had issued warnings to students.[63] A survey of program directors for surgical residencies found that 33 percent of respondents who reviewed applicants' social media presence had lowered a student's standing on the rank list due to his or her postings. The percentage of programs screening applicants in this manner was low (17 percent), but survey respondents anticipated that it will increase.[64] A variety of sources have created tips for maintaining an acceptable online presence. *Forbes* magazine recommends performing a personal audit, deleting questionable postings, updating privacy settings, and reviewing them intermittently.[65] A physician-specific guideline gives a brief set of "Dos and Don'ts."

DO respect patient confidentiality.

DON'T blur professional boundaries.

DO be open about conflicts of interest.

DON'T make abusive or gratuitous comments about individuals online.

DO identify yourself by name when posting as a physician on publicly accessible social media.

DO use appropriate channels to raise concerns rather than social media.[66]

How should physicians apply these guidelines to themselves? How should health systems use these guidelines when considering hiring, disciplining, or dismissing a physician or other health care professional? What other guidelines should be considered? What are the potential hazards for medical students, physicians, and other health care professionals who do not follow these guidelines?

A. Electronic Patient Portals

Electronic patient portals are electronic communication platforms that provide patients with different degrees of access to their health information stored in an EHR and managed by the health care system. Patients are granted access to the EHR via the portal to select clinical information such as laboratory test results or treatment plan summaries. In addition, electronic patient portals may provide patients the ability to electronically request medication refills, schedule appointments, and communicate through a secure messaging system with their care teams. Health care professionals must evaluate thoughtfully how these messages are received and responded to in a timely manner. Initiating communication with patients through this means creates an expectation that the provider will receive it and incorporate transmitted information into the patient's care. Critical information that is not attended to due to a staff member's absence from the office or being tied up in other patient care or administrative activities can result in patient harm. Well-defined and efficient processes need to be established to receive, review, and respond to patient portal requests in a timely manner. The processes must include clearly defined roles, criteria for nurse and physician review, protocol for internal communication among team members, and timely communication back to patients.

In chronic disease management such as diabetes and congestive heart failure, electronic patient portals have been reported to enhance physician-patient communication and improve patient satisfaction, compliance with prescribed treatments, disease management, and patient outcomes.[11,12] In addition, electronic patient portals have the potential to improve efficiency of care, reduce the frequency of patient clinic visits, and reduce the cost of care. Additional possible benefits include improved coordination of care by allowing patients to monitor various processes, such as the accuracy of their listed medications.

Despite the positive impact of electronic patient portals, several challenges and barriers limit their effectiveness and widespread use. Only a minority of patients are currently using electronic patient portals when available, possibly because of low computer literacy or low motivation among less ill patients. There are also concerns about patients viewing new clinical information outside of the context of the complete clinical picture. Patients may experience confusion or distress when they view abnormal test results before a physician or other health care professional is able to explain the results. One solution to this challenge is to delay the release of the clinical information to patients until after they have been reviewed by the clinician or after the patient meets with the provider; however, this approach may prevent the patient from having timely access to the information. Another challenge is that the documents and information are presented in a medical clinician-centric rather than a patient-friendly language. Therefore, the information presented in the electronic portals may not be understood by patients. This may limit the effectiveness of the communication. Additional limitations of electronic patient portals include the cost of technology, the security of the information, the liability of the providers, and the potential that the increased access to physicians will translate to increased nonreimbursed physician effort.

B. Social Media

More than 80 percent of Americans seek health information online.[13] The adoption of social media, especially social networking, by health care systems and professionals may lead to a more patient-centered health care system and may enhance patient engagement, health information exchange, and the communication between patients, health care providers (physicians, nurses, pharmacists), and health care administrators. Social media is used in different ways and for multiple purposes by the health care system; the following are three examples:

1. Health care systems are utilizing social media to engage their patients and the community at large in customer service, promotion and advertisement, and provision of news and information and fundraising.

2. Physicians use social media primarily for professional purposes. Physicians use social media to network with other colleagues, seek expert advice, listen to experts, and research new medical developments. In addition to professional development, physicians use social media to interact with patients and support groups around patient education, health monitoring, health behavior, and medication adherence.

3. Patients and support groups are the most frequent users of social media. They use social media for a wide variety of reasons, including education, networking, seeking support, finding information, access to care, and searching for research participation. In addition, patients are utilizing social media and online applications to monitor their health, track their progress, and set health-related goals. Social media may be beneficial for patients with chronic diseases, cancer, complex care needs, and rare diseases as well as aid patients with general wellness, prevention, and lifestyle modification. There is more evidence that the use of Internet-based interventions may have a positive impact on weight loss, tobacco cessation, and physical activity.

Although the use of social media has many promising benefits, numerous challenges remain. Health care systems, physicians, and patients are faced with challenges regarding confidentiality, privacy, personal identity, professionalism, and information inaccuracy.

Physicians need to ensure a strict and clear separation between their personal and professional presence on social media. Interactions between patients and their physicians online present challenges given the lack of regulation that takes into account professional and ethical considerations. Privacy of patients and physicians may be compromised during these online interactions.

Patients also face the threat of finding false information that may lead to confusion, poorly informed decisions, or harm. In addition, sharing of sensitive private information online may have negative repercussions on patients in regard to their employment or their insurance cost and coverage.

Social media is a promising platform for more effectively engaging patients, the community, physicians, and health care systems in improving health and the quality of care. However, these entities need to develop methods to regulate the use of social media taking into consideration privacy, professional, and ethical concerns.

CASE STUDY 3

One of the tenets of the Jehovah's Witnesses' faith is a prohibition against receiving blood products. During earlier eras, patients of this faith were often barred from receiving potentially lifesaving procedures due to concerns that this restriction would put patients at risk without physicians having the ability to rescue with traditional interventions. Elective or semi-elective surgeries, some chemotherapies, and other therapies were deemed "too risky." Some hospitals and physicians, however, chose to work closely with this faith group to explore the options and identify new approaches. *The New Yorker* magazine in 2015 ran a three-part series chronicling advances in "bloodless medicine" and described how Englewood Hospital and Medical Center of New Jersey is providing advanced care while respecting patients' beliefs.[60] Extremely complex operations, including lung transplantations, have been successfully performed without the otherwise routine use of transfusion in highly selected patients. The Institute for Patient Blood Management and Bloodless Medicine and Surgery at Englewood Hospital and Medical Center has become an international leader in this field and trains health care professionals and administrators in the care of patients without transfusion. Their advances have enhanced care for patients in circumstances in which blood is not available, not only when it is religiously prohibited. In addition, less reliance on transfusion in general reduces transfusion-related infections and other complications for all patients.

What health systems science principles come into play in this situation? How have they been applied? What can be learned from this situation that may be applied to other challenges in health systems science? What interventions might be counterproductive to efforts to better serve Jehovah's Witnesses?

IV. ORGANIZATIONAL CULTURE

Interacting with the external population is a significant component of most leaders' work, but the greater portion is typically the internal community. As complex microcosms with multiprofessional teams, ambiguity, and competing demands, health care organizations require leaders who are able to balance missions while adhering to strong principles. Like all entities, practices, hospitals, and health systems are composed of people. Creating, fostering, and managing the culture of an organization is critical to its success. Commonly attributed to Peter Drucker, the quote that "Culture eats strategy for lunch" highlights the power of this dimension. In

medicine, culture is grounded in the professional behavior of staff entrusted with the safety, privacy, and care of vulnerable individuals. While there are codes of professional behavior, operationalizing these codes falls to leaders as does ensuring that the organizations themselves function in ethical ways. The concept of a **"Just Culture"** has been identified as critical to patient safety.

Health care organizations serve the communities in which they are situated. In addition to providing patient care, they are businesses that, though mostly not-for-profit, depend on being selected by their customers. As the industry becomes more competitive, institutions typically ramp up their advertising and outreach, modify their services, and make other changes with the goal of enhancing their share of the health care market. Leaders are tasked with creating environments that are welcoming and respectful without compromising their missions. Demonstrating receptiveness and flexibility, along with awareness of issues that may impact patients and their families can lead to enhanced patient care, adherence to treatment, and satisfaction. Insensitivity to patient wishes or preferences can impair both the patient experience and the organization's bottom line. Quality, safety, and effectiveness of care are impacted by the engagement of patients, and failure to address needs leads to nonadherence with recommendations. Health outcomes can be negatively impacted by these factors as well. Taking on the challenge of service to a population's needs can lead to exciting and creative advances that improve health care in general.

Well-intended health care organizations may lack the nuanced knowledge to provide sensitive care to patients who have suffered discrimination either in their medical care or other aspects of their lives. As our society becomes more respectful and receptive to individuals whose lives are not lived in the most prevalent part of the spectrum of normal variation, we must adapt. Care for transgender individuals presents an opportunity for excellence in cultural competence, as many have previously been treated with abasement and humiliation and faced physicians and other health care professionals who refuse to care for them. Because of prior unpleasant interactions, many transgender individuals avoid health care encounters and may present with advanced disease. Hospital computer systems, policies, and traditions may not be prepared to respectfully manage patients in transition of their gender expression. Forethought, training, and the development of new procedures are necessary to create an environment that is supportive. Planning is essential for appropriate handling of changes in name and gender identification as well as bathroom availability and labeling, patient room assignment, and other issues. Legal documentation may not match the patient's presenting gender either by choice or by barriers within the state's laws. The publication *Creating Equal Access to Quality Health Care for Transgender Patients: Transgender-Affirming Hospital Policies* provides guidance and model policies.[14]

V. TEAMWORK

Delivering care to a patient requires a complex network of professionals: physicians, other health care professionals, and supporting staff who are all semi-autonomous and interdependent. At a basic level, a simple clinic visit requires the coordinated work of a receptionist, a medical assistant, a nurse, a physician, and possibly a pharmacist, a physician assistant, and a social worker. However, the visit would not be possible without the work of environmental services, maintenance personnel, supply delivery personnel, and a clinic manager. The level of complexity increases when a patient has to navigate multiple settings and interact with multiple teams. For example, if a medication is prescribed in clinic, the patient will have to interact with the dispensing pharmacy, which has its own complex network of individuals to deliver the medication. An even more complex situation occurs if a patient is referred to a consultant clinic and then is asked to undergo an imaging study and obtain blood studies. The highest complexity occurs when patients are admitted to the hospital from clinic or the emergency department and undergo diagnostic tests and therapeutic interventions and then are discharged to another setting such as home or a subacute facility for convalescence. The physician and the nurse play a central role in the health care delivery process; however, they are only a part of the system.

Unless the members of the delivery network are able to function and interrelate to each other as a functional team, the patient will suffer and health care delivery will be suboptimal. Health care professionals working in highly functional teams tend to have higher job satisfaction and less burnout. Health care errors, unintentional patient harm, and health care inefficiencies are often attributed to aspects of team dysfunction such as poor coordination of care, poor communication among team members, and lack of mutual respect. On the other hand, health care delivery systems can design teams and workflows to facilitate the optimal interactions among the entities within the network and improve the care for patients.

Case Study 4

Serving the health care needs of the Amish population depends on enhanced understanding and respect for their belief systems and willingness to meet them within the boundaries of their community. Leaders at Lancaster General Hospital in Pennsylvania made a commitment to addressing the Amish population within their region. They engaged a research firm and conducted focus groups to identify the needs, utilization, and barriers to care. In respect for their faith, women and men met in separate groups. Examples of important concepts identified included reliance on natural products, willingness to engage the English health care system only for illness, and lack of acceptance of preventive care. Barriers to care included transportation, confusion about costs and billing, and a lack of factual information about health care. Scheduling multiple appointments at a time was viewed as a way to mitigate the transportation barriers.

Other institutions have improved care delivery to the Amish community through respectful, culturally sensitive initiatives. There is an increased prevalence of hemophilia among the Amish. This disorder is lifelong, debilitating, expensive to treat, and best managed through prevention and rapid intervention for bleeding. Especially in children, inadequate dental care can be a preventable source of bleeding and complications. Distrust of prescription medicine, lack of cultural acceptance of preventive care, cost, and complexity are barriers to successful treatment. Akron Children's Hospital manages the largest hemophilia B population in the world. Irene Boehlefeld, BSN, RN, CPON, a nurse educator, worked with leaders of the Amish community on a task force that ultimately led to the development of a home infusion training program for affected families, establishment of a community-based dental clinic, training of nurses to apply fluoride as part of a visiting dental van program, and creation of a culturally appropriate educational curriculum for the schools. As a result of this program, there were significant improvements in rates of factor infusion within 1 hour of the start of bleeding, number of home infusion patients, and completion of training logs. Additional benefits have included enhanced trust and relationships between the community and providers.[61]

What health systems science principles did health system administrators, physicians, and other health care professionals utilize when delivering care to this population? What additional steps can a health system, physician, or other health care professional take to improve care to this population? What are the potential pitfalls to programs such as these?

A. Impact on Quality of Care and Health Professional Satisfaction

A study by Baggs and colleagues examined provider self-reports of collaboration at three intensive care unit (ICU) sites and found that both medical nurse reports of collaboration and unit-level reports of collaboration were positively associated with patient outcomes.[15] Shortell and coworkers collected data from 17,440 patients, all nurses on all shifts, physicians, residents, and ward clerks/secretaries across 42 ICUs and found that caregiver interaction (culture, leadership, coordination, communication, and conflict management) was significantly correlated with lower risk-adjusted length of stay, higher evaluated technical quality of care, and greater evaluated ability to meet family member needs.[16] Benzer and colleagues correlated patient data from 223 primary care clinics with provider organizational climate survey data and reported relational climate as a strong predictor of high-quality diabetes care.[17] Leykum and coworkers found significant associations between reciprocal learning (intrateam learning and problem solving that occurs through conversation and reflection among team members) and chronic disease care in 40 small primary care practices.[18] Gittell and colleagues found associations between **relational coordination** (defined as coordination among team members that occurs through frequent, high-quality communication supported by relationships based on shared goals, shared knowledge, and mutual respect) and improved quality of care, reduced postoperative pain, and decreased lengths of hospital stay in a nine-hospital study of orthopedic patients.[19]

Risser and colleagues report the findings of a retrospective study of claims files, using a convenience sample drawn from eight participating hospitals. Fifty-four cases were reviewed by physician-nurse teamwork-trained pairs to identify whether the absence of teamwork contributed to the medical error in each case.[20] The pairs judged over one-half of the deaths in the malpractice cases to be avoidable under conditions of better teamwork. Donchin and coworkers studied the rate of errors in a medical-surgical ICU of a university hospital over a 4-month period and concluded that a significant number of the errors could be attributed to physician-nurse communication.[21]

Aiken and colleagues compared risk-adjusted mortality rates for Medicare beneficiaries cared for at 39 hospitals characterized by nurses as having a positive work environment (defined as level of status, autonomy, and relationships with physicians).[22] They found a 5 percent lower risk-adjusted mortality rate for these hospitals when compared with the 195 hospitals selected as matched controls. Uhlig and coworkers studied the introduction of a new "interdisciplinary care team" model that included a collaborative communication protocol and daily team rounds at each patient's bedside and reported a 56 percent reduction in risk-adjusted mortality for cardiac surgery patients.[23] Neily and colleagues analyzed Veterans Health Administration (VHA) quality improvement data and structured interviews to determine whether correlations existed between a VHA team training program and surgical mortality; they found a 50 percent greater decline in the risk-adjusted surgical mortality rate in the training group when compared to the nontraining group.[24] Kim and coworkers conducted a population-based retrospective cohort study of statewide hospital organizational survey and hospital discharge data in 112 acute care hospitals.[25] They found (after adjusting for patient and hospital characteristics) that daily rounds by an interprofessional team were associated with significant reductions in the odds of death.

In addition to the compelling link between high-functioning teams and quality of care, numerous studies link collaborative workplace culture with increased job satisfaction, lower levels of burnout, and decreased turnover. Baggs and colleagues found that higher levels of physician-nurse collaboration in decision making around patient care correlated with increased nurse satisfaction.[26] Vahey and colleagues conducted cross-sectional surveys of 820 nurses and 6212 patients from 40 units in 20 urban hospitals across the United States and found that nurses reporting a positive working environment (including good relationships between physicians and nurses) also reported significantly lower burnout.[26a] Shortell and coworkers collected data from 42 ICUs and found significant associations between caregiver interaction and lower nurse turnover.[27]

B. Creating and Sustaining High-Functioning Teams

As demonstrated in the studies discussed earlier, teamwork significantly influences patient outcomes, including quality, safety, and mortality, as well as efficiency of care delivery and health care provider job satisfaction. As health care organizations seek to improve care, reduce cost, and reduce provider burnout and turnover (also associated with decreased efficiency), development of effective care teams is critical. Yet while the evidence linking teamwork to key outcomes is robust, the development of collaborative, high-functioning interprofessional teams in health care remains a complex and challenging task for many reasons, including differing perceptions of collaboration; the need for shared and clear goals, communication, and tasks; and barriers to team collaboration.

1. Differing Perceptions of Collaboration

Makary and colleagues surveyed operating room personnel in 60 hospitals using the Safety Attitudes Questionnaire and found that ratings of teamwork differed substantially by operating room caregiver type, with physicians rating the teamwork of others as "high" or "very high" and nurses rating the teamwork as "mediocre."[28] Thomas and coworkers surveyed physicians and nurses working in ICUs in two teaching and four nonteaching hospitals and found that 33 percent of nurses rated the quality of collaboration and communication with the physicians as high or very high, in contrast to the 73 percent of physicians who rated collaboration and communication with nurses as high or very high.[29] O'Leary and colleagues surveyed nurses, primary care hospital physicians, and medical subspecialty consultants on four general medical units on the quality of communication and collaboration with their own and other disciplines.[30] Survey results indicated that the majority of physicians rated collaboration with nurses as high or very high, but a minority of nurses rated collaboration with physicians as high or very high.

2. Factors That Influence the Quality of Team Collaboration

Effective **interdisciplinary teams** are composed of members with particular skills and capacities who intentionally and successfully collaborate to accomplish well-defined, shared goals, and are supported by facilitating organizational structures and administrative policies. The Pew-Fetzer Task Force report, *Health Professions Education and Relationship-Centered Care,* outlines four core capacities that are essential for the development of effective interdisciplinary teams: 1) self-awareness, 2) knowledge of other health professions, 3) team-building abilities, and 4) understanding of team dynamics.[30a] Lanham and colleagues analyzed data sets from four National Institutes of Health studies of primary care practices and identified seven key relationship characteristics that together are associated with high-performing teams: 1) trust, 2) openness, 3) performing individual tasks with an understanding as to how they relate to the larger group tasks, 4) respectful interaction, 5) appreciation of diversity of perspectives, 6) social and task relatedness, and 7) rich and lean communication.[30b]

D'Amour and colleagues explored links between factors influencing collaboration within health care teams and distinguished three major categories of determinants that influence successful collaboration: 1) macrostructural determinants or determinants outside the organization; 2) determinants within the organization; and 3) interpersonal determinants.[31] Determinants outside the organization include social determinants, such as power differences among professionals; cultural systems that may foster individualism; professional systems that may foster autonomy; and educational systems that may or may not educate professionals with knowledge of the values and perspectives of other professions. Determinants within the organization include organizational structures and hierarchies; organizational values such as openness, fairness, and interdependence; administrative support that encourages and rewards collaborative practice; and team resources such as time and space to meet.

Interpersonal determinants are those that individual health care professionals and trainees must learn to effectively contribute to high-functioning teams. These attitudes and skills include a willingness to collaborate, ability to build trust, skills in communication, and knowledge that enables mutual respect among team members.

Gittell and colleagues have identified a specific construct of team interactions that they term *relational coordination.*[32] The theory of relational coordination asserts that work involving multiple roles and tasks is most effectively carried out through high-quality communication and high-quality relationships that support each other and together enable high-quality coordination of work. The communication domain in this construct includes four dimensions: accuracy, timeliness, frequency, and problem solving. The relational domain includes the three dimensions of shared goals, shared knowledge, and mutual respect. Gittell's research has found associations between relational coordination and improved quality of care, reduced postoperative pain,[19] reduced length of stay, lower total cost of hospitalization, better quality outcomes for medical patients,[33] increased quality of life for long-term care residents,[34] and improved job satisfaction for physicians and other health care professionals.[34] Gittell also found important correlations related to role definition, including associations between boundary spanning (the ability to perceive flexible job boundaries and crossover between roles to achieve shared goals), shared knowledge (an understanding of the roles of others and how those roles relate to one's own), and relational coordination.[35]

Research on the efficacy of interdisciplinary teams has identified several barriers to health care teamwork. In the primary care setting, Shaw and coworkers interviewed members of the interdisciplinary teams in 21 practices and found that lack of shared or identifiable goals, hierarchical structures, and poor team communication were impediments to effective teamwork.[36] Wittenberg-Lyles conducted ethnographic observation of interdisciplinary team meetings for five teams in a Midwest hospice and found that the introduction of psychosocial information by the case managers created tension in the team and clearly deviated from the standard biomedical format.[37] Thomas and colleagues surveyed physicians and nurses working in ICUs in six hospitals and found that relative to physicians, nurses reported that it is difficult to speak up, disagreements are not appropriately resolved, more input into decision making is needed, and nurse input is not well received.[38] Weber and coworkers analyzed taped recordings of physician and nurse interactions on ward rounds in two general internal medicine wards and found that they were physician-led and physician-centric, while nurses do not contribute substantially to what is said.[39]

3. Knowledge of Other Health Professions

All of the models of effective teamwork outlined earlier identify knowledge and/or appreciation of the roles, tasks, or perspectives of other team members as factors influencing effective teamwork. Yet many health care providers have little knowledge of the education, roles, or practices of other health care professionals. Health professions education is commonly siloed into separate schools or training programs with little shared clinical or content education and differing professional languages. Processes that enable team members to better understand the unique contributions of each team member to the shared work increases shared knowledge and mutual respect and improves work processes as each provider develops an enhanced understanding of how his or her own work activities fit with those of his or her colleagues.

4. Systems That Support Teams

Team-supporting systems help teams to clearly understand their shared mission and goals, which furthers the abilities of team members to carry out their individual work within the larger perspective of the team. These systems promote a culture of collaboration and coordination rather than hierarchy and an orientation toward group problem solving. A culture explicitly oriented to promote and reward team success enhances the motivation for members to share responsibility, maintain an openness to others' ideas, trust, empathize, and act generously. Systems that recognize that the strength of the group is greater than any one individual actively encourage multiple perspectives and foster appreciation of diversity. Systems that value interprofessional communication will foster opportunities to bring diverse team members together for collaboration and communication. Effective health care teams require both individual members who possess key teamwork capacities and a systems infrastructure that facilitates effective team development and interactions.

Health care systems have designed and developed health care teams and supporting systems to improve the quality, safety, and efficiency of the care they provide. We will review the development of **accountable care teams, rapid response systems,** and EHRs as applications of these concepts.

Accountable care teams are a model of collaborative inpatient unit-based practice.[40] Each team is composed of an interprofessional group of providers who assume accountability for the clinical, service, and financial outcomes of the patients on their respective inpatient unit. This model has been developed and implemented since 2012 at Indiana University Health Academic Health Center in Indianapolis.[40] The model is founded on three principles: enhancing interprofessional collaboration, enabling data-driven decisions, and providing accountable leadership.[40] The implementation of the model was based on eight interventions rooted in the principles of the Accountable Care Teams.

In order to enhance interprofessional collaboration, this health center implemented geographical cohorting of patients and providers. Before the model was implemented, the **hospitalists** covered patients on multiple different units and worked independently of the nurses. In the accountable care team model, each hospitalist is localized to one specific unit and provides care only to patients on that unit. An interdisciplinary team including a **case manager,** clinical nurse specialist, pharmacist, nutritionist, and social worker are also assigned to one specific unit. Learners (residents as well as pharmacy and medical students) are embedded in the team. The unit-based hospitalist collaborates with the **nurse manager,** and they are jointly accountable for the outcomes of patients on their unit.

Interprofessional collaboration also included bedside collaborative rounding. Unit-based providers round on their patients with the bedside nurse guided by a customizable script. It also involved a daily huddle. The hospitalist, learners, and the interdisciplinary team for the unit meet each weekday to discuss each patient's quality of care, discharge planning, and needs for a safe transition out of the hospital. Additionally, each unit has a white board at the nursing station that captures the components of the daily huddle discussion pertaining to quality of care, discharge planning, and safe transition. Guidelines delineating responsibilities for providers of each specialty were developed in order to facilitate the co-management of patients between the unit-based hospitalist and the surgical or medical specialists.

Data-driven decisions were enabled through a monthly review of unit-level data. A unit-specific data dashboard was developed to track key metrics including quality and safety metrics, length of stay, patient satisfaction scores, re-admission rates, and costs. The data are reviewed monthly in interdisciplinary meetings, and improvement plans are developed in order to meet the goals. The unit's nurse manager and physician leader also conduct patient rounds weekly focusing on the patient's experience and opportunities for improvement.

Accountable leadership is provided by designating unit-based physician leaders who are committed to serve each unit for at least 1 year as a resource for both medical and operational problem solving. The leader collaborates closely with the unit's nurse manager, and they are both responsible for their unit's quality, efficiency, and patient experience outcome trends.

Within 12 months of the implementation of the accountable care team model, the units adopting all components of the intervention were able to improve the quality and safety of care provided and the patient and provider satisfaction as well as the efficiency of the care delivery. These units were able to achieve a statistically significant reduction in their patients' length of stay and their variable direct cost adjusted for severity of illness. The rate of re-admission remained stable overall. The units adopting the model had fewer safety events and unintended patient harm. Patient satisfaction improved with geographic cohorting of patients and physicians. Team members reported that they were more engaged and satisfied with their job after implementation of the model.

Rapid response systems are interprofessional teams that are developed to intervene when patients show early signs of clinical deterioration on general hospital wards in order to reduce the rate of "failure to rescue," the incidence of cardiopulmonary arrest, and hospital mortality.[44,45] "Failure to rescue" is a failure to react promptly or adequately escalate care when a patient's condition is unexpectedly deteriorating. Patients commonly show signs and symptoms of deterioration for hours before cardiopulmonary arrest. When these arrests occur outside of the ICU setting, the outcomes are poor, with only 15 percent of patients surviving the event. Cardiopulmonary arrests have a common set of antecedent signs and symptoms, however they are often unrecognized by health care providers due to infrequent assessments of vital signs, lack of clearly defined triggers, individual and subjective interpretation of clinical condition by the clinical staff, delays in physician notification, a long chain of command for escalation (nurse to charge nurse, to intern, resident, fellow, and then to attending physician), unavailability of the nurse or physician because they are busy with other tasks, failure to attend to and assess the patient's deteriorating condition, suboptimal response to the urgency of the symptoms, and failure to seek help or advice. Overcoming these barriers to an effective and timely recognition and response to a clinical deterioration may reduce the chance of a cardiopulmonary arrest and death. Rapid response teams generally have the following four components:

1. The **Afferent limb** is designed for identifying a patient deterioration and activating the rapid response team using predefined trigger criteria. These criteria usually include vital signs and general concern expressed by a clinician or family member. The afferent limb empowers bedside clinicians to trigger the response team, bypassing the traditional hierarchy and expeditiously delivering the necessary expertise and equipment to the bedside.

2. The **Efferent limb** is the rapid response team. The response team is most frequently composed of ICU-trained personnel and equipment. Team composition varies based on the local needs. Most rapid response teams do not include a physician and are usually led by advanced practice providers, nurses, or respiratory therapists.

3. The quality improvement component provides a feedback loop by collecting and analyzing data from events to guide improvement of prevention and response.

4. The administrative or governance component is in charge of coordinating resources, purchasing equipment, and coordinating the education of hospital staff regarding the rapid response process.

Rapid response systems were initially introduced in the 1990s in Australia, and then the Institute for Healthcare Improvement introduced the concept in the United States. Since then, these systems have been associated with improved outcomes such as reduced anxiety among nursing staff, increased interdisciplinary teamwork, decreased cardiac arrests outside of ICUs, and a reduction in hospital mortality.

Computerized physician order entry (CPOE) is the process by which a physician enters medical orders directly into an EHR and manages the results of these orders.[46,47] The Institute of Medicine has identified the implementation of CPOE as an opportunity to improve medication safety, reduce ordering errors, and enhance compliance with guidelines, therefore improving patient safety. Sometimes the CPOE system is supported by a decision support system, making the system capable of alerting physicians about drug interactions, inappropriate dosages, and other drug-related problems. In addition, CPOE may reduce order duplication, reduce the time required to complete clinical tasks, and reduce the time that nurses spend on reviewing, verifying, and correcting clinical instructions. CPOE and EHRs provide the ability to coordinate patient care among team members and across different teams, facilities, or health care settings. The electronic transfer of patient health information is especially important when information is needed quickly, for example, when a patient presents at the emergency department or when the patient transitions from an inpatient to an outpatient setting. In addition, the electronic exchange of data is faster, more efficient, more complete, and more accurate than traditional written, faxed, or phone communications.

Although CPOE may have significant positive impact on coordination of care and patient safety, if its implementation is not planned well, it may have negative impacts on clinical workflow and collaboration between physicians and nurses. The clinical workflow can be disrupted by the use of CPOE systems because of asynchronous communication among team members, problems with human-computer interactions, change in the sequence and dynamics of clinical activities, and reduced clinical situation awareness.

VI. PROFESSIONALISM

Medical professionalism has been defined by many individuals and organizations. One of the more widely used definitions was formulated by the Accreditation Council for Graduate Medical Education. Professionalism is "a commitment to carrying out professional responsibilities and an adherence to ethical principles. Residents are expected to demonstrate: compassion, integrity, and respect for others; responsiveness to patient needs that supersedes self-interest; respect for patient privacy and autonomy; accountability to patients, society and the profession; and sensitivity and responsiveness to a diverse patient population, including but not limited to diversity in gender, age, culture, race, religion, disabilities, and sexual orientation."

Professionalism is a desired behavior of not only individual practitioners, but also of organizations that have been entrusted with the care of vulnerable individuals. There are many opportunities for tension between institutional goals and the ideals espoused earlier. Balancing the needs of the individual versus the needs of the system can be one of the most challenging tasks that health care professionals, including leaders, face. Extensive utilization of limited resources for the care of a single patient may make them unavailable for others. On more than one occasion, one of the authors has been asked to determine which of several patients in need can receive platelets for transfusion when they are in short supply. Developing an infrastructure to support decision making that is based on medical need rather than bias is one of the ways that a system can enhance professionalism.

A. Balancing Finance and Ethics

While most health care clinics or hospitals are not-for-profit, they still must function as businesses. Leaders in these institutions are entrusted with "keeping the lights on" and are increasingly selected for their financial acumen. Reimbursement for delivered care is complex and ever-changing; operating margins (defined as the ratio of dollars remaining after costs and operating expenses have been paid) are shrinking, and expectations by patients and communities are high. In this complicated environment, where multiple stakeholders are impacted by each decision, it is particularly important to center decisions in a manner that reflects professionalism.

The margin determines the ability to pursue activities. This is often summarized as "no margin, no mission." For example, choosing to deliver a costly therapy that may benefit a small handful of patients has to be weighed against a less expensive treatment that may prevent disease for large numbers of patients. If the hospital is unable to contain operating expenses, there may not be money for either. Politically, selecting not to provide services on the basis of cost can be unpopular. These kinds of decisions might best be decided by society at large, but often this is not the case. Rather, insurance companies and health care organizations must craft decisions aided by published guidance from professional organizations and the judgment of their leaders. Because they answer to more than one constituency, executives rarely face simple choices. In a particular health care delivery situation, the ethical constructs of altruism, beneficence, nonmaleficence, truth telling, and justice may come into conflict with the perceived best interests of the institution.

Creutzfeldt-Jakob disease (CJD) is a highly contagious prion disease affecting the brain. It is not destroyed by the techniques normally used to sterilize surgical equipment between patients. At present, it is not treatable and usually rapidly fatal. In order to minimize the risk for transmission from one individual to another, when the presence of CJD is suspected, protocols for diagnostic brain biopsies will use either disposable equipment or more expensive and prolonged sterilization. These cases are typically scheduled at the end of the surgical day to allow sufficient time for operating rooms to be intensively cleaned prior to their use for the next patient. Rarely the diagnosis is an unexpected finding on pathologic specimens, and investigation determines that patients were treated with surgical instruments that were not adequately sterilized. This is described as an *iatrogenic exposure*. When this is uncovered, it is usually days to weeks after the incident.

Hospital leaders are faced with a decision about disclosing CJD exposure to affected patients, potentially triggering emotional harm or expensive lawsuits. Some argue that since there is no intervention that can alter the patients' outcome, informing patients may trigger severe emotional trauma and may expose the hospital to financial harm from legal action. One published study interviewed 11 individuals who had been notified about being exposed to CJD. Using quantitative techniques, attitudes, and responses to the disclosure were evaluated. There was no evidence of lasting psychological harm in this limited study. Most subjects reported that their anger and fear were short-lived, and they coped by pushing the concern to the back of their minds. Adherence to prevent forward transmission was variable. "The two exceptions had been notified of surgical exposures after media reports: they questioned hospital practices and still felt angry."[48]

Although CJD exposure is an extremely serious exposure, there have been many other larger-scale examples of inadvertent exposure to harm including inadequately cleaned endoscopic equipment and examples of errors (such as incorrect hormone receptor tests performed on breast cancer pathologic specimens) that have impacted large numbers of patients and likely caused some of them tangible harm.

In the event of such complex decision making, there is a risk that leaders will make choices based on their own self-interests. If a hospital suffers the financial and public relations fallout from disclosing a large-scale medical error, it is common for leadership to be penalized and/or lose their jobs. The VHA has formulated a process that may aid leaders. VHA directive 2008-002, "Matrix to Aid in Adverse Event Disclosure Decisions for Large Scale Events," outlines an inclusive process to identify and involve all stakeholders in decision making, using surrogate decision makers where necessary to stand in for the patients' best interests. Ethicists are part of the multidisciplinary advisory panel that uses a structured set of questions to examine the situation in as transparent, comprehensive, and fair way as possible.[49] A 2010 *New England Journal of Medicine* article evaluates this and other approaches to making such decisions.[50]

Unfortunately, this situation is not as rare as one would hope, with at least two widely publicized disclosures of CJD exposure in 2013 and 2014.[51,52] The leaders of Forsyth Hospital in North Carolina were praised for the forthright and compassionate way in which they handled this disclosure.[53] Although no organization wants to deal with the publicity, potential litigation, and harm to reputation that can follow acknowledgment of errors, there is the possibility that timely, accurate, and compassionate disclosure can enhance trust.

A culture of professionalism is essential to the delivery of high-value care. Aligning physician and organizational understanding and behavior is a critical step. Mission statements and codes of conduct have been used to formalize expectations, but cannot succeed unless they are universally applied and adherence to them enforced equitably. Education and opportunities for professional development around this content is essential to creating a community that supports these goals.

Some organizations have developed programs that provide support for physicians who are challenged by adherence to these expectations. When remediation or disciplinary actions are applied inconsistently, they can undermine the establishment of a professional environment; when high-revenue generators are observed to be held to the same behavioral standards as other physicians, these guidelines reinforce professionalism. Ensuring equity in these matters falls to institutional leaders.

B. The Disruptive Physician

This chapter has discussed the importance of ensuring that organizations function in alignment with ethical and professional principles, as leaders' decisions can have a dramatic impact on the function of the system. Beyond their own clinical microsystem, an individual physician's behavior can significantly interfere with the system's delivery of safe, effective, compassionate, and cost-conscious care. There are many examples of the impact that criminal behavior can have on an institution, and physicians are not immune from the temptations that can lead to felonious acts. Physicians have access to information, drugs, and individuals in ways that can be abused for personal gain. In addition, physicians are humans and are subject to the same medical frailties as anyone else. Depression, anxiety disorders, and substance abuse by a physician can negatively impact the delivery of care. This section will focus on the "disruptive physician." There is some overlap with mental health and substance abuse, but the issue is much broader than mental health and substance abuse alone.

There are many definitions of disruptive behavior by physicians, but they generally include elements of intimidation, outbursts (angry or threatening), passive behaviors of nonparticipation in activities that impact patient safety, and/or refusal to perform routine tasks. This may include things like failure to complete charting, nonresponse to pages, or treating peers, patients, or staff with condescension. Other individuals may exhibit these behaviors, but historically, many institutions have accepted or explained away these actions by physicians, especially those seen as "rainmakers" (those who generate significant income). A survey by the American College of Physician Executives (renamed the American Association for Physician Leadership in 2014) found that 38 percent of physicians surveyed believed that "physicians in my organization who generate high amounts of revenue are treated more leniently when it comes to behavior problems."[54] In the last several decades, it has been recognized that disruptive behavior impacts health care delivery and patient safety. The Joint Commission has begun to address this issue by requiring demonstrated compliance with standards to achieve accreditation. In 2008, they issued a Sentinel Alert Bulletin that explained the rationale for two new leadership standards.[55]

EP 4: The hospital/organization has a code of conduct that defines acceptable and disruptive and inappropriate behaviors.

EP 5: Leaders create and implement a process for managing disruptive and inappropriate behaviors.

An important part of the impact of disruptive physicians was described by a survey on workplace intimidation conducted by the Institute of Safe Medication Practices (ISMP). In this survey of 2095 hospital-based health care providers (1565 nurses, 354 pharmacists, 176 others), a direct connection between intimidating behavior and overriding patient safety practices was seen. Seventeen percent of respondents had felt pressured to accept a medication order despite concerns about its safety on at least three occasions in the previous year, 13 percent had refrained from contacting a specific prescriber to clarify the safety of an order on at least 10 occasions, and 7 percent said that in the previous year they had been involved in a medication error where intimidation played a part. Sixty-four percent of pharmacists and 34 percent of nurses reported that, during the past year, they had assumed that a medication order was correct and safe rather than interact with a particular prescriber.[56] Health care systems have an obligation to identify and solve the issue of disruptive physician behavior (Table 13.1).

In addition to issues of patient safety, an individual physician's disruptive behavior can negatively impact other aspects of health care systems. An institution that does not effectively address disruptive behavior experiences higher staff turnover, lower patient satisfaction, and increased medical errors. One attempt to quantify the cost of disruptive behavior was published in 2013. The authors estimated costs based on the prevalence of particular behaviors and the financial impact attributed to them. In a 400-bed academic hospital, the cost due to medication and procedural errors, along with staff turnover, exceeded $1 million.[57]

In some cases, individuals identified as disruptive report that they were acting as "whistle blowers," trying to address a concern and escalating their actions until a response is elicited.[58] Health systems must provide opportunities for those impacted by policies to have a say in their construction and implementation. In addition, maintaining robust and non-punitive pathways for providers and staff to raise concerns may also reduce this issue. In turn, physicians and other health care providers must be self-aware about the impact their behaviors can have on their colleagues and the broader health care community. Providing stress management, anger management, and other supportive care services can be an important component of reducing disruptive behaviors.[59]

VII. CHAPTER SUMMARY

Evidence-based medicine helps define the best options based on current science. This chapter reviewed several methods employed to support translating that information into practice. Clinical practice guidelines and pathways provide specific and concrete algorithms for decision making. Monitoring adherence to these algorithms allows health care leaders to give feedback to practitioners frequently operating outside of these guidelines. Formularies are another mechanism to support moving evidence into operations. When implemented well, formularies limit the ability to provide care outside of that supported by the best evidence unless a rational justification is given.

Expanding modalities of communication present both challenges and opportunities. Striving to "meet people where they live" includes communicating with them in the way they prefer. We have discussed some of the advantages and perils

Table 13.1 The Joint Commission's Recommended System Approach to Disruptive Behavior

1. Educate all team members—both physicians and nonphysician staff—on appropriate professional behavior defined by the organization's code of conduct. The code and education should emphasize respect. Include training in basic business etiquette (particularly phone skills) and people skills.
2. Hold all team members accountable for modeling desirable behaviors, and enforce the code consistently and equitably among all staff regardless of seniority or clinical discipline in a positive fashion through reinforcement as well as punishment.
3. Develop and implement policies and procedures/processes appropriate for the organization that address:
   - "Zero tolerance" for intimidating and/or disruptive behaviors, especially the most egregious instances of disruptive behavior such as assault and other criminal acts. Incorporate the zero tolerance policy into medical staff bylaws and employment agreements as well as administrative policies.
   - Medical staff policies regarding intimidating and/or disruptive behaviors of physicians within a health care organization should be complementary and supportive of the policies that are present in the organization for nonphysician staff.
   - Reducing fear of intimidation or retribution and protecting those who report or cooperate in the investigation of intimidating, disruptive, and other unprofessional behavior. Non-retaliation clauses should be included in all policy statements that address disruptive behaviors.
   - Responding to patients and/or their families who are involved in or witness intimidating and/or disruptive behaviors. The response should include hearing and empathizing with their concerns, thanking them for sharing those concerns, and apologizing.
   - How and when to begin disciplinary actions (such as suspension, termination, loss of clinical privileges, reports to professional licensure bodies).
4. Develop an organizational process for addressing intimidating and disruptive behaviors that solicits and integrates substantial input from an interprofessional team including representation of medical and nursing staff, administrators, and other employees.
5. Provide skills-based training and coaching for all leaders and managers in relationship-building and collaborative practice, including skills for giving feedback on unprofessional behavior, and conflict resolution. Cultural assessment tools can also be used to measure whether or not attitudes change over time.
6. Develop and implement a system for assessing staff perceptions of the seriousness and extent of instances of unprofessional behaviors and the risk for harm to patients.
7. Develop and implement a reporting/surveillance system (possibly anonymous) for detecting unprofessional behavior. Include ombuds services and patient advocates, both of which provide important feedback from patients and families who may experience intimidating or disruptive behavior from health professionals. Monitor system effectiveness through regular surveys, focus groups, peer and team member evaluations, or other methods. Have multiple and specific strategies to learn whether intimidating or disruptive behaviors exist or recur, such as through direct inquiries at routine intervals with staff, supervisors, and peers.
8. Support surveillance with tiered, nonconfrontational interventional strategies, starting with informal "cup of coffee" conversations directly addressing the problem and moving toward detailed action plans and progressive discipline, if patterns persist. These interventions should initially be nonadversarial in nature, with the focus on building trust, placing accountability on and rehabilitating the offending individual, and protecting patient safety. Make use of mediators and conflict coaches when professional dispute resolution skills are needed.
9. Conduct all interventions within the context of an organizational commitment to the health and well-being of all staff, with adequate resources to support individuals whose behavior is caused or influenced by physical or mental health pathologies.
10. Encourage interprofessional dialogues across a variety of forums as a proactive way of addressing ongoing conflicts, overcoming them, and moving forward through improved collaboration and communication.
11. Document all attempts to address intimidating and disruptive behaviors.

From The Joint Commission. Behaviors that undermine a culture of safety. http://www.jointcommission.org/assets/1/18/SEA_40.PDF. Published July 9, 2008. Accessed March 13, 2016.

of opening new channels such as patient portals. Physicians and other health care professionals need to ensure that they do not create risks for themselves or patients by making assumptions about communication being completed when it has merely been initiated. We explored how social media can be used as an effective tool to disseminate information or gather opinions and discussed some cautionary information about hazards of health care professionals having a social media presence.

Having a diverse society poses unique challenges to health care providers, and this chapter explored examples of challenges raised by providing health care services to individuals with diverse backgrounds and beliefs that do not always align with the prevailing views of modern medicine. Adapting to the needs of unique communities can better care for all patients.

Medicine is a team sport, and providing care today requires an understanding of how effective teams function. This chapter includes two examples of formal teams that have been designed to enhance health care quality. Accountable care teams foster interprofessional collaboration and collegiality. Rapid response systems have demonstrated significant improvements in patient survival and other metrics through enhanced teamwork.

In new and unique ways, health care professionals face challenges to their professionalism. These challenges may take the form of crises, such as the identification that patients may have inadvertently been exposed to infectious disease risks, such as CJD through medical procedures, or that errors that impact patients' health may have occurred. Balancing the potential liabilities of disclosure against the ethical imperatives to protect patient's autonomy can be difficult. Other formidable conflicts can require weighing financial realities with community clinical health imperatives. Institutions can also face the challenge of dealing with disruptive professionals, staff, and clients and prepare through formulating appropriate responses.

This chapter reviewed examples of the systems-level impact of a variety of domains. Leaders are presented with opportunities to excel in providing service to diverse communities through innovation and sensitivity. Operationalizing the best evidence in medicine can enhance patient safety, and failing to do so can be detrimental to both patients and organizations. Fostering excellence in teamwork and communication can raise the quality of care delivered, as well as enhance the satisfaction of patients and staff. While mastering all of these areas can seem a daunting task, awareness of their importance is a first step.

QUESTIONS FOR FURTHER THOUGHT

1. In order to keep up with modern times, a practice is trying to increase its accessibility by setting up a Twitter account. Can you identify any challenges that this might raise?
2. A complaint is brought to the attention of the chief medical officer of a hospital alleging that a physician is continuously texting during surgery (she has her cell phone wrapped in a sterile bag to maintain "scrub"). Can you identify any concerns that this raises?
3. A patient is in need of a surgical intervention due to a life-threatening condition. The patient's culture does not accept direct discussions of death, fearing that speaking about it brings it to pass. How can informed consent be obtained in this context?
4. As a member of an interprofessional working group that is responsible for improving care for patients with mental health challenges in the ambulatory care setting in your institution, you observe that the group and all of its subcommittees are headed by physicians. Is this likely to help or impair the success of the work?

Annotated Bibliography

Azar J, Adams N, Boustani M. The Indiana University Center for Healthcare Innovation and Implementation Science: bridging healthcare research and delivery to build a learning healthcare system. *Z Evid Fortbild Qual Gesundhwes*. 2015;109(2):138–143.
  This article provides an overview of the translation of health care advances from research to clinical practice.
Medical Defense Union. Ethical social networking. http://www.themdu.com/guidance-and-advice/journals/good-practice-october-2013/ethical-social-networking. Published October 2013. Accessed January 24, 2016.
  This article reviews the ethical challenges that arise in the use of social media by health care professionals.
Shapiro J, Whittemore A, Tsen LC. Instituting a culture of professionalism: the establishment of a center for professionalism and peer support. *Jt Comm J Qual Patient Saf*. 2014;40(4):168–177.
  This paper outlines key elements for the support of professional behavior in the physician workplace.

References

1. Patel P, White DL, Deswal A. Translation of clinical trial results into practice: temporal patterns of β-blocker utilization for heart failure at hospital discharge and during ambulatory follow-up. *Am Heart J*. 2007;153(4):515–522.
2. Lenfant C. Clinical research to clinical practice—lost in translation? *N Engl J Med*. 2003;349(9):868–874.
3. McGlynn EA, Asch SM, Adams J, et al. The quality of health care delivered to adults in the United States. *N Engl J Med*. 2003;348(26):2635–2645.
4. Azar J, Adams N, Boustani M. The Indiana University Center for Healthcare Innovation and Implementation Science: bridging healthcare research and delivery to build a learning healthcare system. *Z Evid Fortbild Qual Gesundhwes*. 2015;109(2):138–143.
5. Institute of Medicine (now Health and Medicine Division). Clinical practice guidelines we can trust. http://iom.nationalacademies.org/Reports/2011/Clinical-Practice-Guidelines-We-Can-Trust.aspx. Published March 23, 2011. Accessed March 13, 2016.
6. National Comprehensive Cancer Network. NCCN clinical practice guidelines. http://www.nccn.org/. Accessed March 13, 2016.
7. American Society of Clinical Oncology Institute for Quality. http://www.instituteforquality.org/. Accessed March 13, 2016.
8. Adelson KB, Qiu YC, Evangelista M, Spencer-Cisek P, Whipple C, Holcombe RF. Implementation of electronic chemotherapy ordering: an opportunity to improve evidence-based oncology care. *J Oncol Pract*. 2014;10(2):e113–e119.
9. Dellit TH, Owens RC, McGowan JE, et al. Infectious Diseases Society of America and the Society for Healthcare Epidemiology of America guidelines for developing an institutional program to enhance antimicrobial stewardship. *Clin Infect Dis*. 2007;44(2):159–177.
10. Nuila F, Cadle RM, Logan N, Musher DM. Members of the Infectious Disease Section of the Michael E DeBakey VA Medical Center. Antibiotic stewardship and *Clostridium difficile*–associated disease. *Infect Control Hosp*. 2008;29(11):1096–1097.
11. Beard L, Schein R, Morra D, Wilson K, Keelan J. The challenges in making electronic health records accessible to patients. *J Am Med Inform Assoc*. 2012;19(1):116–120.
12. Kruse CS, Bolton K, Freriks G. The effect of patient portals on quality outcomes and its implications to meaningful use: a systematic review. *J Med Internet Res*. 2015;17(2):e44.
13. Chou W-YS, Hunt YM, Beckjord EB, Moser RP, Hesse BW. Social media use in the United States: implications for health communication. *J Med Internet Res*. 2009;11(4):e48.
14. New York City Bar, Lambda Legal, Human Rights Campaign. *Creating Equal Access to Quality Health Care for Transgender Patients: Transgender-Affirming Hospital Policies*. http://hrc-assets.s3-website-us-east-1.amazonaws.com//files/assets/resources/transgender-affirming-hospital-policies.pdf. Accessed March 13, 2016.
15. Baggs JG, Schmitt MH, Mushlin AI, et al. Association between nurse-physician collaboration and patient outcomes in three intensive care units. *Crit Care Med*. 1999;27(9):1991–1998.
16. Shortell SM, Zimmerman JE, Rousseau DM, et al. The performance of intensive care units: does good management make a difference? *Med Care*. 1994;32(5):508–525.
17. Benzer JK, Young G, Stolzmann K, et al. The relationship between organizational climate and quality of chronic disease management. *Health Serv Res*. 2011;46(3):691–711.
18. Leykum LK, Palmer R, Lanham H, et al. Reciprocal learning and chronic care model implementation in primary care: results from a new scale of learning in primary care. *BMC Health Serv Res*. 2011;11:44.
19. Gittell JH, Fairfield KM, Bierbaum B, et al. Impact of relational coordination on quality of care, postoperative pain and functioning, and length of stay: a nine-hospital study of surgical patients. *Med Care*. 2000;38(8):807–819.
20. Risser DT, Rice MM, Salisbury ML, Simon R, Jay GD, Berns SD. The potential for improved teamwork to reduce medical errors in the emergency department. The MedTeams Research Consortium. *Ann Emerg Med*. 1999;34(3):373–383.
21. Donchin Y, Gopher D, Olin M, et al. A look into the nature and causes of human errors in the intensive care unit. *Crit Care Med*. 1995;23(2):294–300.
22. Aiken LH, Smith HL, Lake ET. Lower Medicare mortality among a set of hospitals known for good nursing care. *Med Care*. 1994;32(8):771–787.
23. Uhlig PN, Brown J, Nason AK, Camelio A, Kendall E, John M. Eisenberg Patient Safety Awards. System innovation: Concord Hospital. *Jt Comm J Qual Improv*. 2002;28(12):666–672.
24. Neily J, Mills PD, Young-Xu Y, et al. Association between implementation of a medical team training program and surgical mortality. *JAMA*. 2010;304(15):1693–1700.
25. Kim MM, Barnato AE, Angus DC, Fleisher LF, Kahn JM. The effect of multidisciplinary care teams on intensive care unit mortality. *Arch Intern Med*. 2010;170(4):369–376.
26. Baggs JG, Ryan SA. ICU nurse-physician collaboration & nursing satisfaction. *Nurs Econ*. 1990;8(6):386–392.
26a. Vahey DC, Aiken LH, Sloane DM, et al. Nurse burnout and patient satisfaction. *Med Care*. 2004;42(suppl 2):1157–1166.

27. Shortell SM, Zimmerman JE, Rousseau DM, et al. The performance of intensive care units: does good management make a difference? *Med Care*. 1994;32(5):508–525.

28. Makary MA, Sexton JB, Freischlag JA, et al. Operating room teamwork among physicians and nurses: teamwork in the eye of the beholder. *JACS*. 2006;202(5):746–752.

29. Thomas EJ, Sexton JB, Helmreich RL. Discrepant attitudes about teamwork among critical care nurses and physicians. *Crit Care Med*. 2003;31(3):956–959.

30. O'Leary KJ, Ritter CD, Wheeler H, Szekendi MK, Brinton TS, Williams MV. Teamwork on inpatient medical units: assessing attitudes and barriers. *Qual Saf Health Care*. 2010;19(2):117–121.

30a. Tresolini CP, Inui TS, Candib LM, et al. *Health Professions Education and Relationship-Centered Care*. San Francisco: The Pew-Fetzer Task Force; 1994.

30b. Lanham H, McDaniel R, Crabtree B, et al. How improving practice relationships among clinicians and nonclinicians can improve quality in primary care. *Jt Comm J Qual Patient Saf*. 2009;35(9):457–466.

31. D'Amour D, Ferrada-Videla M, San Martin Rodriguez L, et al. The conceptual basis for interprofessional collaboration: core concepts and theoretical frameworks. *J Interprof Care*. 2005;19(1 suppl):116–131.

32. Gittell JH. Brandeis University. Relational coordination: guidelines for theory, measurement and analysis. https://www.researchgate.net/public ation/228668390_Relational_Coordination_Guidelines_for_Theory_M easurement_and_Analysis. Published 2009. Accessed March 13, 2016.

33. Gittell JH, Weinberg DB, Bennett AL, Miller JA. Is the doctor in? A relational approach to job design and the coordination of work. *Hum Resource Manag J*. 2008;47(4):729–755.

34. Gittell JH, Weinberg D, Pfefferle S, Bishop C. Impact of relational coordination on job satisfaction and quality outcomes: a study of nursing homes. *Hum Resource Manag J*. 2008;18(2):154–170.

35. Gittell JH. Organizing work to support relational co-ordination. *Int J Hum Resource Manag*. 2000;11(3):517–539.

36. Shaw A, de Lusignan S, Rowlands G. Do primary care professionals work as a team: a qualitative study. *J Interprof Care*. 2005;19(4):396–405.

37. Wittenberg-Lyles EM. Information sharing in interdisciplinary team meetings: An evaluation of hospice goals. *Qual Health Res*. 2005;15(10):1377–1391.

38. Thomas EJ, Sexton JB, Helmreich RL. Discrepant attitudes about teamwork among critical care nurses and physicians. *Crit Care Med*. 2003;31(3):956–959.

39. Weber H, Stockli M, Nubling M, Langewitz WA. Communication during ward rounds in internal medicine. An analysis of patient-nurse-physician interactions using RIAS. *Patient Educ Couns*. 2007;67(3):343–348.

40. Kara A, Johnson CS, Nicley A, Niemeier MR, Hui SL. Redesigning inpatient care: testing the effectiveness of an accountable care team model. *J Hosp Med*. 2015;10(12):773–779.

41. Deleted in review.

42. Deleted in review.

43. Deleted in review.

44. Jones DA, DeVita MA, Bellomo R. Rapid-response teams. *New Eng J Med*. 2011;365(2):139–146.

45. Winters BD, Weaver SJ, Pfoh ER, Yang T, Pham JC, Dy SM. Rapid-response systems as a patient safety strategy: a systematic review. *Ann Intern Med*. 2013;158(5 Pt 2):417–425.

46. Niazkhani Z, Pirnejad H, Berg M, Aarts J. The impact of computerized provider order entry systems on inpatient clinical workflow: a literature review. *J Am Med Inform Assoc*. 2009;16(4):539–549.

47. Niazkhani Z, Pirnejad H, Van der Sijs H, de Bont A, Aarts J. Computerized provider order entry system—does it support the inter-professional medication process? *Methods Inf Med*. 2010;49(1):20–27.

48. Elam G, Oakley K, Connor N, et al. Impact of being placed at risk of Creutzfeldt-Jakob disease: a qualitative study of blood donors to variant CJD cases and patients potentially surgically exposed to CJD. *Neuroepidemiology*. 2011;36(4):274–281.

49. Veteranclaims's blog. VA's Directive 2008-002, Disclosure of Adverse Events to Patients. https://veteranclaims.wordpress.com/2010/07/27/vas-directive-2008-002-disclosure-of-adverse-events-to-patients/. Accessed March 13, 2016.

50. Dudzinski DM, Hébert PC, Foglia MB, Gallagher TH. The disclosure dilemma—large-scale adverse events. *N Engl J Med*. 2010;363(10):978–986.

51. FoxNews Health. 18 North Carolina hospital patients potentially exposed to rare brain disease. http://www.foxnews.com/health/2014/02/11/nc-hospital-apologizes-for-exposure-to-disease.html. Published February 11, 2014. Accessed March 13, 2016.

52. Catholic Medical Center. Possible patient exposure to Creutzfeldt-Jakob disease announced. https://www.catholicmedicalcenter.org/news-detail/possible-patient-exposure-to-creutzfeldt-jakob-disease-announced/28.aspx. Accessed March 13, 2016.

53. Powers & Santola, LLP. Differences in mistake disclosure from hospital to hospital. http://www.powers-santola.com/blog/2014/03/differences-mistake-disclosure-hospital-hospital/. Accessed March 13, 2016.

54. Keogh T, Martin W. Managing unmanageable physicians. *Physician Exec*. 2004;30(5):18–22.

55. The Joint Commission. Behaviors that undermine a culture of safety. Sentinel Event Alert. http://www.jointcommission.org/assets/1/18/SEA_40.pdf. Published July 9, 2008. Accessed March 13, 2016.

56. Institute for Safe Medication Practices. Intimidation: practitioners speak up about this unresolved problem (part 1). http://www.ismp.org/Newsletters/acutecare/articles/20040311_2.asp. Published March 11, 2004. Accessed March 13, 2016.

57. Rawson JV, Thompson N, Sostre G, Deitte L. The cost of disruptive and unprofessional behaviors in health care. *Acad Radiol*. 2013;20(9):1074–1076.

58. My Health Law Attorneys. The disruptive physician. http://www.myhealthlawattorneys.com/#!The-Disruptive-Physician/c1seg/C614CC79-EE29-40F1-A7E8-B873E9F9E8BC. Published September 19, 2014. Accessed March 13, 2016.

59. Shapiro J, Whittemore A, Tsen LC. Instituting a culture of professionalism: the establishment of a center for professionalism and peer support. *Jt Comm J Qual Patient Saf*. 2014;40(4):168–177.

60. Schaffer A. How Jehovah's Witnesses are changing medicine. *The New Yorker*. August 12, 2015. http://www.newyorker.com/news/news-desk/how-jehovahs-witnesses-are-changing-medicine. Accessed March 13, 2016.

61. Akron Children's Hospital. Addressing barriers to care in the Amish community. https://www.akronchildrens.org/cms/addressing_barriers_to_care_in_amish_community/. Accessed March 13, 2016.

62. Kinsey MJ. What happens in the hospital doesn't stay in the hospital. *Slate*. January 10, 2014. http://www.slate.com/articles/technology/future_tense/2014/01/doctors_on_social_media_share_embarrassing_photos_details_of_patients.html. Accessed January 24, 2016.

63. Chretien KC, Greysen SR, Chretien JP, Kind T. Online posting of unprofessional content by medical students. *JAMA*. 2009;302(12):1309–1315.

64. Go PH, Klaassen Z, Chamberlain RS. Attitudes and practices of surgery residency program directors toward the use of social networking profiles to select residency candidates: a nationwide survey analysis. *J Surg Educ*. 2012;69(3):292–300.

65. Symonds M. 5 Social media tips to protect your future from your online past. *Forbes*. March 14, 2014. http://www.forbes.com/sites/mattsymonds/2014/03/14/5-social-media-tips-to-protect-your-future-from-your-online-past/#7c43edce59ab. Accessed January 24, 2016.

66. Medical Defense Union. Ethical social networking. http://www.themdu.com/guidance-and-advice/journals/good-practice-october-2013/ethical-social-networking. Published October 2013. Accessed January 24, 2016.

14

The Use of Assessment to Support Learning and Improvement in Health Systems Science

Richard E. Hawkins, MD, Karen E. Hauer, MD, PhD, and Kimberly D. Lomis, MD

LEARNING OBJECTIVES

1. List key behaviors that will promote success in acquiring the knowledge, skills, and attitudes intrinsic to health systems science.
2. Describe the elements of self-regulated learning and how they may be used to support lifelong learning.
3. Describe how informed self-assessment, feedback seeking, and reflection can identify learning and improvement needs and lead to enhanced learning and performance.
4. Understand the core principles of assessment and how they help guide selection and optimal use of assessment methods.
5. Describe the various methods used in the assessment of health systems science domains and how they may be used to identify learning and improvement needs.

This chapter focuses on the use of assessment in driving and measuring learning and improvement in health systems science (HSS). The chapter begins by describing the need for students to take the initiative in defining their assessment, learning, and improvement needs and provides a list of key steps that will help students in developing the knowledge, skills, and attitudes intrinsic to HSS. The concept of **self-regulated learning** is introduced as the means by which learners can adjust their behaviors to achieve their learning goals. During self-regulated learning activities, learners direct their thoughts, feelings, and actions toward controlling their academic and clinical performance. Key elements of self-regulated learning include goal setting, self-efficacy, attributions of learning outcomes, self-assessment, feedback seeking, and reflection. To be effective, self-assessment needs to be informed by external data or feedback; without this information, learners and physicians typically self-assess inaccurately. With external data or feedback, assessment then becomes a driver and a measure of learning. Core principles of assessment are delineated in order to help learners understand how they may be best applied in measuring their knowledge, skills and, ultimately, their performance in practice. Although learners may not control which assessments are used within their educational programs, understanding how they are used and the results generated by them will help learners get the most out of assessment in supporting their self-regulated learning. A variety of assessment methods that will be commonly used to assess knowledge, skills, and performance in HSS domains are reviewed.

I. INTRODUCTION

The preceding chapters of this text encourage the reader to view the delivery of health care from the perspective of a system. Most learning occurs in the context of a system as well, either in a structured, educational environment, or in a clinical workplace environment. In order for students to optimize performance, they need to understand the system in which they learn and are assessed. The intent of this chapter is to empower students by providing guidance on tracking their own performance.

Each individual within a system must strive to develop the personal knowledge, skills, and attitudes requisite for patient care. However, to accomplish learning or care delivery, a **high-performing system** also relies upon meaningful interactions among members. This demands that each individual possess greater awareness of the collective performance goals and develop a broader set of competencies.[1]

This chapter offers two major perspectives to assist students. HSS is a relatively new content area, so motivated students will need to take more ownership for their own learning and assessment. The first section of the chapter provides strategies for adapting to the less structured learning environment of the clinical workplace, although many of these strategies will also be effective in structured learning contexts. This section offers tips to develop successful self-regulated learning habits that will be necessary throughout one's medical career. Because more medical schools will soon begin to directly address HSS, the second section of this chapter describes a variety of frameworks used in formal educational programs to assess a student's performance. A stronger understanding of the rationale for the common assessment methods that are used to measure performance will enhance student success in both HSS and in other competencies.

Provided are "keys to success" (Table 14.1), which integrate content from this chapter into actionable steps that students can practice.

II. STUDENT-DIRECTED ASSESSMENT STRATEGIES FOR THE CLINICAL WORKPLACE

Students participating in the **health care delivery system** quickly recognize that the educational process is less structured in the workplace than in traditional classroom environments. Learning strategies that serve students well in other contexts are insufficient to promote success in the workplace. The scaffolding that was provided earlier in their education (such as uniform lecture notes and published learning objectives) is withdrawn, and the learner must assume more self-direction in setting and achieving individual learning goals. Additionally, since HSS is a relatively novel area of expertise for physicians and other health care professionals, students may encounter inconsistent role modeling in the workplace. By actively engaging in this domain, they can become change agents in the health care system.

The modern health care environment is dynamic and rapidly evolving, demanding that physicians continuously update their knowledge and skills to keep pace with scientific advances and changes in systems of care. Physicians in practice are expected to monitor their knowledge and skills, take action to address personal gaps, and stay current with new developments in the field.[2,3] Each physician must engage in repeated cycles of learning: seeking meaningful evidence about one's performance, identifying gaps, creating goals, pursuing resources, and re-assessing. The concepts of lifelong learning and self-direction of one's learning are increasingly emphasized for physicians and trainees.[4,5] Despite the attention to these skills, it remains challenging for students, residents, and practicing physicians to implement them. There is a natural tendency for students who are eager to be accepted into the system, to focus their energies on *appearing* to perform well. True growth requires a willingness to openly acknowledge one's limitations and actively pursue learning opportunities. This strategy can be daunting, but it is critical to the delivery of safe and effective patient care.

Table 14.1 Keys to Success in Health Systems Science*

1. Be aware of your personal perspectives on learning and how you define success.
2. Strive for a growth mindset.
3. Take ownership of your learning and performance.
4. Seek feedback from multiple sources and perspectives.
5. In addition to personal performance, consider how well you contribute to the system, help your teams attain their desired results, and support positive patient outcomes.
6. Be cognizant of the criteria by which you are formally assessed.
7. Critically review evidence about your performance (informed self-assessment).
   - Be familiar with the value and limitations of various assessment methods.
   - Consider whether a given assessment aligns with the intended outcome.
   - Consider reliability and validity when weighing data about your performance.
   - Seek advice from a mentor to interpret feedback, especially if evidence seems contradictory.
8. Identify areas in need of improvement and areas of strength to build upon.
9. Set goals and identify resources for learning.
10. Protect time to reflect upon performance and to follow through on goals.
11. Re-assess by reviewing subsequent performance evidence.
12. Seek opportunities to contribute to the teaching and assessment of HSS at your institution.

*Since HSS is an emerging content area, you may need to take initiative to understand whether you are developing the necessary knowledge, skills, and attitudes in this domain.

A. Self-Regulated Learning as the Basis for Lifelong Learning

The process of how learners and physicians engage in ongoing learning can be understood through the lens of self-regulated learning theory, which describes the processes by which individuals adjust their behaviors to achieve goals.[6] Self-regulation comprises one's thoughts, feelings, and actions that are directed toward achievement of goals.[7] Self-regulated learning describes a cycle of control of one's academic and clinical performance through the following:[8]
1. Goal-directed behavior
2. The use of specific strategies to attain goals
3. Adapting and modifying behaviors or strategies to optimize learning and performance

Self-regulated learners therefore take charge of their own learning through strategies that involve their thoughts and actions. They actively monitor their own learning rather than passively waiting to be told what and how to learn. Though many people believe they are learning and growing, making these behaviors as intentional and habitual as possible can maximize learning. Self-regulated learning behaviors can be fostered from the beginning of medical school.

The three components of self-regulated learning translate to three phases or steps that a student follows during a learning activity:
1. **Before:** Before a learning activity, the student prepares by reading the assignment or gathering information about the activity and sets goals and plans to achieve those goals.
2. **During:** During the activity, the student uses strategies to focus and optimize learning. These can entail when and where to study, with whom to study or practice, how to

Table 14.2 Examples of the Dimensions of Attribution in Self-Regulated Learning

Dimension of Attribution	Why Student Achieved a Certain Learning Result	
Locus of control	**External:** My score is due to the difficulty of the assignment or the help I got from my friends or my teachers.	**Internal:** My score is due to the amount of effort I applied, the strategy I used to learn the material, and understanding of the material on the text.
Stability	**Stable (ability):** My grade is due to my intelligence; I am always going to be good at certain things but not others.	**Unstable (modifiable with effort):** My grade is due to the time I spent studying. When I worked harder or wrote brief quizzes for myself on the material, my performance improved.
Controllability	**Uncontrollable:** Outcomes due to luck. I did not learn because my attending was too hard on me.	**Controllable with effort:** I worked very hard in my peer group and learned all of the material.

From Graham S. A review of attribution theory in achievement contexts. *Educ Psychol Rev*. 1991;3(1):5–39.

participate in a small group, and what strategies to use (e.g., quizzing, rehearsing).

3. **After:** After an activity, the student reviews what happened and reflects on what worked well and what could have worked better. This reflection informs the next attempt with the same or a similar learning activity.

Teachers can create an environment that invites self-regulated learning behaviors by helping the student to understand the desired performance, guiding the student toward that performance, and motivating the student. The three steps of self-regulated learning require specific skills and attitudes that will be described in the following sections with examples from medical education.

1. Goal Setting

The first phase of self-regulated learning includes setting a goal for what is to be accomplished. Based on this goal, the student can begin goal-directed behavior. Students' goal orientation varies based on the goals to which they aspire. Students with mastery-oriented goals want to improve, learn materials, and develop skills. Students with performance-oriented goals want to earn high scores or good grades, win awards, or avoid public failure. Mastery goals are better for learning because they are associated with internal motivations, greater effort, and willingness to attempt challenges and new learning experiences. Useful goal setting involves goals that are achievable and measurable within a defined timeframe, so that the student or the teacher can know if the goal was accomplished. There are the following different kinds of goals:

- **Process goals:** Process goals are the steps taken to achieve an outcome. For medical students, process goals could include how much or when to study for an examination, how to practice cardiac auscultation and seek feedback during a clerkship, or learning a mnemonic for a patient handoff.
- **Outcome goals:** Outcome goals are the end product the student seeks. Outcome goals can include a course grade, acceptance to a residency, or successfully leading a team briefing.

In general, process goals are more helpful for early learners because they clearly define the steps that need to improve. However, over the long run, a balance of process goals and outcome goals is effective.

2. Self-Efficacy

Self-efficacy entails one's belief in one's own ability to accomplish something. Strong self-efficacy increases one's performance of that action (i.e., if you believe you can do something, you are more likely to succeed). In medical education, carefully designed early clinical experiences can promote the self-efficacy that is critical to self-regulated learning. These experiences should expose students to the people and practices of the clinical context and provide opportunities to contribute successfully later during their clinical rotations. This occurs through providing students with clear roles and opportunities to build the necessary knowledge and skills. This situation could occur in an early preceptorship in which first-year medical students see patients and help the interprofessional staff or physicians with clinical tasks.

3. Attributions

In the third phase of self-regulated learning, students reflect on how they did and interpret why their performance played out as it did. In this phase, students engage in attribution by identifying the primary reasons for the results they achieved. Attributions can be understood in these dimensions as outlined in Table 14.2.[9]

The attributions that best promote learning and self-regulated learning behaviors are internal, unstable, and controllable. The student who will achieve the best performance will believe that performance in clinical settings or on examinations is due to the effort or approach used to study and learn the knowledge and skills. For example, a student may note that her efforts during the pediatrics clerkship, which entailed setting and following a reading schedule and practicing her patient sign-out skills with her resident, led to improvements in her team's evaluation of her performance.

Carol Dweck's work on growth mindsets builds on this information about attributions.[10] In order to fulfill their potential, students should have a growth mindset, believing that their potential to improve is within their control. Students should focus on their efforts and study strategies rather than worrying, "Am I smart enough?" when faced with a challenge. Teachers and clinical supervisors should praise students' effort and persistence and the strategies they use and choices they make rather than their ability or intelligence.

B. Self-Assessment and Feedback Seeking

To engage in self-regulated learning, students must set goals that are appropriate for their learning needs. To identify those goals, students must be able to assess how they are doing and what improvements are needed. This process of individually evaluating one's performance is called *self-assessment.* For example, a student preparing for the MCAT reviews his or her prior performance on practice tests to decide how much to study for each section. It is often said that physicians are poor self-assessors. Studies have shown that low-performing students or physicians may overrate their performance (due to poor insight) and high-performing students or physicians may underrate their performance (due to their tendency to perpetually aim for higher and better performance).[11–13]

This illustrates the need for evidence-based self-assessment, also known as *informed self-assessment.*[14] From the student's perspective, it is possible to engage in informed self-assessment by seeking and reviewing any performance information available. It is important for students to begin by asking supervisors of expectations up front, and then, after some time working together, soliciting honest and specific constructive feedback on ways to improve. A student can ask for feedback, scores, and written comments from assessments, that is, after being observed presenting or seeing patients in a clerkship, after taking a written examination, or after interacting with a small group of peers. Observing a peer or student slightly ahead in the curriculum can also serve as a source of information about ways to do things differently and better.

Fortunately, there are strategies to improve the accuracy of self-assessment.

- **Clarity and understanding of the expected level of performance:** The first is defining the performance expectation. For a student self-assessing how well he or she used evidence-based practice methods in addressing a difficult patient problem, he or she would want to know which skills and behaviors were expected, such as developing a good clinical question, searching and appraising the literature, and applying the best available evidence to the patient's problem, and how those will be assessed.
- **Feedback:** Students who receive feedback from a preceptor or by watching a video of their performance with standardized patients are more likely to rate themselves similarly to the ratings provided by a faculty or standardized patient. Students should seek feedback from their supervising attending and resident physicians as well as their advisors and mentors to improve their understanding of their own performance and therefore their self-assessment, which can guide their learning planning.
- **Experience:** More experience with a skill may improve self-assessment due to greater understanding of what is expected, more prior practice, or more opportunities for feedback.
- **Assessment:** Test-enhanced learning describes the learning benefit of taking tests. Testing can improve self-assessment when it is coupled with feedback on performance. Students learn more when they are regularly tested compared to when they continue to study without being tested. Taking a test requires the student to recall information, and this process strengthens memory. This effect is particularly strong if the test requires the student to retrieve information (as with a short-answer or fill-in-the-blank examination) rather than just recognizing it (as with a multiple-choice examination).[15]
- **Mentoring:** Many medical schools pair students with a faculty member who will serve as a mentor in the learning process. This individual may be called a *mentor, coach, advisor,* or *master.* Regardless of the title, a faculty mentor can be very helpful in guiding a student through the process of self-regulated learning. The mentor may help set learning goals, provide information about expected performance, offer feedback, or critique the student's reflections on performance. Students should seek mentorship from trusted faculty to guide them in this process.

C. Reflection

Reflection on one's performance should occur during each phase of self-regulating learning. Before an activity, the student reflects upon what he or she has learned in the past and considers how to prepare for the activity. During the activity, reflection occurs in real time as the students monitor their performance and make needed adjustments. Reflection occurs most prominently after the activity as the student self-assesses, reviews information about expected benchmarks for performance and feedback received on the performance, and identifies the gap between actual and ideal performance.

D. Awareness of Team Performance

The heightened acknowledgment of health care delivery as a team process mandates assessment of performance at the level of the team in addition to evaluating individual members. How does a team know it is working well? Students certainly have experience in managing group projects in classroom or extracurricular settings, but often assume that assessing the function of their clinical teams is beyond their scope. Due to the nomadic nature of clinical assignments, students may feel more like guests rather than true members of the team. This section will highlight why and how students should engage in assessing team performance.

As novices to the health care delivery system, students learn by closely observing the activities of others. Students may thus identify important issues that other busy team members fail to notice. Not limited by preconceived ideas about how things are done, students are in a unique position to question existing processes and to notice inefficiencies that may have evolved unintentionally. Many students would hesitate to raise such questions, assuming that the more established team members know better. However, if one accepts that complex care delivery systems are prone to error, the student should consider such observations to be potential contributions to the team's success. Indeed, it is a student's duty to improve the system in which he or she learns and works. With careful phrasing, a student's inquiry can be posed in a manner that is not confrontational and communicates the intent to enhance team outcomes.

A first step to judging the success of a team is to clarify common goals. This may not be straightforward since the goals of the individuals within each team often differ significantly. Clinical care teams are composed of members at varying stages of development across a mix of professions, each with differing individual outcomes expected from a given clinical placement. Gaining clarity about what success looks like for the team is important, and remaining focused on meeting the needs of patients is fundamental. Residents are often tasked with directing the daily work of clinical teams. A resident who is just developing management skills and challenged by frequent changes in team membership may not have established a habit of orienting each member as they rotate onto the team. Students should take the initiative to clarify their supervisors' expectations at the beginning of each clinical placement and routinely seek guidance from all members of the team.[16] That will enable them to actively pursue opportunities to contribute meaningfully to the team's function.

True teamwork is difficult to attain; there is a difference between working next to one another versus truly working together. The clinical workplace is demanding, placing many pressures on individuals and on the team. Maintaining productive, positive interactions among team members requires active management; any interpersonal conflicts or unprofessional behaviors should be addressed openly.[17] This, too, can be intimidating for students to tackle. Gaining the maturity and confidence to address interpersonal challenges is essential to a student's full development as a professional. It is helpful to approach such conversations with the goal of optimizing team performance rather than viewing this as simply a personal issue. It is less threatening to use phrasing that reports an observation about behavior rather than passing judgment: "This is what I observed; can you help me understand?" All team members can serve as role models in the workplace (either good or bad). Helping one another maintain professional standards enhances the working/learning environment and, thereby, improves the quality of care that is delivered.

Increasingly, formal team briefings and debriefings are being instituted to address the issues outlined earlier. A huddle at the start of a clinic session or before beginning a procedure can clarify expectations and roles for each member. Similarly, a brief review at the end of a session confirms whether goals were met and can help address any problems that arose. Students who routinely reflect on how they can best contribute will feel empowered to participate in these structured discussions. Since students will rise quickly into leadership roles as residents, practicing these strategies as students will help them become more effective team leaders in the future.

Case Study 1

Joe, a second-year medical student, meets with his advisor to review his performance in the school's competency domains. His scores and comments from his preceptors indicate that his communication skills are consistently below the expected benchmark and below the class mean. Peer feedback comments include a few concerns about his quiet nature and hesitancy to speak up in small group despite seeming to be well-prepared with notes and diagrams. One peer wrote, "Joe sometimes doesn't say anything in small group." With his advisor, Joe reflects on the reasons that he seems quiet and nonparticipatory and how he could change that (internal, unstable, controllable attributions). Joe sets the process goals that he will make at least two comments in each small group session and seek feedback from his preceptor on his communication skills at every clinical session. He follows through on each of these goals and reflects on how he performed during and after each small group and

preceptorship. Using his scores at the next advisor meeting, Joe is pleased to see improvement and then sets new goals for continued improvement in his learning.

One year later, Joe is midway through his core clerkships and again meeting with his advisor to review his progress. In his first clerkship, Joe again felt hesitant to speak up in the context of the fast-paced surgical service. However, he recognized this challenge within the first 2 weeks and focused on the process goals of asking one question and offering one suggestion during each day's interdisciplinary rounds. Comfortable with this approach, he applied it through all of his clerkships. He also notes in his multisource feedback from nursing that he is commended for checking in with his patients' nurses regularly. He and his advisor noted that his communication scores were all above the mean. Asked to set a goal for the remainder of his clerkships, Joe identifies his desire to contribute more to the team's work. "I can read and learn on rounds and do an H & P, but I want to help the team more with discharge planning like a sub-intern would do." He considers how to adapt his skills and sets the goals to write orders and participate in discharge planning with his interns. To accomplish these goals, Joe and his advisor decide that he will review standard admission and discharge orders with his team and in his pocket clerkship guide and ask his team to be allowed to write these orders for all of his patients and to receive feedback. His team enthusiastically agrees to this plan. Joe seeks feedback on each order set, so that he can apply the improved methods with the next patient. He is pleased to receive feedback at the end of the rotation on his proactive approach and teamwork with the interns and hospital discharge coordinator.

What educational strategies did Joe take advantage of to improve his medical school experience and eventually provide better care for patients? What attributions of self-regulated learning is Joe using? What assessment methods is Joe using? What assessment methods are his instructors using? What role is peer teaching and assessment playing in this situation?

III. ASSESSMENT WITHIN EDUCATIONAL PROGRAMS

Educational systems employ a variety of assessment methods to ensure that students gain the knowledge, skills, behaviors, and attitudes that are consistent with the program's educational goals and objectives. Students who have a basic understanding of the rationale behind specific assessment methods employed will be better positioned to use assessment results to improve personal performance. This section outlines basic principles and common tools used in measuring student performance.

Assessment plays an important role in supporting student learning by providing feedback on progress in achieving learning objectives. Specific feedback from assessment can identify strengths and weakness and help target learning and improvement efforts. Trustworthy assessment methods are necessary to provide the high-quality feedback supporting the deliberate practice and mastery learning that have been shown to lead to high levels of performance and positively affect patient care practices and health outcomes.[18] As students think about how to apply assessment information toward learning or improvement efforts, it will be helpful to understand some core principles about assessment. Early in medical school, course or clerkship directors or faculty will make many of the decisions about assessment methods. However, as a student traverses the educational continuum and moves into the practice environment, he or she will be making more of the decisions about which assessments are used to guide his or her learning and improvement efforts and how results will be reported to various clinical, administrative, and regulatory authorities. In addition, there may be times when it is necessary or appropriate for the student to pursue additional self or external assessment methods to support or optimize learning efforts. The next two sections will promote understanding of the strengths and limitations of various assessment methods, how they impact learning, and how faculty make decisions about student progress. Even though students may not own much of the responsibility for their assessment in medical school, understanding how and why certain approaches are being used should help in using the results more effectively in meeting learning goals.

A. Core Principles of Assessment

1. Assessment Is an Essential Component of an Educational Program and Should Be Closely Linked to Program Learning Objectives and Activities (Curriculum) Designed to Help Students Meet Those Objectives

Learning is enhanced when program or course objectives are clear and well understood by learners and faculty, when the educational experiences (the curriculum) are well designed to optimize learner achievement, and when a sound assessment plan is in place that provides feedback to learners regarding their performance and determines whether objectives are being met.[19] As stated earlier, self-assessment is enhanced when learning and performance goals are clearly understood. Assessment data can also be aggregated across all students in a particular course or clerkship to provide feedback to educational program leaders on the overall quality and success of the program in ensuring that learners meet program objectives. Good assessment, then, provides feedback to learners and to program leaders to guide ongoing improvement efforts at both the learner and program level. Although a student may not be aware of how program leaders use assessment data to improve educational processes, it is obviously in his or her best interest that such data are used to support continued improvement of the educational program.

Assessment is a critical driver for learning, both by providing feedback on learners' performance to help them grow and improve (assessment *for* learning or *formative* assessment) and by providing motivation to demonstrate on higher-stakes assessments the performance level necessary to move to the next step along the educational continuum (assessment *of* learning or *summative* assessment). As described earlier, the process of assessment itself enhances learning by requiring retrieval of knowledge or skills as part of the assessment activity. Another reason for using assessment data to target learning needs, also mentioned earlier, is based on research showing that learners (within and outside the medical profession) are not able to accurately appraise their knowledge, skills, and abilities in the absence

of external, objective data (such as test scores, ratings by faculty, medical record review). The prevailing opinion among experts in medical education and assessment is that self-assessment should be informed or guided by the use of external data that accurately reflect learner strengths and areas for improvement.[14,20]

2. The Assessment Method Should Be Appropriate for the Competency Being Assessed

One of the ways educators think about the development of knowledge, skills, and attitudes, and their subsequent integration into clinical practice is through the lens of **Miller's pyramid** (Fig. 14.1). George Miller was a highly respected medical educator who designed this pyramid to help faculty and educational program leaders understand the progressive and developmental acquisition of clinical competence and how they might apply, in a valid manner, different assessment tools across the levels of the pyramid.[21] For many complex skills or competencies, a certain level of knowledge *(knows)* must be present to begin mastering that skill or competency. For example, learning how to function effectively on a health care team will require some knowledge about the concept of mutual performance monitoring and its importance to successful team functioning. Next along the developmental trajectory is *knowing how* to apply that knowledge in practice, for example, how to provide feedback to a team member to facilitate self-correction. Possession of the requisite knowledge base and understanding how to apply that knowledge in practice are essential for the next step, demonstrating or *showing how* the skills are executed in practice. Lastly, the ability to perform a skill or demonstrate mastery of a competency does not necessarily mean that the physician or other health care professional will properly do so in the actual practice of medicine, so assessment of what one actually *does* in practice is the top level of Miller's pyramid.

It is important to understand how different assessment methods target different levels in Miller's pyramid and how this match influences the validity of assessment results. Measuring knowledge base, for example, may be best accomplished by examinations with multiple-choice questions

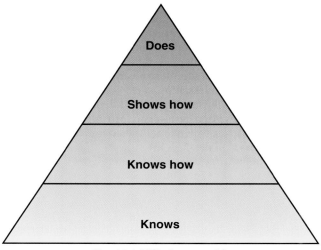

Fig. 14.1 Miller's pyramid.

(MCQs) or more open-ended question formats such as fill-in-the-blank or essay questions. An open-ended question, requiring a narrative response, or case-based discussion with a question-and-answer exercise would be a good approach to assess how someone applies their knowledge *(knows how)* in different situations. Demonstration of skills, or showing how, is best measured with some form of direct observation, either in a simulated setting or in a real clinical context. Common methods for assessing what one actually does in practice include medical record audits, measurements of actual patient outcomes, and indirect observational methods such as multisource feedback where patients, peers, and/or other professional colleagues provide feedback based on their interactions and observations of student behaviors in different contexts.

The previous paragraph describes assessment methods that are good matches for certain domains of competence. However, other methods may not be good choices for a variety of reasons. For example, while multiple-choice tests may provide appropriate information about a student's knowledge regarding good communication practices or professional obligations to patients and society, such tests will not allow for accurate (valid) impressions regarding actual communication skills or professional behaviors. Communication and interpersonal skills would be better assessed by direct observation of a patient encounter, either using a standardized patient *(shows)* or by feedback from the patients encountered during clinical rotations *(does)*. As another example, quality of care measurements or patient outcomes do not necessarily provide valid and cost-efficient measurement of knowledge and/or communication skills. Many factors such as the availability of resources in the health care system, patient preferences, and actions by other health care professionals impact quality and outcome measures in such a way that quality of care measurement itself may not be useful in providing feedback on individual physician knowledge and skills.

CASE STUDY 2

You are a subintern on the internal medicine service. You receive sign-out from another subintern at the end of the day. The patient is a 60-year-old woman with COPD and CHF admitted with pneumonia. As you listen to the sign-out from your fellow subintern, you notice that he presents the information in a way that is disorganized and incomplete. You are not sure whether your team should resend blood cultures if the patient spikes another fever, and the subintern's verbal sign-out mentions different antibiotic doses than those documented in the patient's chart. You are surprised because this subintern always scores high on written tests in the core clerkships.

What is the key lesson about the difference between performance on a written test versus providing care for real patients? What assessment method might have identified this subintern's skill deficiencies earlier?

The subintern providing sign-out may be able to demonstrate adequate knowledge on written examinations, but a different assessment method could have identified his lack of competency in sign-out. For example, a standardized patient encounter can realistically simulate a patient sign-out encounter and characterize specific actions that are done or not done. The checklist used for scoring can serve as the basis of feedback to the learner to inform future learning.

3. The Assessment Method Should Lead to Reliable and Valid Results

In deciding which assessment tool to select to meet a student's learning or improvement needs, or to understand the meaning behind assessment results when others have chosen the assessment method, there are a few basic properties of assessments and their results that would be helpful to understand. Understanding these properties can help the student select which method is best for measuring a particular skill, how much he or she trusts the results, and then determine how best to use the feedback it provides. Traditionally, medical educators have focused most of their attention on the validity and reliability of assessment results, but the educational value and cost-effectiveness of assessment are also important to consider.[22]

Determining the **validity** of a particular assessment method involves seeking information about whether the results of that assessment method provide accurate information about what is being measured. If assessment results are known to lead to valid impressions about a particular aspect of competence or performance, then the student can trust and act on the feedback based on the assessment result. Determining the validity of a test, to a certain extent, can be made by asking and answering two simple questions. Does the assessment method match the task or competency being measured, and do the assessment results provide accurate information regarding the skill or competency being assessed? As in the previous example, a student could assume that a multiple-choice examination will provide a reasonably valid measure of knowledge in a particular area (e.g., foundations of patient safety), but he or she probably would not trust the same examination results as a valid measure of his or her ability to lead a time out in the operating room or disclose a medical error to a patient, both important skills related to patient safety. Rather, scores and feedback based on a simulated operating room experience involving a time out or based on ratings from an observed encounter with a standardized patient while disclosing a medical error would be more likely to yield valid results for these skills. As another example, patients and other health care providers can be expected to provide valid feedback on a student's patient-centered and interprofessional communication, but may not be able to provide valid assessment of his or her diagnostic or procedural abilities in the absence of specific training in these areas.

Like validity, the **reliability** of an assessment result is important. Reliability refers to the consistency or reproducibility of an assessment result and whether the same result would occur if the assessment were administered at some future time or in different circumstances. A critical determinant of reliability in assessments used in medical education is how deeply or extensively important content is covered (often referred to as *sampling*) by the assessment. For the previously mentioned multiple-choice examination, its reliability will increase as the number and breadth of questions increases in each specialty area. A test with 20 or more questions in each specialty area that broadly samples the types of cases that are typically seen in that specialty will be more reliable than a test with just a few questions in each area.

The same principle of sampling applies to the reliability of assessments targeting skills and competencies other than medical knowledge, such as communication and patient management skills. It is well known that physician performance will vary to some degree depending upon a specific patient's presenting complaint or diagnosis. For example, a physician may be able to competently manage a patient with chest pain, but less able to evaluate a patient with symptoms of depression. Therefore, in order to get a reliable impression regarding that physician's overall patient management skills, a reasonable number of different cases are necessary. Research on tools commonly used to measure patient management skills (chart audit or case-based discussion) or communication skills (standardized patient encounters or direct observations of real patient encounters) suggests that a sample of at least 8 to 12 different cases are required to formulate accurate impressions about the competence or skills being measured.

Reliability is most important when making overall judgments about competence or performance in order to make decisions about passing or failing a course or clerkship, readiness to advance to the next year, or graduate from medical school. This is why end of clerkship or end of year Objective Structured Clinical Examinations (OSCEs) generally include 8 to 12 cases that cover a broad sample of clinical content in the specialty area or across specialty areas, respectively. The need for highly reliable results is less critical when a student is being assessed on an individual patient case for the purpose of providing feedback to improve his or her knowledge or skills. Here, reliability may not be as important as the educational value of the case and the quality of the feedback provided. Observation and feedback based on a single patient encounter, one team-based exercise, or a review of one entry in an electronic health record (EHR) may be very helpful in identifying learning or improvement opportunities, even though it cannot be used alone to determine whether the student would pass the clinical rotation.

For some assessments, both reliability of the overall assessment and high-quality feedback are attainable and underscore their utility in certain contexts. For example, multisource feedback, which involves getting feedback based on the observations of a variety of different raters in a variety of different contexts, is a good method for assessing professionalism or teamwork. Multiple observations and ratings of student performance by different health care professionals can provide a reliable assessment of his or her overall interprofessional communication skills and respectful behaviors toward her colleagues, while at the same time, narrative comments that reflect a specific observation of a critical event or difficult interaction with a colleague or patient may provide a powerful learning experience. The reliability and validity of tools used to assess knowledge, skills, behaviors, and competencies in HSS will be discussed further in the following section.

Case Study 3

You are a third-year medical student on your ob-gyn clerkship. You are enjoying a great working relationship with your intern and senior resident. You have learned a lot caring for two patients in labor over your first week and have been reading regularly from the recommended textbook. However, you are concerned that you've only directly participated in two patients' care so far. You'd like to get involved earlier and with more patients to gain more experience on labor and delivery. You are not sure how to do this without

interfering with other people's work or seeming to step on toes. The fast pace of the labor and delivery floor can be intimidating to you as a student.

What educational tools can this medical student use to gain more experience in labor and delivery and provide care for more patients? How might feedback from physicians and other health care professionals in this setting help this student achieve his or her goals?

Your clerkship director stated at the clerkship orientation that you need to complete Multisource Feedback Forms. Specifically, you are expected to obtain four feedback forms completed by nurses, midwives, or nurse practitioners during the clerkship. You decide to hand these forms to these interprofessional staff early in the rotation to see if you can gain any insight into how to become more involved. Although these forms are not used to determine your clerkship grade, you find that you gain valuable feedback from them. Multiple staff comment on their forms that you seem pleasant but quiet, and that they wish you would speak up more and ask for opportunities to participate. Based on this information, you become involved in more patients' cases and find the clerkship to be more satisfying and educational for you.

B. Assessment of Knowledge, Skills, and Practice Performance in Health Systems Science

As discussed in Chapter 2, HSS is organized into core, crosscutting, and linking domains. Although the domains are organized as separate concepts within the HSS curriculum framework, there is much overlap and interdependence between them during educational and clinical experiences. Examples of this overlap include the following:

- A solid foundation of knowledge regarding *health care structure and processes* is essential to understanding how to effect positive change within health care systems to improve the quality or reduce the cost of care. Effective change in health care systems will also involve applying the knowledge and skills in the *health systems improvement* and *value-based care* domains.
- Acquisition of knowledge and skills in the *clinical informatics and health information technology* domain will enable physicians to collect, review, and use information about their patients to make health care decisions that are based on the best available clinical evidence *(evidence-based medicine and practice)*. At the same time, adherence to professional values and ethical principles regarding patient confidentiality will guide appropriate use of patient data in a manner that is consistent with their best interests and protects their privacy *(professionalism and ethics)*.
- Knowledge and understanding regarding how health care is financed and patient care interventions reimbursed *(health care policy, economics, and management)* will help physicians manage their patients and provide the highest-quality and least costly care to the community or patient population they serve *(population and public health, value-based care)*.

Reflecting back on how competence is developed as illustrated in Miller's pyramid, each domain begins with a core set of knowledge *(knows)* and principles that must be learned and then applied *(knows how)* in the context of delivering patient care services in our health care systems. Mastery and then application of the knowledge and principles of each domain supports the development of the skills and behaviors constituting the practice of HSS (the *shows* and *does* of Miller's pyramid).

In the first example earlier in the chapter, health system structures and health care delivery processes are the targets of initiatives to improve the quality or efficiency of health care through application of a **Plan-Do-Study-Act (PDSA) cycle.** As a student learns about PDSA cycles, he may first be tested to see if he *knows* what the individual steps are, then he may be asked in a small-group case-based discussion to describe a PDSA approach to improving care processes for a selected patient presentation or condition to see if he *knows how* to apply it in a clinical context. Later, in one of his clinical clerkships, he may be tasked by his preceptor to identify a patient care problem and develop a PDSA cycle to *show how* he can apply it in a real clinical setting. Later, when he is a resident or practicing physician, hospital-based or practice-based initiatives designed to measure the quality of care delivered by him or his health care team will provide feedback on how he is monitoring and improving patient care quality *(does)*.

1. *Assessment of Knowledge in Health Systems Science Domains*

As discussed earlier, MCQ examinations are a valid and reliable means of broadly assessing knowledge in a given content area. Course and clerkship directors have begun developing and administering examinations in HSS content areas over the last several years as educational leaders have become aware that these domains are becoming increasingly important to cover in undergraduate medical education. Recent articles describe the use of locally developed assessments or the adaption of nationally available assessments to address knowledge and knowledge application in **quality improvement, patient safety, evidence-based practice,** and **teamwork.**[23–28] It turns out that it is difficult to write good MCQ items in some of the HSS content areas, such as patient safety and teamwork. This is because, in many clinical instances, the correct answer is so obvious that it is difficult to find plausible distractors (alternate answers that are incorrect). In other instances, it may be difficult for item writers to agree on the right answer in content domains that are rapidly evolving.

Also, unlike in basic or clinical science content areas, in some domains course or clerkship directors may not have **National Board of Medical Examiners (NBME)** subject examinations or **United States Medical Licensing Examination (USMLE)** results to use as part of their assessment of HSS knowledge domains. The USMLE and NBME subject examinations do not provide broad coverage of HSS content areas for several reasons. One reason, as mentioned earlier, is that it is difficult to write high-quality items in some of the HSS domains. Secondly, USMLE and NBME subject examinations tend to focus on testing stable knowledge for which a solid evidence base exists to help write items with a clearly correct answer. The evidence base in some of the HSS domains is less mature than in the basic and clinical science areas. Lastly, the USMLE (from which many of the subject items originate) focuses on knowledge that is important for the competent physician to know in order to provide safe and effective care

for individual patients (a very important factor for licensing authorities). For some of the HSS content domains, such as health care policy, leadership, or scholarship, a direct relationship to safe or effective patient care practices may not exist to warrant inclusion in the licensing examination.

The fact that much HSS content is not covered in NBME subject examinations or USMLEs creates a tension that was raised in Chapter 2 (see Fig. 2.3). Student motivation for learning is substantially influenced by what is covered in NBME subject examinations that often contribute to final course and clerkship grades and in the USMLE, which plays a role in the residency selection process. Likewise, medical education leaders appreciate the importance of USMLE scores and often prioritize their teaching and assessment based on USMLE content outlines, as well as reports of student performance from previous examinations. Although faculty and students will understand and buy in to the importance of leadership, health systems improvement, value-based health care, and so on, these domains may not be perceived as a high priority when time and resources are limited for study and assessment.

This is not to say that HSS content will not be taught or assessed by faculty, and it is likely that this content area will continue to grow and increase in perceived importance. In recognition of the increasing importance of HSS in medical education, this textbook is one of the first efforts to organize HSS domains into a coherent educational product. Many of the authors of this textbook are from medical schools that are members of the American Medical Association's Accelerating Change in Medical Education Consortium, which is collaborating with the NBME to develop a subject examination in HSS. Furthermore, the NBME has begun work to increase licensing examination coverage of some HSS content areas such as patient safety and evidence-based medicine. While these trends and initiatives evolve, the strongest rationale for prioritizing the learning and assessment of HSS content and a source of motivation for self-regulated learning will be student and faculty perceptions regarding its importance to patients and the public.

The review questions at the end of each chapter are useful in assessing a student's grasp of the knowledge and principles addressed in each chapter, and the authors would advise students to take advantage of these exercises and discuss them with faculty and peers. The examinations being developed in HSS domains such as quality improvement, patient safety, and evidence-based practice will also be helpful in providing feedback in HSS areas. Another way to assess knowledge in HSS in a manner that also facilitates and reinforces learning is through the activity of writing questions for self-assessment, peer assessment, or for other assessment purposes. There are examples published in the medical education literature of students who received training in item writing then writing high-quality questions for use in self-assessment as well as for use in tests administered in their schools.[29–31] While solving questions is associated with enhanced learning, a solid knowledge base itself is an important prerequisite to writing good items.[29] Students report that item writing not only enhances their learning; they also feel that the process may improve their test-taking ability.[30]

In addition, the act of writing questions has been shown to require the cognitive strategies that are foundational to self-regulated learning.[31] Students engaged in generating test items assume an element of ownership for their own learning and assessment and the metacognitive and critical-thinking processes required for good item writing are core abilities of self-regulated learning.[31] In terms of learning goals related to item writing, improving student knowledge base in HSS domains constitutes an important outcome goal. The item-writing activity itself is a process goal, while honing the cognitive skills involved in good item writing may be viewed as a separate learning goal in support of student self-efficacy in becoming a skilled lifelong learner.

The benefits of question development to learning extends beyond the use of MCQ formats. In fact, as mentioned earlier, open-ended question formats may have a more significant effect on learning by requiring a more challenging process for retrieving information from memory.[15] The development of open-ended questions using prompts such as signal words (*who, what, when, where, how,* and *why*) as seen at the end of each chapter in this book or generic question stems (Table 14.3) are known as *comprehension-fostering* or *comprehension-monitoring self-regulatory cognitive strategies*.[32] King described research she and others have done on the use of guided

student-generated questions using generic question stems to enhance learning in high school and adult education.[33] Developing and answering questions that involve insertion of specific content into generic question stems results in levels of comprehension and recall that are greater than that which results from answering independent lecture review questions provided by others, unstructured small group discussion, or unguided question writing or answering.[33]

King attributes the enhanced learning to the use of high-level cognitive activities (analysis, application, inference, generalization, evaluation, and explanation) involved in developing and answering the questions and the degree of student autonomy that characterizes the process. Increased learning is seen when such questions are self-generated or generated by peers. However, guided peer-generated questions yield superior comprehension and recall, perhaps because there is a higher level of motivation to successfully answer peer questions, gaps in learning are more likely to be identified in discussion with peers, or the quality of the explanation may be better

Table 14.3 Using Generic Question Stems for Student-Generated Questions in Health Systems Science (numbers in parentheses following questions refer to chapters from which questions were drawn)

What is a new example of …?	**What do we already know about the determinants of population health outcomes, and what is the contribution of health care? (10, 11)**
What is a new example of risk stratification in effective population management? (3)	*What do we already know about cultural competence that will enhance the ability of our health care system to interact effectively with diverse patient populations? (13)*
What is a new example of care transition that should be anticipated and managed properly because new types of health care providers are engaged in patient care activities? (5)	**How does … tie in with what we learned before?**
What is a new example of a formulary-related design process that is intended to reduce variation, improve safety, and/or reduce cost in medication prescribing? (13)	*How does the list of things that health care providers can do to promote high-value care tie in with what we learned in our clinical clerkships? (4)*
How would you use … to …?	*How do the qualities of good communication as a cross-cutting competency in HSS tie in with what we learned regarding patient-physician communication? (13)*
How would you use a cause-and-effect diagram to evaluate a "near miss"? (5)	**Explain why …**
How would you use the concept of patient-centeredness to describe important leadership attributes? (8)	*Explain why different stakeholder groups have conflicting perspectives that impact health care costs. (4)*
How would you use an electronic patient portal to improve population health? (10, 11)	*Explain why it is critically important to measure health care quality from the perspectives of different parties, including patients, health care plans, hospital leadership, and policy developers. (6)*
How would you use a partnership with a community agency/resource/ service to address a social determinant that has a negative impact on a particular population? (11)	*Explain why consistent interoperability standards are necessary for optimal use of EHRs within and across our health care systems. (9)*
What would happen if …?	*Explain why it is important to consider external, organizational, team, and personal factors when trying to improve the function of a health care team. (13)*
What would happen if health care provider education was more effective in preparing graduates to deliver high-value, cost-conscious care? (4)	**Explain how …**
What would happen if physicians declined leadership roles in our health care systems, allowing nonphysician administrators and executives to assume all such positions? (8)	*Explain how accountable care organizations use different financial models to improve health care value. (3)*
What would happen if all provisions of the Affordable Care Act were implemented successfully in terms of health inequity? (12)	*Explain how standardization and constraint methodologies might prevent medical errors. (5)*
What are the strengths and weaknesses of …?	*Explain how the input-process-output heuristic helps understand the contributions of individual factors, task-related factors, and team processes to the outcomes of team-based care. (7)*
What are the strengths and weakness of using big data in prioritizing quality improvement projects? (3, 4, 9)	*Explain how scientific evidence, social strategy, and political will influence policy generation. (12)*
What are the strengths and weakness of using clinical registries in performing quality improvement projects? (6)	**How does … affect …?**
What are the strengths and weaknesses of electronic patient portals in care for patients with chronic illness? (13)	*How does professional identity formation impact one's ability to participate effectively in interprofessional education and on health care teams? (7)*
What do we already know about …?	*How does full disclosure of a medical error to a patient impact his or her emotional response and likelihood of pursuing malpractice litigation? (5)*
What do we already know about data-gathering errors and cognitive bias that increase the likelihood of diagnostic error? (5)	*How does the use of computerized provider order entry (CPOE) affect the quality, safety, and efficiency of health care? (9, 13)*
What do we already know about professionalism, communication, and relationship management that will help us serve as effective leaders? (8)	

Continued

Table 14.3 Using Generic Question Stems for Student-Generated Questions in Health Systems Science (numbers in parentheses following questions refer to chapters from which questions were drawn)—cont'd

How does the Affordable Care Act affect access to health care for US citizens? (12)

What is the meaning of …?

What is the meaning of the Swiss Cheese model of system failure? (5)

What is the meaning of flattening the hierarchy in team-based care? (5)

What is the meaning of "hotspotting"? (10)

What is the meaning of the social gradient of health? (11)

Why is … important?

Why is a registry important in facilitating effective population management? (3)

Why is it important to have a systems view when trying to reduce or prevent medical errors? (5)

Why is it important to ensure accurate phrasing of the clinical question when completing a literature search? (9)

Why is service learning important in learning about the impact of socio-ecological determinants of health? (11)

What is the difference between … and …?

What is the difference between structure, process, and outcome measures in evaluating health care quality? (3)

What is the difference between an adverse event, a medical error, and a preventable adverse event? (5)

What is the difference between a team and a clinical microsystem? (3, 7)

What is the difference between population health and public health? (10)

How are … and … similar?

How are normalization of deviance in systems-based practice and lapses in professionalism in patient care similar? (5)

How are the health care structure and process priorities of accountable care organizations and patient-centered medical homes similar? (10)

How are the Triple Aim and the three core aims of health care reform (health policy trifecta) similar? (12)

How are the personal attributes that impact team function and the characteristics of a highly functioning team similar? (13)

What is the best …, and why?

What is the best way to transfer responsibility of care for a patient from one provider to another, and why? (5)

What is the best way for physicians to influence the determinants of population health that do not relate directly to health care, and why? (10, 11)

What is the best way to (re-) structure our health care reimbursement and incentive process to improve population health, and why? (10)

What are some possible solutions to the problem of …?

What are some possible solutions to the problem of high costs in health care? (4)

What are some possible solutions to the problem of suboptimal uptake of evidence-based safety interventions, such as surgical time outs? (5)

What are some possible solutions to the problem of increasing cost of health insurance premiums? (12)

Compare … and … with regard to …

Compare the use of administrative data with data obtained by chart abstraction with regard to their most appropriate use in measuring health care quality. (6)

Compare Lean and Six Sigma with regard to their roles in addressing patient experience versus medical error–related improvement goals. (6)

Compare "predictive analytics" and "business intelligence" with regard to their respective uses in shaping health care delivery practices. (9)

What do you think causes …?

What do you think causes the "storming" behaviors encountered during team formation and performance? (7)

What do you think causes the racial and ethnic difference in health outcomes for patients with diabetes and high blood pressure? (10, 11)

What do you think causes better outcomes for both patients and providers when care is delivered by high-functioning teams? (13)

Do you agree or disagree with this statement …? Support your answer.

Do you agree or disagree that there is a significant disconnect between the quality of care in the United States and our annual expenditure on health care services? Support your answer. (4)

Do you agree or disagree that, although systems thinking identifies system flaws as the predominant reason for medical errors, individual health care providers may also be accountable for preventable adverse events? Support your answer. (5)

Do you agree or disagree that health care systems should not be reimbursed for patient health care needs resulting from adverse events (such as a nosocomial infection or unexpected re-admission? Support your answer. (10)

when responding to peers. Writing questions for self-study or for peer assessment and learning activities could be done as part of the before, during, or after phase of a self-regulated learning activity as described earlier. Table 14.3 includes the generic question stems described by King and colleagues into which is inserted content from the HSS chapters. Although the research on using generic questions stems across the continuum of education generally involves some training by faculty,[32,33] answering the questions in Table 14.3 and generation of questions on one's own will likely serve to increase student comprehension and recall of HSS content.

2. Assessment of Skills Acquisition and Practice Performance

Various assessment methods may be used by faculty and course and clerkship directors to provide feedback on student development and acquisition of skills and behaviors in HSS and also to ensure that students have met learning objectives relative to these attributes. Some of these methods

may be usable by students in a self-directed manner to gather feedback on their clinical performance, such as peer assessment, multisource feedback, or some forms of simulation. Most assessments of HSS in educational settings will be one of three different types: assessment of a work product created through the application of student knowledge, skills, or behaviors; assessment of student performance using various forms of simulation; or assessment of performance by direct observation during clinical rotations. Later, when physicians or other health care professionals are in clinical practice and presumed to have demonstrated acquisition of the competencies necessary for safe and effective patient care, assessment will use various methods to ensure that they continue to exercise the skills and behaviors that they have acquired. Most assessment in clinical practice involves measurement of provider compliance with evidence-based processes of care and patient health outcomes and may also involve gathering feedback from professional peers based on observation of performance in different contexts. During graduate medical education, assessment methods will include a mix of those used in undergraduate education and in practice as learners traverse the developmental continuum and begin to provide actual patient care in indirectly supervised situations.

For the most part, assessments that are used to provide feedback regarding learner progress or determine whether learner progress meets expectations measure the *shows how* level of Miller's pyramid. Assessments of quality of care and patient outcome focus on the *does* level of the pyramid, where the individual being assessed is not immediately aware that the assessment is taking place.

While it may be possible to limit assessment to domains of HSS when measuring HSS knowledge or its application, that will not usually be the case with performance assessment targeting the top two levels of Miller's pyramid. Assessment of performance with regard to HSS will often occur in patient care contexts where student or resident skills and behaviors will likely reflect those relevant to direct patient care as well as the HSS domains targeted by the assessment. For example, a standardized patient case designed to assess teamwork will measure a team member's knowledge of each other's roles, ability to manage conflict, and interprofessional communication; such a case will also bring into play the patient care and communication skills exercised by team members. Direct observation of a conversation with a patient about the cost-effectiveness of a particular treatment requires application of knowledge regarding the Triple Aim and high-value, cost-conscious care, but requires that a student's professional attitudes and interpersonal skills be appropriately applied to engaging in informed decision making with the patient.

While the measurement aspects of performance assessment of HSS in the clinical workplace may be complicated by the simultaneous exercise of direct patient care competencies, this is actually a desirable situation from the standpoint of learner achievement and competence development. This textbook focuses primarily on HSS, as coverage of HSS domains has been significantly lacking across the continuum of medical education and practice. However, in clinical practice, direct patient care and HSS competencies are integrated in the daily care of patients. High-quality patient care demands that physicians have a sound knowledge base, communicate effectively with patients, and exercise their professionalism while remaining cognizant about the need to be judicious in their use of critical system resources, address system variables that impact quality and safety, leverage information technology, and work effectively within teams to deliver effective, patient-centered care. Assessment of performance in the clinical workplace has been increasingly focused on the integration of different competencies in authentic patient care situations. Because much of this learning and assessment occurs in real clinical settings during the process of clinical work, it is referred to as *work-based assessment*.

The following sections describe different assessment methods that learners will encounter throughout the continuum of medical education. These assessments will be used for the purpose of facilitating learning and improvement and also to help course, clerkship, and program directors make decisions about the adequacy of learner progress. The purpose in describing these assessments is to foster understanding of their purpose and use so that learners may get the most out of their application and begin to think about assessment methods they may choose to use themselves, either in parallel to course assessments or later after completion of training. Table 14.4 lists examples of assessments of different HSS domains that focus on

Table 14.4   Examples of Methods Used to Assess Skills and Practice Performance in Health Systems Science Domains

Domain	Skill or Behavior	Example of Method for Assessing Skill Acquisition	Example of Method for Assessing Performance in Practice
Clinical informatics: EHR	Create usable notes	Review of note entries into virtual or real EHR	Audit of EHR documentation as part of a quality improvement (QI) project
Clinical informatics: EHR	Graph, display, and trend vital signs and laboratory values over time	Review of electronic report of patient panel data for HbA1c levels in diabetic patients	Audit of EHR documentation of HbA1c levels as part of a QI project
Clinical informatics: patient privacy	Protect patient privacy and security	Direct observation of EHR use to ensure appropriate use of security features and adherence to HIPAA regulations	QI project using process measure to ensure use of HIPAA authorization forms signed by all new patients
Clinical informatics: communication	Respond to patient questions using electronic media	Standardized patient inquiry about a medication side effect through simulated electronic patient portal (remote)	Patient experience of care survey question regarding the clarity of physician advice regarding medication use
Evidence-based medicine: literature search	Search, find, and apply knowledge-based information to patient care	Review of search details to ensure accurate clinical question and articles relevant to patient problem and context	QI project using process measure to ensure medication use consistent with current standards
Evidence-based medicine: clinical guideline	Apply an evidence-based clinical guideline	Case-based discussion and assessment of student application of a selected clinical guideline for a clinical problem	QI project using measurement of compliance with an evidence-based clinical guideline
Leadership: communication	Communication skills and relationship management in leading a patient-centered team meeting	Direct observation of leading a team meeting to plan a patient discharge and outpatient management	Multisource evaluation from the team members
Patient safety: medication error	Safe prescribing or order writing (or entry)	Review of order entry into virtual or real medical record using case-based discussion	QI project using process measure—documentation in medical record of patient medication allergies

Continued

Table 14.4 Examples of Methods Used to Assess Skills and Practice Performance in Health Systems Science Domains—cont'd

Domain	Skill or Behavior	Example of Method for Assessing Skill Acquisition	Example of Method for Assessing Performance in Practice
Patient safety: medication error	Medical reconciliation	Direct observation of medical reconciliation by clinical preceptor	QI project using process measure—documentation of updated allergy list
Patient safety: surgical error	Informed decision making	Direct observation of informed consent discussion with preoperative patient	Patient experience of care survey focusing on adequacy of informed consent process
Patient safety: surgical error	Lead or participate in a time out in the operating room (OR)	Team-based operating room simulation and debrief with faculty	Multisource feedback including operating room nurse input on frequency and quality of time outs
Patient safety: transition of care	Handoff of patient care	Direct observation of patient sign-out to on-call team	Patient experience of care survey regarding quality of follow-up after hospital discharge
Population health: public health	Identify community partners to reduce the impact of chronic disease	Clinical skills examination case—student uses Behavioral Risk Factor Surveillance System (BRFSS) data to identify potential community-based interventions	Outcome measure focusing on health outcomes in patients with chronic disease with social determinants (diagnosis of Type 2 diabetes, weight loss, blood pressure control)
Population health	Apply patient problems to populations	Encounter with standardized patient with suboptimal chronic care management—develop a process to assess care of similar patients in the community	Assess QI projects for alignment with community or system priorities
Population health: analytics	Use wearable technology to gather data about a population of patients	Direct observation of a student instructing a patient in ambulatory blood pressure monitoring	QI project using wearable technology to monitor patient exercise and heart rate
Population health: quality and safety	Analyze an adverse event from a population perspective	Clinical skills examination case of hospital re-admission—assess factors that led to re-admission	Outcome measure focusing on re-admission rates for selected conditions or procedures
Quality improvement	Use the appropriate type of quality measure	Case-based discussion to determine the best measure to use to identify and resolve a potential gap in care quality	Patient experience of care measure to gather feedback from patients regarding coordination of care during recent hospitalization
Quality improvement	Apply the Model for Improvement	Case-based discussion to assess ability to develop a clear AIM statement for a QI project	Measures of improvement to determine if the correct changes are made to close a gap in care quality
Quality improvement	Understand how and when to apply different quality improvement methods	Case-based discussion to assess ability to apply a PDSA cycle, Lean methods, or DMAIC process (Six Sigma) to measuring and improving a care process	Multisource feedback from team members regarding leadership and/or meaningful participation in developing and implementing different tools used in QI projects
Teamwork: personal qualities	Demonstrate good communication skills and knowledge about other health care professionals	Team-based simulation assessing communication with team members and knowledge about their roles and abilities	Multisource feedback from team members regarding communication skills and awareness and respect for their roles
Teamwork: leadership	Demonstrate leadership behaviors	Team simulation to assess ability to lead a team briefing and demonstrate the appropriate skills and behaviors	Multisource feedback to clinical staff regarding leadership behaviors
Socio-ecological determinants of health	Consider socio-ecological factors when evaluating patients	Clinical skills examination case of patient with poorly controlled diabetes and blood pressure—considers socio-ecological reasons for health status	QI project with process measures that review documentation of dietary patterns, physical activity, employment, education, race/ethnicity, and health literacy
Socio-ecological determinants of health	Identify community resources	Clinical skills examination case of patient whose health needs could be met with community resource	QI project with process measure that assesses referrals to community-based services

assessment of learner acquisition of the relevant knowledge, skills, and behaviors and also examples of assessment that may be used later to measure performance in practice. It is very likely that students will encounter or have already experienced several of these during their educational experiences.

a. ASSESSMENT OF WORK PRODUCTS

Examples of work products that may be assessed or serve as a stimulus for assessment include notes or orders written in an EHR, a report from a literature search, a written description of a quality improvement or safety activity such as a PDSA cycle or event analysis, or analysis of a database regarding a particular patient population question or problem. These notes, reports, or analyses may themselves be assessed, or they may serve as the substrate or stimulus for assessment, for example, as part of a case-based discussion exercise based on a patient note. In addition, assessment of some nontraditional competencies might involve the use of more unconventional methods such as field notes, reflective essays, or written project reports based on community or health system experiences.[34] Because such methods are often less structured, qualitative, or subjective in nature, they are less likely to be used as summative measures compared to more traditional tools such as MCQ examinations or OSCEs.

One domain in which EHR notes, various reports or analyses, and/or case-based discussion might be used is in the assessment of evidence-based practice. That is because evidence-based practice consists of multiple stages (asking a clinical question, searching the literature, appraising the literature, applying the evidence to the clinical question, and reviewing the process and outcome of the exercise), each requiring related but different skill sets for which different methods might be best suited.[35] There are only a few validated approaches to assess the complete range of skills composing the individual steps of evidence-based practice.[35,36] A case-based discussion after a patient encounter or based on an EHR note is one approach to assessing the quality of clinical query that leads to the literature search. A printout of the actual search itself might be directly assessed, while literature appraisal may be summed up in a report for assessment purposes. Application of the retrieved evidence to the patient problem could be the target of a reflective essay or a case-based discussion.

b. ASSESSMENT USING SIMULATION

Simulation-based assessment methods vary in their level of complexity, the extent to which they include technology-based methods, and fidelity to actual patient care. There are several advantages of simulation-based methods in medical education: they are available when needed to meet learner needs, and the difficulty can be adjusted based on learner level or standardized across learners to ensure fairness in assessment. Their use can guarantee that learners have some exposure to important clinical material when real patient experiences may be limited. Another important advantage of simulation-based methods is that there is no risk to patient safety when they are used to teach or assess procedural skills or difficult communication skills such as delivering bad news to a patient. Challenges to using simulation-based methods include their potential cost, the need to make sure that the skills and behaviors assessed are consistent with good clinical care, and the difficulty that some learners may have in suspending reality during simulated clinical scenarios.

A common low-tech simulation method used in medical education is role-playing, which is often used in teaching and assessing acquisition of data gathering and communication skills and will be useful in assessing similar tasks at the nexus of direct patient care and systems-based practice. Examples include role-playing scenarios involving counseling a patient about the cost-effectiveness of different therapies, disclosing a medical error, or holding a team briefing. While many role-playing activities are directed by faculty, there is no reason that such experiences cannot be conducted within

a peer-based learning and/or assessment session. A helpful literature collection on the value of peer-based learning and assessment is summarized in a later section.

The use of simulated patients (also referred to as *standardized patients* in selected contexts) for learning and assessment is widespread in medical education, and a robust evidence base supports their use for assessing a broad range of data-gathering, communication, and interpersonal skills. They are also a well-suited method for assessing integration of direct patient care skills and system-related skills. Simulated patient exercises may be supplemented with a range of clinical materials (e.g., medical records, diagnostic results, and web-based content provided by "patients") and assessment formats (virtual EHRs with patient notes and computerized provider order entry [CPOE], computerized manikins, and other technology-based simulation) that require integration of various competencies to effectively manage.

Simulated patient and other clinical content and assessment formats may be combined in clinical skills examinations or OSCEs to assess broadly across HSS domains or may be used to focus in depth on a particular domain such as patient safety. Varkey described the use of a multiple-station OSCE to assess fellow performance in the practice-based learning and improvement as well as systems-based practice competencies, which overlap with many of the HSS domains. Cases included assessment of the following: planning of a quality improvement activity, performance of a root cause analysis, evidence-based medicine, knowledge about insurance, prescription writing, team collaboration, and negotiation skills.[37]

Actors that simulate patients can also play the role of other members of the health care team to support learning and assessment of teamwork skills. As long as the simulations are realistic in representing real clinical situations, students feel that they provide effective ways of teaching and assessing their teamwork skills.[38] The use of standardized assessment instruments in team-based simulation facilitates the delivery of effective feedback on important team skills and behaviors such as leadership, structured and closed-loop communication, situational awareness, assertiveness, conflict resolution, and mutual support.[24,39]

c. ASSESSMENT USING DIRECT OBSERVATION IN THE WORKPLACE

Direct observation of performance in the workplace, as part of workplace-based assessment (WBA), is currently an intense area of research and development. Efforts are underway to optimize the reliability and validity of different assessment methods targeting a wide variety of skills and behaviors that are demonstrated during authentic clinical situations. Many of the skills and behaviors within HSS domains, including those listed earlier as the focus of simulation-based assessment, are natural targets for assessment in the workplace (some are listed in Table 14.4). A number of HSS domains could be assessed in real clinical settings by observing faculty, residents, or peers, including the following examples: handover of a patient to a colleague who is on-call or receiving the patient in a different hospital location, informed decision making with a patient regarding the risks and benefits of a surgical procedure, counseling a patient who requests a diagnostic test that is expensive and not clinically indicated, disclosing a medical error to a patient's family, and working with a health care team to discharge a patient from the hospital.

Reliability and validity of WBA will depend upon the extent to which the relevant skills and behaviors in each domain are well-defined, observable, and measurable, the extent to which observers are aware and agree on standards of performance for those skills and behaviors, and the availability of instruments that might help structure and guide the assessment process. For some of the HSS domains listed earlier, the standards are agreed upon (such as informed decision making), but for others (such as teamwork and patient handover) there is not yet uniform agreement on the essential skills and behaviors in that domain. However, there is enough known about the individual qualities of "teamness" for different observers to help students identify ways to enhance their teamwork skills and behaviors.

There is much work being done in WBA to capture some of these domains, in particular teamwork. For example, the teamwork mini-clinical evaluation exercise (T-MEX) was developed to directly observe and assess medical student collaboration in health care teams.[40,41] The T-MEX focuses on student competence in developing supportive team relationships, self-awareness and responsibility, and safe communication in different team-based care contexts, such as team meetings, discharge planning, and handovers.

Assessment using the T-MEX instrument is intended to provide focused feedback to facilitate reflection and informed self-assessment.[40,41] Another example is an instrument developed to assess intern sign-out of a patient to the night float team.[42] The instrument uses a mnemonic (SIGN-OUT) to assess intern performance. Aggregate data from the intern assessment was used for program evaluation and led to both curricular modifications and system-level changes to improve the safety of the sign-out process.[42]

d. ASSESSMENT USING MULTISOURCE FEEDBACK

Multisource feedback (MSF), also often referred to as 360-degree feedback, is an approach that is widely used in business and industry and is increasingly being used in medical education and clinical practice. In medical education and practice, MSF involves gathering information from peers and other health care professionals based on their observations of the learner in different contexts. Such observations are generally considered to be more indirect as the individual being observed may be less aware (or unaware) that the observation is taking place. An important assumption is that the learner behaviors may be more representative of their authentic clinical behaviors than when they are more conscious of being observed as they would be during a simulation exercise.

One area in which MSF may be especially useful is in the assessment of teams and individuals within teams. Assessment and feedback by members of the health care team (residents, peers, nurses, administrative staff, and patients) can yield reliable feedback that has been found acceptable to both the assessors and the students receiving feedback.[43] While numerical ratings of an individual's performance on a team may provide feedback that is useful, narrative descriptions that stem from specific interactions or events that are based on observed behaviors may be especially helpful in identifying opportunities for change or improvement. Residents, peers, nurses, and administrative staff are able to provide specific comments on a student's team performance based

on the different contexts in which performance is observed and based on their role and perspectives on the team.[44]

E. PEER-BASED LEARNING AND ASSESSMENT

The use of peer assessment is common across the continuum of medical education and practice from assessment of various tasks and behaviors in basic science courses to assessment of the clinical performance of physicians in practice. In medical education contexts, one of the more common uses of peers is in the assessment of professional behaviors.[45,46] However, peers may also provide reliable and valid assessment of specific clinical tasks (performing a literature search), other competencies (interpersonal skills), or complex clinical interactions (diagnostic evaluation of a patient).[45,47-50] Peer assessment is often, but not universally, well received by those receiving feedback from their peers.[51] Those who receive peer feedback may experience both cognitive and emotional reactions that may have a more significant impact on attitudes and behaviors.[52]

Research also shows that assessing one's peers has beneficial impact on the professional behavior and learning outcomes of the assessors themselves.[47-49,51,53] In addition to a positive impact on immediate learning outcomes, engagement in providing peer assessments may help instill the attitudes and skills that will serve students well as future lifelong learners engaged in professional self-regulation.[51] Making judgments about peers' performance may lead to more critical thinking about clinical competence in general and provide useful insights about the learner's own performance.[46] Lastly, in many education programs, faculty resources may be limited and student peer assessment may be able to fulfill an important function within an assessment program as students are well-positioned to observe their peers in many different contexts.[47,51] In particular, peers may be able to offer relevant observations regarding difficult to assess domains such as leadership, initiative, work ethic, respect, collaboration, and teamwork.[49]

There are some potential risks involved in peer assessment in medical education. Some individuals do not appreciate assessment by their peers and will resist the assessment and devalue the feedback received.[52] Although, with training, most individuals can learn to provide specific, constructive feedback, occasional negative, inappropriate, or harmful comments are conveyed.[45] An institutional culture that endorses the importance of peer feedback and offers a safe environment may mitigate some of the potential adverse consequences.[53] It may be useful for faculty to help monitor, if not filter, feedback and be available should students need assistance in responding to inappropriate feedback.[45] Based on research in peer assessment, there are a few guidelines that should be followed in developing a peer assessment process that will optimize the quality of the assessment and feedback.[45,50-52]

1. The reliability of peer assessments is enhanced when based on multiple observations by multiple different observers. Therefore, whenever possible, feedback should ideally be based on repeated observations in different contexts.
2. Transparency is important to obtain buy-in from those being assessed and those providing the assessment. The purpose of the assessment, expected levels of performance, the criteria used to perform the assessment, and potential outcomes of the assessment should be clearly communicated to all parties.

3. Some training is generally required for assessors. They should know and understand the performance objectives against which assessments will be based, how to use any rating instrument (checklist, rating scale) that may be required, and how to provide constructive feedback if that will be their responsibility.

4. Opportunities for qualitative feedback should be available. Narrative comments that describe specific, observed behaviors in association with discrete events are likely to lead to reflective learning and corrective behavior.

Experts who have written about peer assessment generally suggest that, in order to optimize the validity of assessment results, it should occur in a low-stakes setting and ratings should be provided anonymously.[45,48,50] A high-stakes assessment might result in inflated (lenient) ratings and less useful feedback, and known relationships between assessors and assessees might serve to raise, or perhaps lower, peer ratings. On the other hand, some students feel that feedback is more meaningful when it is signed by the individual providing the assessment.[52]

This section has focused on the role of peer assessment in furthering the knowledge, skills, and attitudes of those assessing their peers and those being assessed. However, students can contribute to educational programs in other ways, including helping to develop educational content and materials and contributing to research, monitoring, and evaluation of educational programs and interventions.[54] Peer teaching is commonly used in medical education as a supplement to other curricular activities. Peers at the same academic level or from a higher academic level ("near-peers") may be selected or volunteer to perform various teaching functions.[55,56] Peers or near-peers are often at or near the same knowledge and skill level as the other students they are teaching, can better understand their needs, and can explain concepts in a manner that may be more easily understood and in a context in which they are less anxious, more comfortable revealing their weaknesses, and asking questions.[55–59] In many cases, students who have read this book and completed the end-of-chapter questions will have acquired a knowledge and understanding of health systems principles and practices that many of their faculty or more senior students and residents do not have the opportunity to experience. Thus students become a source of expertise that can meaningfully contribute to developing and prioritizing learning content and teaching and assessment approaches in this emerging third science.

Similar to peer assessment (which itself may play a role in peer teaching) both the teacher and the learner may benefit significantly from the activity.[55,56] Learning material to teach others invokes a learning or mastery goal orientation that requires a higher level of information processing and deeper learning than that which usually occurs in preparing for an examination. Techniques that students may use to prepare for teaching such as verbalization, recitation, and rehearsal tend to consolidate and increase the durability of learning.[55,56] In addition, the role and responsibilities of being a teacher may positively impact a learner's confidence, motivation, and attribution style, enhancing self-efficacy and self-determination.[55,56] Lastly, engagement in teaching or coaching colleagues will allow learners to acquire skills and attitudes (including leadership, supervisory skills, and confidence) that will serve them well in caring for, counseling, and educating their patients as well as interacting with various professional colleagues in the health care systems.[56]

F. ASSESSMENT OF PERFORMANCE IN PRACTICE

Physicians and other health care professionals in clinical practice are expected to become involved in assessing the quality of care delivered as individual practitioners and/ or within health care teams. This will often be driven by requirements to maintain board certification or other credentials or comply with federal, institutional, or practice plan-level obligations. Very likely, providers will have technical support or resources (such as clinical registries) provided by their practices, hospitals, or professional societies to help them meet quality measurement requirements. During clinical rotations in medical school or other health professions schools, students may have an opportunity to help with a quality improvement activity in which residents or attending staff are also involved. Later, these students will become residents who will most likely be expected to develop, lead, or participate in quality-improvement projects.

As described in Chapter 6, assessment of health care quality involves assessment of structures, processes, and outcomes. The ultimate measure of quality of care provided by an individual or a health care team is the health outcomes of their patients. Examples of commonly used outcome measures are mortality after a myocardial infarction, hospitalizations in children with cystic fibrosis, and postoperative infections. While outcome measures are undeniably important yardsticks reflecting health care quality, there are significant limitations to their use as a marker of individual performance. One limitation relates to the fact that patient complexity and illness severity may vary across providers and practices, and risk-adjustment will be necessary to account for these differences if comparisons are made between providers or important credentialing decisions are based on the results. Another challenge to outcomes-based assessment is that patients are often cared for by teams or by multiple physicians, and attribution of specific outcomes to a particular physician may be difficult. Attribution may be less of a limitation when measuring team-based outcomes.

Measurement of processes of care is less susceptible to attribution problems and complexity differences and is commonly used in quality improvement activities. In using process measures, it is important to select those that correlate with clinical outcomes, such as using β blockers in patients with myocardial infarction or perioperative antibiotics in selected surgeries. Challenges to the use of process measures in quality assessment are inconsistencies in how well such measures are documented in the medical record and the often unknown impact of patient preferences on their use.

IV. CHAPTER SUMMARY

This chapter provided perspectives on assessing student performance in HSS. Since systems science is a relatively new area of focus in medicine, there is a significant role for student-directed processes of self-assessment and self-regulated learning. Additionally, as educational programs increasingly incorporate assessments of this critical aspect of clinical practice, students who understand how they are being assessed and are able to integrate assessment results into their learning and improvement plans and activities are more likely to succeed.

QUESTIONS FOR FURTHER THOUGHT

1. What key behaviors will enhance student acquisition of the knowledge, skills, and attitudes intrinsic to health systems science?
2. What are the attributions in self-regulated learning, and how can the way in which students attribute various learning outcomes impact their learning process and development of competence?
3. What is meant by *reliability*, and how does the importance of the reliability of assessment results vary depending on whether the assessment purpose is to provide feedback to guide learning or to make pass/fail decisions regarding a course or clerkship?
4. What assessment methods could be used for assessing acquisition of skills in quality improvement? What methods could be used for assessing performance of quality improvement in clinical practice?
5. Peer teaching and assessment has been shown to benefit those being taught and assessed. How does peer teaching and assessment benefit students who are teaching or providing the assessment?

Annotated Bibliography

Chen JY. Why peer evaluation by students should be part of the medical school learning environment. *Med Teach.* 2012;34(8):603–606.

Finn GM, Garner J. Twelve tips for implementing a successful peer assessment. *Med Teach.* 2011;33(6):443–446.

Furmedge DS, Iwata K, Gill D. Peer-assisted learning—beyond teaching: how can medical students contribute to the undergraduate curriculum? *Med Teach.* 2014;36(9):812–817.

These three articles provide a rationale for involving peers in teaching, assessment, and other activities involved in undergraduate medical education. They help define the roles that learners may play and provide useful advice in establishing peer-assisted learning and peer-assessment programs.

Hickson GB, Pichert JW, Webb LE, Gabbe SG. A complementary approach to promoting professionalism: identifying, measuring, and addressing unprofessional behaviors. *Acad Med.* 2007;82(11):1040–1048.

Using a program that tracks unsolicited patient complaints to identify team members who would benefit from coaching regarding professionalism, Hickson's group has noted that many physicians demonstrating unprofessional behaviors self-correct after an "awareness" intervention. Additionally, systematic intervention improves patient safety and the work environment for all. The group is now advocating that team members address (or report) unprofessional behaviors promptly. Table 2 outlines potential actions a resident might take upon observing an incident and the potential drawbacks of each. The description of a "cup of coffee conversation" offers a validated approach to share concerns with a colleague.

Miller GE. Invited reviews: the assessment of clinical skills/competence/performance. *Acad Med.* 1990;65(suppl 9):S63–S67.

This often-cited article was actually an invited review regarding the state-of-the-art of standardized patients for assessing clinical competence. While many new assessments have since been developed and studied and the concepts of health systems science and "systems-competencies" were not yet anticipated, this article helped many to understand the developmental nature of clinical competence and performance and the principles underlying the reliability and validity of assessment approaches.

Sandars J, Cleary TJ. Self-regulation theory: applications to medical education: AMEE Guide No. 58. *Med Teach.* 2011;33(11):875–886.

This comprehensive and readable review defines the three phases of self-regulated learning: 1) goal-setting and planning for learning activities, 2) application of learning and practice strategies, and 3) reflection on their learning. Multiple examples from medical education in the classroom and in clinical settings show how self-regulated learning behaviors can improve students' performance.

Sklar DP. Integrating competencies. *Acad Med.* 2013;88(8):1049–1051.

In this editorial, Dr. Sklar, editor of Academic Medicine, *uses a patient vignette to illustrate the need for physicians to possess a breadth of competencies and an awareness of the larger health care delivery system in order to successfully care for patients.*

Telio S, Ajjawi R, Regher G. The "educational alliance" as a framework for reconceptualizing feedback in medical education. *Acad Med.* 2015;90(5):609–614.

Telio and colleagues advocate for a shift in our thinking about feedback as a unidirectional (teacher to student) process. They advocate instead for a "dialogue occurring within an authentic and committed educational relations that involves seeking shared understanding of performance and standards, negotiating agreement on action plans, working together toward reaching the goals, and co-creating opportunities to use feedback in practice."

References

1. Sklar DP. Integrating competencies. *Acad Med.* 2013;88(8):1049–1051.
2. Campbell C, Silver I, Sherbino J, Cate OT, Holmboe ES. Competency-based continuing professional development. *Med Teach.* 2010;32(8):657–662.
3. Shaughnessy AF, Slawson DC. Are we providing doctors with the training and tools for lifelong learning? *BMJ.* 1999;319(7220):1280.
4. Accreditation Council for Graduate Medical Education. ACGME program requirements for graduate medical education in internal medicine. http://www.acgme.org/portals/0/pfassets/programrequirements/140_internal_medicine_2016.pdf. Published 2011. Accessed November 6, 2016.
5. Royal College of Physicians and Surgeons of Canada. The CanMEDS framework. http://www.royalcollege.ca/rcsite/canmeds/canmeds-framework-e. Published 2014. Accessed November 6, 2016.
6. Zimmerman BJ, Bandura A, Martinez-Pons M. Self-motivation for academic attainment: the role of self-efficacy beliefs and personal goal setting. *Am Educ Res J.* 1992;29(3):663–676.
7. Zimmerman BJ. Self-efficacy: an essential motive to learn. *Contemp Educ Psychol.* 2000;25(1):82–91.
8. Sandars J, Cleary TJ. Self-regulation theory: applications to medical education: AMEE Guide No. 58. *Med Teach.* 2011;33(11):875–886.
9. Graham S. A review of attribution theory in achievement contexts. *Educ Psychol Rev.* 1991;3(1):5–39.
10. Dweck C. *Mindset: The New Psychology of Success.* New York: Random House; 2006.
11. Davis DA, Mazmanian PE, Fordis M, Van Harrison R, Thorpe KE, Perrier L. Accuracy of physician self-assessment compared with observed measures of competence: a systematic review. *JAMA.* 2006;296(9):1094–1102.
12. Langendyk V. Not knowing that they do not know: self-assessment accuracy of third-year medical students. *Med Educ.* 2006;40(2):173–179.
13. Dunning D, Heath C, Suls JM. Flawed self-assessment implications for health, education, and the workplace. *Psychol Sci Public Interest.* 2004;5(3):69–106.
14. Sargeant J, Armson H, Chesluk B, et al. The processes and dimensions of informed self-assessment: a conceptual model. *Acad Med.* 2010;85(7):1212–1220.
15. Brown PC, Roediger HL, McDaniel MA. *Make It Stick.* Cambridge, MA: Harvard University Press; 2014:23–45.
16. Telio S, Ajjawi R, Regher G. The "educational alliance" as a framework for reconceptualizing feedback in medical education. *Acad Med.* 2015;90(5):609–614.
17. Hickson GB, Pichert JW, Webb LE, Gabbe SG. A complementary approach to promoting professionalism: identifying, measuring, and addressing unprofessional behaviors. *Acad Med.* 2007;82(11):1040–1048.

18. McGaghie WC, Issenberg B, Cohen ER, Barsuk JH, Wayne DB. Medical education featuring mastery learning with deliberate practice can lead to better health for individuals and populations. *Acad Med.* 2011;86(11):e8–e9.

19. Tyler RW. *Basic Principles of Curriculum and Instruction: Syllabus for Education 305.* Chicago, IL: University of Chicago Press; 1959.

20. Galbraith RM, Hawkins RE, Holmboe ES. Making self-assessment more effective. *J Contin Educ Health Prof.* 2008;28(1):20–24.

21. Miller GE. Invited reviews: the assessment of clinical skills/competence/performance. *Acad Med.* 1990;65:S63–S67.

22. Van der Vleuten CP. The assessment of professional competence: developments, research and practical implications. *Adv Health Sci Educ.* 1996;1(1):41–67.

23. Aboumatar HJ, Thompson D, Wu A, et al. Development and evaluation of a 3-day patient safety curriculum to advance knowledge, self-efficacy and system thinking among medical students. *BMJ Qual Saf.* 2012;21(5):416–422.

24. Meier AH, Boehler ML, McDowell CM, et al. A surgical simulation curriculum for senior medical students based on TeamSTEPPS. *Arch Surg.* 2012;147(8):761–766.

25. Mookherjee S, Ranji S. An advanced quality improvement and patient safety elective. *Clin Teach.* 2013;10(6):368–373.

26. Shaneyfelt T, Baum KD, Bell D, et al. Instruments for evaluating evidence-based practice. *JAMA.* 2006;296(9):1116–1127.

27. Singh MK, Ogrinc G, Cox KR, et al. The Quality Improvement Knowledge Application Tool Revised (QIKAT-R). *Acad Med.* 2014;89(10):1386–1391.

28. Tartaglia KM, Walker C. Effectiveness of a quality improvement curriculum for medical students. *Med Educ Online.* 2015 May 8;20:27133.

29. Sircar SS, Tandon OP. Involving students in question writing: a unique feedback with fringe benefits. *Am J Physiol.* 1999;277(6 Pt 2):S84–S91.

30. Harris BH, Walsh JL, Tayyaba S, Harris DA, Wilson DJ, Smith PE. A novel student-led approach to multiple-choice question generation and online database creation, with targeted clinician input. *Teach Learn Med.* 2015;27(2):182–188.

31. Papinczak T, Babri AW, Peterson R, Kippers V, Wilkinson D. Students generating questions for their own written examinations. *Adv Health Sci Educ Theory Pract.* 2011;16(5):703–710.

32. Rosenshine B, Meister C, Chapman S. Teaching students to generate questions: a review of the intervention studies. *Rev Educ Res.* 1996;66(2):181–221.

33. King A. Facilitating elaborative learning through guide student-generated questioning. *Educ Psych.* 1992;27(1):111–126.

34. Smith SR, Goldman RE, Dollase RH, Taylor J. Assessing medical students for non-traditional competencies. *Med Teach.* 2007;29(7):711–716.

35. Thomas A, Saroyan A, Dauphinee WD. Evidence-based practice: a review of theoretical assumptions and effectiveness of teaching and assessment interventions in health professions. *Adv in Health Sci Educ.* 2011;16(2):253–276.

36. Dory V, Gagnon R, De Foy T, Duyver C, Leconte S. A novel assessment of an evidence-based practice course using an authentic assessment. *Med Teach.* 2010;32(2):e65–e70.

37. Varkey P, Natt N, Lesnick T, Downing S, Yudkowsky R. Validity evidence for an OSCE to assess competency in systems-based practice and practice-based learning and improvement. *Acad Med.* 2008;83(8):775–780.

38. Balasooriya C, Olupeliyawa A, Iqbal M, et al. A student-led process to enhance the learning and teaching of teamwork skills in medicine. *Educ Health (Abingdon).* 2013;26(2):78–84.

39. Wright MC, Segall N, Hobbs G, Phillips-Bute B, Maynard L, Taekman JM. Standardized assessment for evaluation of team skills: validity and feasibility. *Simul Healthc.* 2013;8(5):292–303.

40. Olupeliyawa AM, Balasooriya C, Hughes C, O'Sullivan A. Educational impact of an assessment of medical student's collaboration in health care teams. *Med Educ.* 2014;48(2):146–156.

41. Olupeliyawa AM, O'Sullivan AJ, Hughes C, Balasooriya CK. The Teamwork Mini-Clinical Evaluation Exercise (T-MEX): a workplace-based assessment focusing on collaborative competencies in health care. *Acad Med.* 2014;89(2):359–365.

42. Gakhar B, Spencer AL. Using direct observation, formal evaluation, and an interactive curriculum to improve the sign-out practices of internal medicine interns. *Acad Med.* 2010;85(7):1182–1188.

43. Sharma N, Cui Y, Leighton JP, White JS. Team-based assessment of medical students in a clinical clerkship is feasible and acceptable. *Med Teach.* 2012;34(7):555–561.

44. White JS, Sharma N. "Who writes what?" Using written comments in team-based assessment to better understand medical student performance: a mixed-methods study. *BMC Med Educ.* 2012;12:123. http://www.biomedcentral.com/1472-6920/12/123.

45. Finn GM, Garner J. Twelve tips for implementing a successful peer assessment. *Med Teach.* 2011;33(6):443–446.

46. Speyer R, Pilz W, van der Kruis J, Wouter Brunings J. Reliability and validity of student peer assessment in medical education: a systematic review. *Med Teach.* 2011;33(11):e572–e585.

47. Basehore PM, Pomerantz SC, Gentile M. Reliability and benefits of medical student peers in rating complex skills. *Med Teach.* 2014;36(5):409–414.

48. Eldredge JD, Bear DG, Wayne SJ, Perea PP. Student peer assessment in evidence-based medicine (EBM) searching skills training: an experiment. *J Med Lib Assoc.* 2013;101(4):244–251.

49. Spandorfer J, Puklus T, Rose V, et al. Peer assessment among first year medical students in anatomy. *Anat Sci Educ.* 2014;7(2):144–152.

50. Norcini JJ. Peer assessment of competence. *Med Educ.* 2003;37(6):539–543.

51. Chen JY. Why peer evaluation by students should be part of the medical school learning environment. *Med Teach.* 2012;34(8):603–606.

52. Nofziger AC, Naumburg EH, Davis BJ, Mooney CJ, Epstein RM. Impact of peer assessment on the professional development of medical students: a qualitative study. *Acad Med.* 2010;85(1):140–147.

53. Schonrock-Adema J, Heijne-Penninga M, van Duijn MAJ, Geertsma J, Cohen-Schotanus J. Assessment of professional behavior in undergraduate medical education: peer assessment enhances performance. *Med Educ.* 2007;41(9):836–842.

54. Furmedge DS, Iwata K, Gill D. Peer-assisted learning—beyond teaching: how can medical students contribute to the undergraduate curriculum. *Med Teach.* 2014;36(9):812–817.

55. Ten Cate O, Durning S. Dimensions and psychology of peer teaching in medical education. *Med Teach.* 2007;29(6):546–552.

56. Ten Cate O, Durning S. Peer teaching in medical education: twelve reasons to move from theory to practice. *Med Teach.* 2007;29(6):591–599.

57. Lockspeiser TM, O'Sullivan P, Teherani A, Muller J. Understanding the experience of being taught by peers: the value of social and cognitive congruence. *Adv Health Sci Educ Theory Pract.* 2008;13(3):361–372.

58. Ross MT, Cameron JS. Peer assisted learning: a planning and implementation framework: AMEE Guide no. 30. *Med Teach.* 2007;29(6):527–545.

59. Silbert BI, Lake FR. Peer-assisted learning in teaching clinical examination to junior medical students. *Med Teach.* 2012;34(5):392–397.

15

The Future of Health Systems Science

Jeffrey M. Borkan, MD, PhD, Therese M. Wolpaw, MD, MHPE, and Victoria Stagg Elliott, MA

LEARNING OBJECTIVES

1. Understand health systems science (HSS) as dynamic in terms of focus, knowledge, attitudes, and skills.
2. Project how HSS aligns with future trends in medical education and health care.
3. Propose directions that this textbook and its offshoots may take in the future.

This chapter explores the impact that this dynamic third science will have on the education and training of physicians and medical professionals as well as on the US health care system as a whole. This chapter also explores the future directions and forms of dissemination that may shape textbooks like this moving forward.

CHAPTER OUTLINE

I. INTRODUCTION—A BRIEF REVIEW OF THE CONTEXT/CONTENT OF THIS TEXTBOOK

This textbook has sought to provide an overview of health systems science (HSS)—the third medical science in a complementary triad with the basic and clinical sciences. Like these first two sciences, competence in HSS is necessary for practitioners to proficiently serve patients in both current and future health care environments. The domains of HSS range from information technology to health policy, though all are rooted in systems theory, as represented by the bio-psycho-social model.[1] Although there have been many previous efforts to describe the various HSS elements students and trainees need for practice in an evolving health care system (references are reviewed in Chapter 2), this is the first comprehensive effort that provides a broad approach applicable across a continuum of health professions learners.

The authors are building on the literature related to health systems and health care delivery science as well as the work of the HSS interest group of the American Medical Association's Accelerating Change in Medical Education Consortium. This group used a variety of methods to construct a comprehensive set of HSS domains that form the basis of this book's table of contents. Efforts began with systematic literature reviews, in-depth discussions, and elucidation of suggested content areas from all participants at a consortium-sponsored medical education meeting. Further efforts to identify HSS content domains included the analysis of the 32 final consortium grant applications, as well as analysis of relevant sections of the Liaison Committee on Medical Education part II survey questions related to system-based practice. Next, investigators at each consortium member school did "deep dives" into the curricular content and courses at their medical schools (down to the level of individual lectures and seminars) to identify HSS content. This information was then used to identify core, cross-cutting, and linking domains of an HSS curriculum.[2,3] Though gaps likely still exist, this effort produced what we believe is the most thorough and inclusive content review of HSS to date.

II. HEALTH SYSTEMS SCIENCE—A DYNAMIC PARADIGM

Just as the Flexner report[4] heralded the routine adoption of the biomedical dyad model into medical education, the authors of this textbook believe that the time is ripe for the educational model to transform from yesterday's biomedical dyad into today's biomedical and systems triad. We believe that this triad needs to be consistently adopted by US health professional schools and training programs. The basic sciences are essential for a physician or other health care professional to understand the human body and its function. The clinical sciences are essential to translate that understanding into care for the human body. HSS is essential for physicians and other health care professionals to help ensure that patients, communities, and populations achieve optimal health outcomes.

We expect that the subjects explored in this textbook will be expanded upon and added to in an iterative fashion. HSS should not be viewed as a static set of domains and processes. Rather HSS is a dynamic, developmental, contextually-based paradigm that will evolve over time with transitions in focus, curricular objectives, knowledge, attitudes, and skills. Such changes must align with the evolution of the health care system as it transforms from a predominately fee-for-service model to a risk- and value-based model. The gap between the changes in the health care system and changes in health professional education must be as narrow as possible, and the catalyst for transformation may come from either direction. An example of this might be in the area of value-added educational interventions, where students providing particular population-based interventions can change the function and outcomes of the health care system.

When medical education is framed by a triad of HSS, basic science, and clinical science, early learning experiences will be required to introduce all three areas, ideally in an integrated, seamless manner. Learners need to internalize a conceptual framework and role identity that encompasses their development in the science triad. Some medical schools are now implementing early experiences in HSS, reminiscent of the movement in the latter half of the twentieth century to implement early clinical experiences into what was a predominantly basic science curriculum. For example, Penn State College of Medicine has successfully incorporated a core course in HSS that simultaneously pairs conceptual learning in the classroom with experiential learning in the health system. First-year medical students within a couple of months of entering medical school engage in value-added roles by serving as patient navigators across the health care system. Similarly, at the University of California, Davis, a select group of students who are admitted to an accelerated primary care track begin a longitudinal preceptorship experience almost on entry to medical school. They immerse themselves in a practice setting and very quickly identify with their roles as advocates and change agents. At the University of California, San Francisco (UCSF), first-year students are assigned to health care teams. As team members, they learn early clinical skills while simultaneously identifying quality improvement needs they can take on. At the Alpert Medical School of Brown University, students in the dual-degree MD-ScM Primary Care–Population Medicine program participate in the integrated health systems curriculum (with population health, research, and leadership components) throughout their 4 years of study, with clinical experiences tailored for their developmental and curricular stage.

HSS is driving educational change. As noted in previous chapters, nearly all US health professional schools recognize the paucity of HSS training for their graduates. At the same time, these schools recognize the profound importance of this skill set for graduating students if they are to be practice-ready for the health care system they will enter. As the demand for such training increases from students, practitioners, health systems, and regulatory bodies, HSS will have an ever larger and more substantive presence in the curricula of all training and educational programs. Such demands are already driving educational change, and the authors foresee the rapid evolution of both a broader set of HSS content domains and related pedagogic tools. This trend is accelerating as national medical student licensing examinations (e.g., the United States Medical Licensing Examination [USMLE]) are already including HSS content in their tests and will likely include more in the future.

Learners across the full educational spectrum are the adventurers and co-creators of the future of HSS and its alignment with the evolving health care system. This journey to prepare systems-ready caregivers will also involve facilitating the development of systems-ready patients who will increasingly engage in bidirectional communication and shared decision making for their individual decisions and for those involving the scope and direction of the health care system. The simultaneous journeys of learners and patients start with shared access to and utilization of health information data (e.g., portals, open charts, alternate sources of health information) and expand to include direct participation in the decision making about the basket of services offered by insurers (private or governmental), and the development of particular parts of the health care system.

III. HEALTH SYSTEMS SCIENCE AND THE FUTURE OF HEALTH PROFESSIONAL EDUCATION AND TRAINING

Any vision of the future evolution and transformation of health professional education and training must account for a health care environment dominated by rapid change—organizationally, scientifically, and economically. Health professional education must align and change with the evolving needs of the patients, communities, populations served, and the health care system where learners will ultimately become employed. For now, the goal of HSS education may be to develop systems-thinking health care providers who will be ready to take on the Quadruple Aim—which incorporates both the Triple Aim of improved outcomes, better patient experiences, and lower costs,[5] as well as improved provider satisfaction.[6] However, with the interconnected evolution of the health care system and HSS, these priorities will undoubtedly evolve as well. To keep up with the health care needs of society, significant curricular reforms will be required of all health professions disciplines if trainees hope to meet the challenges of providing care in the decades to come. This can only happen with a fundamental change in *agency* for the design of health professional education. By *agency,* we are referring to Bandura's conceptual framework for Human Agency.[7] To be an agent, as defined by Bandura, is to intentionally influence functioning and circumstances. We propose that it is time for shared agency between education leaders and health systems leaders (as well as students and trainees) in the design and outcomes of medical education that would be accomplished through building a shared intention for systems change, visualizing improvement goals and outcomes for the health care system, engaging in a course of action, and making corrective adjustments as necessary. Current forward-thinking dialogue among education and systems leaders about the direction of HSS is discussed in the following sections.

A. Seamless Integration from Undergraduate Medical Education to Graduate Medical Education to Continuing Medical Education and Practice with Shortened Timelines

At this point in time, undergraduate medical education (UME), graduate medical education (GME), and continuing medical education (CME) lack a base of shared goals, vision, curriculum, regulatory bodies, and evaluation methods. The situation is similar in other health professional schools. Reconceptualizing the whole of education, training, and practice as a unified developmental learning continuum will facilitate coordination of training in the full science triad— HSS, as well as in the basic and clinical sciences. This kind of continuum has been successfully envisioned at medical schools, starting with Texas Tech University, where coordination between UME and GME allows shortening of training periods, particularly for students seeking careers in primary care. This accelerated model in which medical school is completed in 3 years is being adopted at a growing list of other medical schools, such as the University of California, Davis, Medical School, New York University School of Medicine, and Penn State School of Medicine.

B. Consideration of New Admissions Criteria

As HSS becomes the third science of medicine, medical schools may need to rethink their admissions processes to ensure that applicants have the capacity to acquire the knowledge, attitudes, and skills required for success in this domain. For example, requirements for admission may well include substantial experience working in teams, a deep respect for the interdependence of knowledge and skill within a health care team, a clear appreciation for patient-centered care, skilled communication ability, and respectful professional and patient interactions. Criteria might also include the ability to function in a setting of uncertainty, resilience, and sufficient adaptive capacity to facilitate functioning in complex adaptive systems. In addition, applicants should have a sense of social responsibility and feel empowerment as change agents. Tools that have sufficient reliability and validity to select such students will need to be developed. The multiple mini-interview format[8] may be an example of a tool that could be amplified in its reach. It has already been employed by an increasing number of medical schools, starting with the Michael G. DeGroote School of Medicine at McMaster University in Canada, to help identify desirable behaviors such as communication skills.[9]

C. Creation of Competency-Based Educational Assessment Tools for Health Systems Science

Competencies, milestones, and entrustable professional activities (EPAs) will need to be constructed and validated for HSS. These must emphasize the key tenets of HSS, encourage lifelong HSS learning, and be translatable into professional behaviors. Uses of competency-based educational outcomes[10] range from guiding learning to feedback, evaluation, and certification. Proposed competencies for optimizing health care delivery and systems science have been forwarded by Lucey.[11]

D. Governance, Public Investment, and Scrutiny

As local, state, and national governments take increasing interest in issues central to HSS, such as health care quality, patient safety, and finances, there will undoubtedly be increased public and legal investment in and scrutiny on the processes and outcomes of health professional education and training. With such investment and scrutiny will come greater expectations for clearly measurable outcomes and accountability on health system issues as disparate as certification and prescribing. Examples already abound and include everything from the federal government's Meaningful Use requirements for electronic health records (EHRs) to the demands of state departments of health for increased training and regulation regarding opioid prescribing. Meaningful Use was instituted as part of the American Recovery and Reinvestment Act of 2009 with the goal to promote the accelerated adoption and significant use of interoperable health information technology and qualified EHRs.[12] Many states have been instituting or plan to institute training and increased regulations on the prescription and monitoring of opioids in an effort to combat the epidemic of addiction and deaths associated with these medications.[13–15] Some of these state efforts mandate specific training for all medical students, residents, and practicing physicians. Efforts such as these will likely increase and will influence the content and instruction of HSS in the future.

E. Advances in Information Technology

Technological advances are changing and will deeply impact health care delivery and HSS.

1. Electronic Health Records

As noted by Tierney and colleagues,[16] although the clinical and operational benefits of EHRs have been lauded by many, "few have considered the effect these systems have on medical education... both the potential benefits and the unintended consequences." Nonetheless, it is becoming increasingly apparent that the near-ubiquitous penetration of EHRs into clinical settings is having broad effects on the communication skills that must be incorporated into health professional education. Health professional schools, however, are lagging in their adaptation of communication skills teaching to new settings and new forms of interaction.[17] When computers are used in provider-patient encounters, they essentially become the "third party" in the consultation room,[18,19] yet students and trainees rarely receive training in how to optimize communication in these settings or how to actively engage patients in the EHR. EHRs can be seen as affecting all six domains of clinical competency introduced by the Accreditation Council for Graduate Medical Education.[16,20] This area is ripe for further guidelines, research, and HSS curriculum development, since it has implications for learning across the full educational continuum training.

2. Expansion of Electronic Health Record Capabilities and Dimensions That Will Positively Impact Health Systems and Health Systems Science

EHRs are rapidly expanding their capabilities in areas that will directly affect health care systems and HSS. These include everything from EHRs' rapidly increasing capacity to integrate and abstract records from multiple sites of care to patient safety features (e.g., drug allergies and drug-drug interactions) to data analytics and patient access to records. The ever-growing capability of EHRs to gather, store, and analyze vast amounts of data for individual patients, physician patient panels, or populations opens up infinite possibilities. This is aided by advances in the science of data management and analysis that will enable everyone from students to physicians to organizations to convert these vast resources into information and knowledge.[21] At New York University School of Medicine, an innovative data analytic project has become part of the standard medical school requirements. Entitled, "Health Care By The Numbers," this curriculum allows students to explore over 4.9 million real patient-level records from the New York State Department of Health Statewide Planning and Research Cooperative System (SPARCS).[22] Patient access to records is becoming much more routine with the use of patient portals, and there are major initiatives that aim to take this to the extreme, opening all records for patient viewing.[23]

There are, however, major gaps in particular EHR capabilities that unless addressed, may deleteriously affect HSS. For example, there is an urgent need for greater EHR accommodation of clinical work flow, interprofessional teams, and decision-support tools. In addition, EHRs could benefit by including system-level variables in addition to the routine categories such as history, physical, allergies, problems, and medications. An example of such a system-level variable might be site of care. This item could focus on whether the care was provided at the right place and time for the patient. Such dilemmas arise frequently in clinical practices regarding ambulatory sensitive conditions. Was the patient with certain diseases or complaints seen appropriately or inappropriately in the emergency department, or could his or her issues have been better addressed in a primary care or similar setting? A next-generation EHR might alert the care team and suggest transferring the patient to the appropriate setting. Similarly, an EHR program for rural hospitals might assist with decisions regarding the need to transfer particular patients to tertiary and quaternary care settings. Other EHR developments might include everything from interactive holograms to natural language processing and artificial intelligence.[24] Hardware and software developments are now making possible the incorporation of wearable technology and smart phone applications into patient care. Further developments are nearly limitless and will affect HSS at every turn.

F. Simulation for Population Health

Simulation is being utilized for an ever-growing number and range of medical educational purposes—from practicing for rare but critical events to practicing interprofessional team care. Future simulation technology, focused at the population or community level rather than individual patient-physician encounters, may be utilized to drive productivity while maintaining patient safety and quality and controlling costs.[25] For example, primary care leaders may be tasked with population health simulations in which they must equitably distribute health care resources to a community while simultaneously balancing restricted budgets.[21]

G. Expansion Beyond Walls

Health professional education is leaving the confines of classroom walls. Online capabilities and advances in information technology have facilitated the expansion beyond the walls of health professional schools and teaching hospitals for the last few decades, and it is expected that this expansion will accelerate. Some, like the editor of *JAMA* Howard C. Bauchner, MD, have suggested that the future of medical education in the United States includes, "No walls, no classes."[26] Such liberation will allow training to occur in varied settings, wherever learning and health care can occur. Students have already voted with their feet in many medical schools where lectures are recorded. Students often watch lectures at home, using higher speeds for sections more easily understood and multiple, slower viewing of sections that are more difficult to conceptualize. Some medical schools accelerate further devolution of the classroom by recording lecturers in studios, without students present. The online learning explosion (from local productions to massive open online courses [MOOCs]) and the "flipped classroom," as well as the expansion and diversification of educational platforms and forums will likely accelerate in the future—influencing the methods and content of learning, including HSS. Similarly, health professional training, to remain aligned with health system needs, will increasingly follow health care wherever it occurs in the community, including in patient homes. The evolution of clinical care for patient populations beyond the hospital and usual clinic settings to accountable care organizations, patient-centered medical homes, community health teams, and through the use of telemedicine and other technologies may further hasten the movement beyond conventional medical school walls. The University of North Dakota School of Medicine and Health Sciences is leading in this area by enhancing medical education through advanced simulation and telemedicine technologies to teach interprofessional competencies along with rural health care skills. Other medical schools are already following in this direction, and more will likely follow.

H. Value-Added Medical Education

Medical schools are developing value-added roles for students and trainees that lead to achievement of the Triple Aim. As suggested by Lin and colleagues,[27] "Change is desperately needed to translate education into better health outcomes for Americans today." Both Lin and colleagues[27] and Lucey[11] as well as others advocate for "value-added medical education," where students' experiential learning experiences can measurably improve health care system processes of care and patient outcomes, adding both value and capacity to the health care system. An example is the novel academic program at Penn State College of Medicine, discussed earlier, that utilizes medical students as patient navigators. This program is a "win-win" for students and patients since the former learn how to navigate the complex health care system through the patient's eyes, while the latter are helped to overcome hurdles including insurance issues, medication concerns, and follow-up.[28] At UCSF, where much of the pioneering work on value-added medical education began, there are programs to improve patient outcomes through medical education,[29] leveraging the talents and commitments of students to add value to the care of patients today. Though these efforts must be supervised to ensure that patients and students truly benefit, they hold promise for further student engagement in the health care system. Another value-added role for medical education involves faculty development. The Brody School of Medicine at East Carolina University (ECU) has established a comprehensive longitudinal core curriculum in patient safety, quality improvement, population health, and team-based care. To execute and facilitate these curricular changes, ECU has established its Teachers of Quality Academy to provide faculty development in the new competencies. Faculty who are trained in this academy in turn train students. They will both be able to bring their quality improvement projects back to their health systems, where implementation should improve patient care for individuals and populations.

I. Patient Safety

Health professional schools will need to further emphasize patient safety—a critical component of HSS—and institute more sophisticated pedagogic methods to ensure its adoption. As noted by Bagian,[30] "[T]here has been growing recognition that improving patient safety must be more systems based and sophisticated than the traditional approach of simply telling health care providers to 'be more careful.'" Rather than reactive, reactionary, or blame-based responses to adverse events, the health system requires system-based approaches to addressing problems that should be instituted with the goal of preventing unintended harm to patients. Tools and skill sets, such as formal root cause analyses and risk mitigation, will need to be acquired, embraced, and practiced by senior clinicians who will serve as role models for their trainees.[30] Our challenge is building that cadre of clinician role models who not only use systems thinking in their patient interactions but also provide a safe environment for learners to practice with guided feedback.

J. Practice-Based Improvement

Similar to patient safety, future health care professionals must be able to engage in practice-based improvement and systems-based improvement if they are to serve as change agents for the health system. Such experiences have been relatively common in student-run clinics, 96 of which are said to be operating in the United States according to the Society of Student Run Free Clinics.[31] However, other opportunities should be encouraged to facilitate students gaining experience in this important HSS domain. The innovative programs at Penn State, UCSF, and ECU discussed earlier are just a few examples of what is possible. The new University of Texas Rio Grande Valley School of Medicine will place medical students at health centers in impoverished rural settlements in unincorporated areas along the US-Mexican border. Students will be taught strategies to support information exchange and empathetic interactions with individuals and diverse groups in multiple settings for numerous preventive health, health maintenance, and health care delivery purposes. This new medical school is in one of the most medically underserved areas of the United States, and its transformative program will improve the local practices and health systems, along with educating the next generation of physicians to be effective in such settings.

CASE STUDY 1

A second-year medical student decides to set up a free clinic in the underserved community near her medical school and pulls together a committee of 20 enthusiastic students and six primary care attendings. They receive free space from a local community agency and plan to operate three evenings per week, with students from the medical, nursing, and social work schools in their area, as well with the help of faculty who will volunteer their time.

What health system issues must she and her colleagues consider and resolve prior to opening and operating the free clinic? What knowledge, attitudes, and skills must they ensure are acquired by students working in the free clinic?

K. Interprofessional Education

Interprofessional collaboration is a rich, essential component of US health care, and it can serve as the foundation for efforts to "broaden the societal reach of academic medicine."[32] However, as noted by Satterfield and Carney:[33]

> Despite policy changes such as the prevention mandate of the Affordable Care Act, medical school curricula spend comparatively little time on behavioral science and often fail to adequately prepare learners for practicing health care in complex interprofessional teams.

The acquisition of HSS competencies can be accelerated by creating opportunities for frequent, meaningful, and varied interprofessional education (IPE) activities in health professional training schools and programs. These might include everything from deliberate learning and practice of team skills to formal evaluation activities (like OSCE) to informal social learning opportunities like interest groups and clubs. IPE activities that involve shared quality improvement projects provide opportunities for expanding two key HSS areas simultaneously. Faculty who have facility and comfort in IPE will be required, since the education system reflects a siloed structure not unlike the health care system. One notable leader in this area is the University of Nebraska Medical Center College of Medicine. This school is engaging with the health care delivery system to enhance IPE and practice in clinical practice environments.

L. Active Discussion of Race in Medicine

Race has often been perceived as a biological variable in the basic and clinical medical sciences, but this understanding is likely to be challenged as more critical thinking emerges as part of HSS training and as social and political movements (such as Black Lives Matter) gain inroads into social consciousness. For example, biological assumptions regarding race are widespread in much of US biomedical research and teaching, although upon closer inspection, the categories are often crude approximations of social categories, rather than genetically informed classifications.[34,35] Despite fairly transparent historical roots in European colonial hegemony, the widespread acceptance of race in medicine has been fairly resistant to change until recently. Research, such as the Tuskegee experiments[36] and more recently by Braun,[37] have poignantly described the deleterious effects of the biologicalization of race. We would expect an acceleration of the diminution of the biologicalization of race in the future—one that would be both shaped by changing social norms and reflected in HSS curriculum.

M. Early Involvement with Patients in Nontraditional Health Settings

Early patient involvement is not new, but what is new is embedding students in nontraditional health care settings, especially on interprofessional teams from early in their training. Early experiential roles with patients, where trainees can see the role-modeling of interprofessional care, are critical. This must involve, however, going beyond observing. Learners need to be immersed in longitudinal patient care exposures as an individual and as part of interprofessional care teams where they can engage in multiple opportunities for practice with feedback. Such immersions should be linked to improving clinical outcomes (as noted earlier), including sustained, substantive application of performance and systems improvement strategies, as well as shared decision making.[32] There are further advantages in immersing students in patient-centered medical homes from the beginning of their education, incorporating integrated clinical, hands-on, and multiple HSS issues as part of the core curriculum.

IV. HEALTH SYSTEMS SCIENCE AND THE FUTURE OF THE US HEALTH CARE SYSTEM

The US health care system is in a period of rapid transformation, buffeted by economic and political demands, as well as demands for greater accountability and achievement of the Triple Aim.[5] Changes in the US health care system in the coming years will accelerate the incorporation of HSS into health professions training as the skill set will become a necessity for physicians and other health care professionals employed by these transformed systems. Training in HSS domains will also enable and empower learners to effect positive changes in the systems in which they currently work to improve quality, efficiency, and patients' experiences of care.

A. Decline of Academic Health Centers and Reductions in Hospitals and Hospital Beds

Academic health centers (AHCs) face an uncertain future[38] as it becomes more difficult to support their interconnected missions of service, research, and education in an environment of decreasing clinical and research dollars. AHCs face

the ever-growing risk of tighter budgets, decreased numbers of beds and services, and even threats of extinction.[39] There is greater likelihood, already occurring in some settings such as those mentioned earlier, that more health professions training will take place in ambulatory, primary care, and community settings, where the connections to elements of HSS are direct and apparent. Such changes are becoming increasingly established in the clinical portions of medical education as evidenced by the ever-growing number of longitudinal integrated clerkships (LICs). Unlike the traditional single discipline, largely inpatient clerkships that have been the norm for the past century, LICs provide students with integrated, longitudinal, and largely ambulatory experiences in the core disciplines with the continuity of patients (often in panels), learners, and mentors. Students in LICs typically follow patients to whatever health care settings they need to access for their care.

CASE STUDY 2

A large academic health center in the Midwest has operated under a fee-for-service model for the last 50 years. During this time, they established large, costly, resource-intensive, specialized medical and surgical services focusing on organ transplant and joint replacements. These units have been profit centers for the academic institution, supporting much of their teaching and research mission. In the meantime, they have developed only a rudimentary primary care network, leaving this to their nonacademic rival across town. In the new health care environment, all the insurers in their state have moved to value-based care with set per-member–per-month payments, supplemented by a quality indicator incentive.

How might these changes affect the resource-intensive services that suddenly become cost centers, and how will the academic health center need to change to ensure its future viability? What population health strategies should be considered?

B. Creation of Clinical Public Health and Clinical Population Health Subspecialties

New and integrated departments and divisions are arising to fill the space between care of individual patients (health care services) and care of the public (public health). Such organizational units tend to originate from partnerships—often between public health, preventive services, and primary care. A classic example is the Clinical Public Health Division at the University of Toronto Dalla Lana School of Public Health.[40] Their mission is, "to engage in innovative research and education programs and service, all aimed at bringing the best science to the creation of the trans-disciplinary approaches, systems, and professionals needed to optimize individual as well as population health in the sustainable health system of the future." Their first goal is, "The development of clinical public health (the integration of primary care, preventive medicine, and public health) activities within the university, associated hospitals and community health centers, and associated public health agencies, aimed at fostering collaborative research, training and knowledge translation programs." Not only are they developing innovative training for all public health students in basic clinical practice and health systems, they are also extending their training to physicians in primary care, addiction medicine, mental health, and even wound care. Other similar programs that aim to impact community and population health are arising throughout the United States, either under the guise of new population risk contracts, accountable care organizations, or the expansion of state or city departments of public health. As forward-thinking academic units form to impact health care delivery to communities and populations, HSS will logically be core to the learning framework.

C. Risk Contracts

Risk contracts, capitation, and value-based financing are expected to expand dramatically over the next decade as insurers, states, and the federal government attempt to control costs. Such arrangements require new HSS skills for physicians and other health care professionals, ranging from the ability to measure, record, and report quality measures to the ability to reduce unnecessary medical expenditures. Medical students and trainees will have to both understand the key concepts, as well as attain the necessary skills to monitor and adjust their own health care provision behaviors.

D. Cost Transparency

The US health care system has been extremely opaque regarding reporting of costs, whether for routine tests or highly specialized procedures. Despite the advancement of efforts to allow consumers to make informed choices, such as health savings accounts, reliable cost data remains difficult and often impossible to access. There has been some notable pilot work, such as at the University of Utah with "radical transparency."[41] Radical transparency involves the creation and distribution of reliable information about the cost and quality of health care—whether it is a CT scan, knee replacement surgery, or cardiology consultation. The University of Utah hospital has used such information to bend the cost curve. As the health care system switches from fee-for-service to capitation, routine assessments and utilization of cost data in clinical decision making will become even more necessary.

V. FUTURE DIRECTIONS THIS TEXTBOOK MAY TAKE

This textbook is meant to be a living document that evolves with the shifts in the social, scientific, and economic context of health systems and health professional education. The authors envision that students, faculty, and patients will engage in thoughtful dialogue that will spur the further evolution and development of HSS.

Elements that may accelerate this iterative process include the following:

- Availability of chapters in various forms and formats
- Online forums
- Periodic updates
- Open content

We also expect that other individuals and groups will work to influence the content and direction of this third science. Stakeholders range from social activists and social movements such as the Beyond Flexner movement or Global Health through Education, Training and Service (GHETS)[42,43] to trainees, health care providers (including interprofessional care groups), social and behavioral scientists, and, of course, patients. We welcome active dialogue as the field evolves.

VI. CHAPTER SUMMARY

HSS, basic science, and clinical science form the science triad that is fundamental to the training of physicians and other health care professionals who will be ready to practice in the health care system they enter. Health professional education must be nimble enough to make continuous adjustments to keep it aligned with the needs of a changing health care system and the needs of the communities and populations served. We return to our earlier statements:

> The basic sciences are essential for a physician or other health care professional to understand the human body and its function. The clinical sciences are essential to translate that understanding into care for the human body. HSS is essential for physicians and other health care professionals to help ensure that patients, communities, and populations achieve optimal health outcomes.

HSS, like our health care system, is a field in evolution. In truth, so too are basic and clinical sciences. Students and trainees, along with their teachers, are the adventurers in the new frontier and co-creators of the future of medical curriculum and the health care system. We invite you to embrace the challenge of dynamically defining the content of HSS while simultaneously developing pedagogic and assessment tools to enhance learning, relevance, and broad acceptability. All health care professions schools and training programs have important contributions to make. Among the greatest challenges at present for HSS is developing the initial cadres of teachers and role models who will guide subsequent generations of learners. Faculty development will be critical to achieve the goals of HSS, as well as promoting culture change within medicine and health care to emphasize key HSS factors. The improvement of the health of the population and the achievement of the Triple Aim and Quadruple Aim depends on achieving these goals.

QUESTIONS FOR FURTHER THOUGHT

1. What are some of the trends in US health care that are currently affecting what should be taught in US medical schools?
2. What is "value-added medical education?" What meaningful roles can students play in our health care systems to facilitate their learning while at the same time contributing to improving health system processes and patient care outcomes?
3. What do you see as the future of the US health care system in 10, 20, and 50 years, and what new knowledge, attitudes, and skills will be required in terms of health systems science?
4. Is the following statement true or false? Patients in most health care markets in the United States can determine the costs of their health care through a combination of online searches and careful examination of their medical bills.

5. What are the potential benefits to physicians and to the health of the public if all physicians master the knowledge and skills and adopt the attitudes intrinsic to health systems science?

Annotated Bibliography

Bodenheimer T. From triple to quadruple aim: care of the patient requires care of the provider. *Ann Fam Med.* 2014;12(6):573–576.
This article builds on the Triple Aim of enhancing the patient experience, improving population health, and reducing costs—tenets that are widely accepted as guideposts to the optimization of health care system performance. The author believes the Triple Aim is insufficient since physicians and other health care professionals report widespread burnout and dissatisfaction, which is associated with lower patient satisfaction, reduced health outcomes, and increased costs. This article recommends that the Triple Aim be expanded to a Quadruple Aim, adding the goal of improving the working lives of physicians and other health care professionals.
Lin SY, Schillinger E, Irby DM. Value-added medical education: engaging future doctors to transform health care delivery today. *J Gen Intern Med.* 2014;30(2):150–151.
Medical student education typically ignores current problems in health care delivery and does not address the pressing societal challenges. Change is desperately needed to translate education into better health outcomes for all people. The authors advocate for "value-added medical education," whereby powerful experiential learning experiences add value and capacity to the health care delivery system. Medical students can be trained and can become involved in a variety of targeted patient care tasks.
Lucey CR. Medical education: part of the problem and part of the solution. *JAMA Intern Med.* 2013;173(17):1639–1643.
High-quality health care requires that medical educators accept a social contract to reduce the burden of suffering and disease through the education of doctors. "Medical schools and residency programs must restructure their views of basic and clinical science and workplace learning to give equal emphasis to the science and skills needed to practice in and lead in complex systems. They must also rethink their relationships with clinical environments so that the education of students and residents accelerates the transformation in health care delivery needed to fulfill our contract with society."
Tierney MJ, Pageler NM, Kahana M, Pantaleoni JL, Longhurst CA. Medical education in the electronic medical record (EMR) era: benefits, challenges, and future directions. *Acad Med.* 2013;88(6):748–752.
This article reviews the effects of electronic medical record use on medical learners through the lens of the six core competencies for medical education promulgated by the Accreditation Council for Graduate Medical Education. The authors examine educational benefits and risks of electronic medical record use, discuss factors that promote successful use when implemented in academic environments, and identify areas for optimization and future research on the role of the electronic medical record in medical education.

References

1. Engel GL. The need for a new medical model: a challenge for biomedicine. *Science.* 1977;196(4286):129–136.
2. Gonzalo JD, Dekhtyar M, Starr SR, et al. Health systems science curricula in undergraduate medical education: identifying and defining a potential curricular framework. *Acad Med.* 2016 April 5. [Epub ahead of print].
3. Gonzalo JD, Baxley E, Borkan J, et al. Priorities and strategies for successful integration and sustainment of health systems science in undergraduate medical education. *Acad Med.* 2016 May 31. [Epub ahead of print].
4. Flexner A. (1910). Medical education in the United States and Canada: a report to the Carnegie Foundation for the advancement of teaching. http://archive.carnegiefoundation.org/pdfs/elibrary/Carnegie_Flexner_Report.pdf. Accessed November 6, 2016.
5. Berwick DM, Nolan TW, Whittington J. The Triple Aim: care, health, and cost. *Health Aff (Millwood).* 2008;27(3):759–769.
6. Bodenheimer T. From Triple to Quadruple Aim: care of the patient requires care of the provider. *Ann Fam Med.* 2014;12(6):573–576.
7. Bandura A. Toward a psychology of human agency. *Perspect Psychol Sci.* 2006;1(2):164–180.
8. Eva KW, Reiter HI, Rosenfeld J, Norman GR. An admissions OSCE: the multiple mini-interview. *Med Educ.* 2004;38(3):314–326.
9. Prep V. How changes to medical school interviews may affect applicants. *US News & World Report.* November 21, 2011. http://www.usnews.com/education/blogs/medical-school-admissions-doctor/2011/11/21/how-changes-to-medical-school-interviews-may-affect-applicants. Accessed April 17, 2016.
10. Norman G, Norcini J, Bordage G. Uses of competency-based education: milestones or millstones? *J Grad Med Educ.* 2014;6(1):1–6.
11. Lucey CR. Medical education: part of the problem and part of the solution. *JAMA Intern Med.* 2013;173(17):1639–1643.
12. Centers for Medicare & Medicaid Services. Electronic health records (EHR) incentive programs. https://www.cms.gov/Regulations-and-Guidance/Legislation/EHRIncentivePrograms/index.html. Accessed April 17, 2016.
13. Centers for Disease Control and Prevention. Injury prevention and control: prescription drug overdose. http://www.cdc.gov/drugoverdose/epidemic/. Accessed April 17, 2016.
14. US Department of Health & Human Services. HHS hosts 50-state convening focused on preventing opioid overdose and opioid use disorder, takes important step to increase access to treatment. http://www.hhs.gov/about/news/2015/09/17/hhs-hosts-50-state-convening-focused-preventing-opioid-overdose-and-opioid-use-disorder.html. Published September 15, 2015. Accessed November 6, 2016.
15. National Institute of Drug Abuse. Overdose death rates. https://www.drugabuse.gov/related-topics/trends-statistics/overdose-death-rates. Revised December 2015. Accessed April 17, 2016.
16. Tierney MJ, Pageler NM, Kahana M, Pantaleoni JL, Longhurst CA. Medical education in the electronic medical record (EMR) era: benefits, challenges, and future directions. *Acad Med.* 2013;88(6):748–752.
17. Hammond MA, Dalrymple JL, Christner JG, et al. Medical student documentation in electronic health records: a collaborative statement from the alliance for clinical education. *Teach Learn Med.* 2012;24(3):257–266.
18. Pearce C, Phillips AM, Trumble S, Dwan K. The patient and the computer in the primary care consultation. *J Am Med Inform Assoc.* 2011;18(2):138–142.
19. Shield RR, Goldman RE, Anthony DA, Wang N, Doyle RJ, Borkan J. Gradual electronic health record implementation: new insights on physician and patient adaptation. *Ann Fam Med.* 2010;8(4):316–326.
20. Accreditation Council for Graduate Medical Education. http://www.acgme.org/. Accessed April 17, 2016.
21. Murdoch TB, Detsky AS. The inevitable application of big data to health care. *JAMA.* 2013;309(13):1351–1352.
22. New York University School of Medicine. http://education.med.nyu.edu. Accessed April 17, 2016.
23. Open Notes. http://www.opennotes.org/. Accessed April 17, 2016.
24. Crico Video. Better, safer care: imagining a medical record of the future. https://www.youtube.com/watch?v=VHMJaV7zJxE. Published November 7, 2012. Accessed April 17, 2016.
25. Walsh K. The future of simulation in medical education. *J Biomed Res.* 2015;29(3):259–262.
26. Bauchner H. *Future of medical education at the American Medical Association.* Chicago: Presentation at CHANGE**MEDED**; October 2, 2015.
27. Lin SY, Schillinger E, Irby DM. Value-added medical education: engaging future doctors to transform health care delivery today. *J Gen Intern Med.* 2014;30(2):150–151.
28. Penn State College of Medicine. Novel academic program uses medical students as patient navigators. https://pennstatemedicine.org/2015/05/08/novel-academic-program-uses-medical-students-as-patient-navigators/. Published May 8, 2015. Accessed April 17, 2016.

29. University of California. San Francisco (UCSF). Improving patient outcomes through medical education—the health professions education pathway to discovery. http://medschool.ucsf.edu/features/improving-patient-outcomes-through-medical-education-health-professions-education-pathway. Published November 5, 2014. Accessed April 17, 2016.

30. Bagian J. The future of graduate medical education: a systems-based approach to ensure patient safety. *Acad Med.* 2015;90(9):1199–1202.

31. Society of Student Run Free Clinics (SSRFC). http://studentrunfreeclinics.org/. Accessed April 17, 2016.

32. Khan AM, Long T, Brienza R. Surely, we can do better: scaling innovation in medical education for social impact. *Acad. Med.* 2012;87(12):1645–1646.

33. Satterfield JM, Carney PA. Agency for Health Research and Quality. Aligning medical education with the nation's health priorities: innovations in physician training in behavioral and social sciences. http://www.ahrq.gov/professionals/education/curriculum-tools/population-health/satterfield.html. Published July 2015. Accessed April 17, 2016.

34. Caulfield T, Fullerton SM, Ali-Khan SE, et al. Race and ancestry in biomedical research: exploring the challenges. *Genome Med.* 2009;1(1):8.

35. Elliott VS. Color-blind? The value of racial data in medical research. *American Medical News.* January 5, 2004. http://www.amednews.com/article/20040105/health/301059952/4/. Accessed April 17, 2016.

36. Brandt AM. Racism and research: the case of the Tuskegee Syphilis study. *Hastings Cent Rep.* 1978;8(6):21–29.

37. Braun L, Fausto-Sterling A, Fullwiley D, et al. Racial categories in medical practice: how useful are they? *PLoS Med.* 2007;4(9):e271.

38. Dzau VJ, Cho A, ElLaissi W, Yoediono Z, Sangvai D, et al. Transforming academic health centers for an uncertain future. *N Engl J Med.* 2013;369(11):991–993.

39. Becker BN, Formisano RA, Getto CJ. Dinosaurs fated for extinction? Health care delivery at academic medical centers. *Acad Med.* 2010;85:759–762.

40. University of Toronto Dalla Lana School of Public Health. www.dlsph.utoronto.ca/. Accessed April 17, 2016.

41. University of Utah School Health Sciences. Health care transformation. http://healthsciences.utah.edu/health-care-transformation/. Accessed April 16, 2016.

42. Beyond Flexner. Beyondflexner.org. Accessed April 17, 2016.

43. Global Health Through Education Training and Service (GHETS). http://www.ghets.org/. Accessed April 17, 2016.

Glossary

Accountable Care Organization (ACO)   A group of hospitals, physicians, and/or other health care professionals who come together to provide coordinated high-quality care. An ACO usually contracts with Medicare, Medicaid, and/or private payers to share in savings achieved while quality goals are maintained or exceeded.

Accountable care teams   Those working with an ACO to maintain or exceed quality goals while reducing health care expenditures. Teams may include physicians, physician assistants, nurses, nurse practitioners, pharmacists, case managers, medical assistants, hospitals, ambulatory care centers, urgent care centers, retail clinics, administrators, and other types of professionals or health entities.

Accreditation Council for Graduate Medical Education (ACGME) competency domains   ACGME's six core competency domains that every physician should have are medical knowledge, patient care, professionalism, interpersonal communication, practice-based learning/personal improvement, and system-based practice/system improvement.

Active failures or **active errors**   Errors involving front-line personnel and occurring as the result of an individual's action. These errors occur as the result of mental lapses, errors in judgment, or procedural violations. Examples include administering the incorrect medication, performing surgery on the wrong site, or ignoring an alarm.

Adverse drug event   Harm caused by a drug. It may or may not be the result of an error.

Adverse event   Harm caused by medical treatment. It may or may not be the result of an error.

Afferent limb   Part of a rapid response system. Usually composed of bedside clinicians empowered to use predefined criteria to trigger the rapid response team, bypassing the traditional hierarchy, in order to expeditiously deliver necessary expertise and equipment to a patient.

Authority gradient   The psychological distance between a worker and a supervisor.

Bias   An inclination of temperament or outlook. A personal and sometimes unreasoned judgment. Can be helpful or harmful.

Bio-Psycho-Social (BPS) model of medicine   A systems thinking approach to all levels of medicine developed by George L. Engel.

Blunt end   The many layers of a health care organization that are removed from direct patient contact, but directly influence what happens to a patient.

Bundled payments   Incorporating expected costs for a typical encounter or episode of care into a single payment.

Case management   A collaborative process of assessment, planning, facilitation, care coordination, evaluation, and advocacy for options and services to meet an individual's and a family's comprehensive health needs. May include the provision of services and goods not traditionally provided in the health care setting that may improve a patient's health.

Case manager   Health care professionals who help provide an array of services to assist individuals and families cope with complicated health or medical situations in the most effective way possible.

Clinical data registries   Collections of data about patients with a similar disease or therapeutic process.

Clinical data warehouses   Central repositories of data where information is integrated together from disparate sources. Typically maintained at the institutional level.

Clinical decision support (CDS)   A component of health information technology that provides clinicians, staff, patients, or other individuals knowledge and person-specific information, intelligently filtered or presented at appropriate times, to enhance health and health care. CDS tools include computerized alerts and reminders to care providers and patients; clinical guidelines; condition-specific order sets; focused patient data reports and summaries; documentation templates; diagnostic support; and contextually relevant reference information, among other tools.

Clinical pathways   Standardized, evidence-based clinical decision tools developed to guide practice at the local level.

Cognitive science   The study of how decisions are made.

Community health needs assessment (CHNA)   A collaborative process between health care organizations and community residents and organizations that uses quantitative and qualitative methods to systematically collect and analyze data to understand health needs within a specific community.

Comparative effectiveness research   Designed to inform health care decisions about drugs, medical devices, tests, surgeries, or ways to deliver care by providing evidence on the effectiveness, benefits, and harms of different options.

Computerized provider order entry (CPOE)   The act of entering medication orders or other physician instructions electronically instead of on paper charts.

Constraint   A limitation in a system requiring an individual to slow down at a critical juncture and complete certain steps or goals in order to proceed with the intended action. Intended to create situational awareness and a recognition that an event has increased potential for harm and all focus should be on preventing such harm.

Core Entrustable Professional Activities for Entering Residency (CEPAER)   Activities defined by the Association of American Medical Colleges that residents should be able to perform on the first day of residency without direct supervision, regardless of specialty choice.

Critical period   A limited time window in an individual's life during which an exposure can have adverse or protective effects on development and subsequent disease outcome.

Data analytics   The extensive use of data, statistical and quantitative analysis, explanatory and predictive models, and fact-based management to drive decisions and actions.

Determinants of health   The multiple factors influencing an individual's health and the health of populations. Determinants can be behavioral, genetic, social circumstances, environmental exposures, and/or health care access.

Diagnostic error   The failure to establish an accurate and timely explanation of a patient's health problem(s) or communicate that explanation to the patient.

Efferent limb   The part of a rapid response system that responds to a situation when alerted by bedside clinicians (the afferent limb). Team composition varies based on the local needs. Most rapid response teams do not include a physician and are usually led by advanced practice providers, nurses, or respiratory therapists.

Electronic patient portal   A secure online tool that gives patients 24-hour access to personal health information.

Error   Not completing a planned action as intended or using the wrong plan to achieve an aim.

Event analysis   A structured method used to analyze serious adverse events. A central tenet is to identify underlying issues that increase the likelihood of errors while avoiding focusing on the mistakes of individuals. May also be referred to as *root cause analysis*. Event analysis is becoming the more common term because adverse events may have more than one cause.

Evidence-based medicine or **evidence-based practice**   Identifying and applying the best available scientific evidence to medical practice and reducing unnecessary variation in health care delivery.

Fee-for-service model   Paying physicians and other health care professionals a fee for each service provided.

Flattening the hierarchy   Creating an environment in which all members of the team feel safe providing input, are valued for speaking up, and are not deprecated for doing so.

Formulary system   An ongoing process through which a health care organization establishes policies regarding the use of drugs, therapies, and drug-related products and identifies those that are most medically appropriate and cost-effective to best serve the health interests of a given patient population.

Health care delivery system   An organization of people, institutions, and resources that delivers health care services to meet the health needs of target populations.

Health care improvement   A broad term that encompasses traditional process and quality improvement and patient safety efforts to close gaps aligned with the six Institute of Medicine (IOM) dimensions of quality.

Health care team   A team of health care professionals who provide diagnostic and therapeutic procedures to a patient.

Health disparities   Differences in health and health outcomes among groups of people.

Health information exchange (HIE)   The mobilization of health care information electronically across organizations within a region, community, or hospital system. HIE may also refer to the organization that facilitates the exchange.

Health Leads   An online instrument developed at Boston Medical Center with support from the Robert Wood Johnson Foundation to lead patients to community and health system resources related to the specific needs that they express.

Health systems science   The study of how health systems deliver care to patients and how patients receive and access that care.

Heuristic   A pattern or "rule of thumb" used to approach a problem.

High-performing system   A system performing dramatically better than other systems as measured by one or more criteria.

High-reliability organizations (HROs)   Organizations that operate in complex, hazardous environments making few mistakes over long periods of time. A key aspect of HROs is a focus on teams.

Hospitalist   An inpatient physician who works exclusively in a hospital.

Individual factors   Aspects of an individual that impact how a patient interacts with the health care system or how a physician or other health care professional provides care.

Institute of Medicine (IOM)   A division of the National Academies of Sciences, Engineering, and Medicine. The Institute of Medicine was renamed the Health and Medicine Division in March 2016.

Institutional context   External regulatory agencies, the medico-legal environment, and financial constraints that impact an institution.

Integrated health care system   A health care system that aligns the incentives of health care professionals in order to deliver value-based care for its patient population.

Interdisciplinary team   A team of health care professionals from a variety of disciplines who coordinate care and base professional relationships on shared goals, shared knowledge, and mutual respect.

Interoperability   The ability of a system, such as an electronic health record, to work with another system.

Interprofessional practice   When multiple physicians and other health care professionals from different disciplines and specialties work together with patients, families, caregivers, and communities to deliver the highest quality of care.

Joint Commission   The accrediting body for health care organizations.

Just Culture   A work culture that allows every employee to advocate for an environment where safety concerns can be addressed in a nonpunitive manner with willingness to address underlying causes.

Lapse   When an action is missed or an individual forgets to do something.

Latent failures or **latent errors**   Errors that result from system or design flaws occurring away from the bedside. Errors may include equipment design flaws, decreased staffing for fiscal reasons, and software interface issues.

Lean   A systematic method of eliminating waste focused on activity that adds value. Originally developed by Toyota.

Learning health system   The presence of standardized interoperable data and systems that not only lead to improved direct care of patients but also to secondary use or re-use of clinical data for quality measurement and improvement, clinical and translational research, and public health.

Malpractice   An instance of negligence or incompetence on the part of a professional.

Mandatory reporting systems   Systems that receive error reports from a designated individual who often is not directly involved in the error. They are typically required for serious events including death, retained foreign object after surgery, radiation overdose, or transfusion error.

Metadata   Data points used to identify data (e.g., who authored a particular clinical note), how data are linked together (e.g., vital signs from multiple records that represent a single patient), or how data have been utilized (e.g., data access and audit logs).

Miller's pyramid   A figure designed by George Miller, a highly respected medical educator, to help faculty and educational program leaders understand the progressive and developmental acquisition of clinical competence and how different assessment tools may be applied.

Mistake   When someone does something he or she thought to be correct, but it was not.

National Board of Medical Examiners (NBME)   Independent, nonprofit organization that develops and manages the United States Medical Licensing Examination (USMLE).

Near miss   An unplanned event or close call that does not reach the patient or cause injury or damage to the patient.

Negligent adverse event   A preventable adverse event that satisfies the legal criteria for negligence where the care provided to the patient does not meet the standard of care an average physician would provide.

Never Event   A largely preventable action such as wrong site surgery or retained sponges that should never occur.

Normalization of deviance   Deviation from standards and policy on a recurrent basis without resistance.

Nurse manager   Registered nurses with the educational qualifications and at least 3 to 5 years of clinical experience qualifying them to effectively supervise nursing units in hospitals, clinics, and other health care institutions.

Objective Structured Clinical Examinations (OSCEs)   Hands-on examinations designed to test competence in skills such as communication, clinical examination, medical procedures/prescription, and other skills required for clinical practice.

Organizational factors   Policies and processes at a health facility or system related to leadership, education, supervision, and availability of equipment or supplies that impact care provided to patients.

Patient factors   Aspects of a patient such as personality, language, culture, and illness complexity that have a direct impact on communication and bias.

Patient handoff   Transferring a patient from one health care setting or professional to another.

Patient registry   An organized system using observational study methods to collect data to evaluate specific outcomes for a population of patients.

Patient safety   A discipline in the health care sector that applies safety science methods toward the goal of achieving a trustworthy system of health care delivery.

Pay for Performance   Payment based on meeting quality measures in care delivery.

Persons approach   An approach that focuses on the errors of individuals at the bedside, such as the physician, nurse, or other caregiver in contact with the patient.

Plan-Do-Study-Act (PDSA) cycle   Part of the Institute for Healthcare Improvement's Model for Improvement. Steps in the PDSA cycle:

Step 1: Plan—Plan the test or observation, including a plan for collecting data.

Step 2: Do—Try out the test on a small scale.

Step 3: Study—Set aside time to analyze the data and study the results.

Step 4: Act—Refine the change, based on what was learned from the test.

Population health   The health outcomes of a group of individuals, including the distribution of such outcomes within the group.

Population management   Management of and payment for health care services for a defined population.

Population medicine   The design, delivery, coordination, and payment of high-quality health care services to a defined group of people.

Precision medicine   Formerly referred to as *personalized medicine*. Identifying which approaches will be effective for which patients based on genetic, environmental, and lifestyle factors.

Predictive analytics   Branch of data mining concerned with the prediction of future probabilities and trends.

Preventable adverse event   An adverse event attributable to error.

Process map   A visual representation of a process showing how a sequence of events leads to a given outcome.

Process measures Measures of the specific steps in a process that lead—either positively or negatively—to a particular outcome.

Quality improvement The combined and unceasing efforts of health care professionals, patients, their families, researchers, payers, planners, and educators to make changes that will lead to better patient outcomes, better system performance, and better professional development.

Rapid response system A tool implemented in hospitals and designed to identify and respond to patients with early signs of clinical deterioration on non-intensive care units with the goal of preventing respiratory or cardiac arrest.

Registry database The file or files derived from a patient registry.

Relational coordination The coordination among team members that occurs through frequent, high-quality communication supported by relationships based on shared goals, shared knowledge, and mutual respect.

Reliability The consistency or reproducibility of an assessment result and whether the same result would occur if the assessment were administered at some future time or in different circumstances.

Root cause analysis A structured method used to analyze serious adverse events. A central tenet is to identify underlying problems that increase the likelihood of errors while avoiding focusing on mistakes by individuals. May also be referred to as *event analysis* because adverse events may have more than one root cause.

SBAR Stands for Situation, Background, Assessment, and Recommendation. A tool to structure conversations at critical junctures in care.

Second victims Physicians and other health care professionals involved in an adverse event, even if they are not primarily responsible.

Self-regulated learning The means by which learners adjust their behaviors to achieve learning goals. Key elements include goal setting, self-efficacy, attributions of learning outcomes, self-assessment, feedback seeking, and reflection.

Sensitive period A time period in an individual's life when an exposure has a stronger effect on development and disease risk than it would at other times.

Sentinel event A patient safety event that reaches a patient and results in death, permanent harm, or severe temporary harm. These events signal the need for immediate investigation and system improvement to prevent further harm.

Shared savings Financial incentives to physicians, other health care professionals, health systems, and medical practices to improve quality while reducing costs.

Sharp end Largely preventable actions such as wrong site surgery or retained sponges that should never occur.

Situational awareness Knowledge of the changing clinical status or environment that enables physicians and other health care professionals to adapt to the emerging situation. Also involves maintenance of a shared mental model, allowing team members to work toward the same goal.

Slip An action that does not occur as planned.

Social gradient of health The concept that health and wealth are typically correlated in a linear, stepwise fashion at all levels of income and class.

Socioeconomic position (SEP) The social and economic factors that influence what positions individuals or groups hold within the structure of a society.

Socioeconomic status (SES) The social standing or class of an individual or group. Often measured as a combination of education, income, and occupation.

Swiss Cheese model Recognizes error as inevitable and that every step in a process has the potential for failure, with each layer of the system serving as a defensive layer to identify and catch the error before harm reaches the patient.

Systems approach Focuses on improving and redesigning the environment and care processes rather than the behavior of a few individuals.

Systems thinking Recognizes and understands the complex interdependencies and relationships within a functional system like health care. Allows the formation of linkages among disparate areas of activity in health care to improve outcomes, patient experience, and value in health care.

Task factors Components of an action that affect its outcome such as the availability and use of clear protocols.

Team science An understanding of teams, their structures, and critical elements.

Teamwork Cooperative or coordinated effort on the part of a group of persons acting together as a team or in the interests of a common cause.

Telemedicine The delivery of health care when the participants are separated by time and/or distance.

Third medical science Health systems science. Basic and clinical sciences are the first two medical sciences.

Transitions of care Times when patients are moved from one setting of care or practitioner to another.

Triple Aim A framework developed by the Institute for Healthcare Improvement describing an approach to optimizing health system performance. It includes the following: Improving the patient experience of care (including quality and satisfaction); improving the health of populations; and reducing the per capita cost of health care.

USMLE United States Medical Licensing Examination.

Validity A determination as to whether the results of an assessment method provide accurate information about what is being measured.

Violation A deliberate, illegal, or otherwise unsanctioned action.

Voluntary reporting systems Systems that receive error reports from physicians and other health care professionals who willingly report adverse events.

Workplace factors Issues in the health care setting that contribute to a physician or other health care professional's ability to carry out a task.

Wrong surgery Procedure performed on the wrong patient or the wrong site; or the wrong surgery was performed.

Index

Pages followed by *b, t,* or *f* refer to boxes, tables, or figures, respectively.

221